Essentials of Oral Histology and Embryology

A Clinical Approach

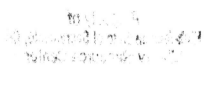

Visit our website at www.mosby.com

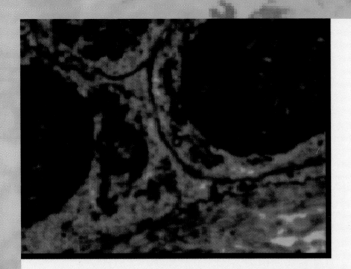

Essentials of Oral Histology *and* Embryology

A Clinical Approach

JAMES K. AVERY, D.D.S., Ph.D.
Professor Emeritus of Dentistry, School of Dentistry
Professor Emeritus of Anatomy, Medical School
University of Michigan
Ann Arbor, Michigan

Edited by

PAULINE F. STEELE, B.S., R.D.H., B.S. (Educ.), M.A.
Director and Professor Emeritus, Dental Hygiene
University of Michigan, School of Dentistry
Ann Arbor, Michigan

SECOND EDITION

with 419 illustrations

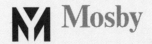 Mosby

A Harcourt Health Sciences Company

St. Louis   London   Philadelphia   Sydney   Toronto

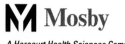

Mosby

A Harcourt Health Sciences Company

Publisher: John Schrefer
Acquisitions Editor: Penny Rudolph
Developmental Editor: Angela Reiner
Editorial Assistant: Stacy Welsh
Project Manager: Patricia Tannian
Production Editor: Gail Stobaugh
Design Manager: Gail Morey Hudson
Cover Design: Teresa Breckwoldt

SECOND EDITION

Mosby, Inc.
A Harcourt Health Sciences Company
11830 Westline Industrial Drive
St. Louis, Missouri 63146

Printed in the United States of America

Library of Congress Cataloging-in-Publication Data
Avery, James K.
Essentials of oral histology and embryology: a clinical approach/
   James K. Avery; edited by Pauline F. Steele—2nd ed.
       p.   cm.
   Includes bibliographical references and index
   ISBN 0-323-00460-1   (alk. paper)
   1. Mouth—Histology.   2. Teeth—Histology.   3. Embryology, Human
I. Steele, Pauline F.   II. Title
   [DNLM: 1. Stomatognathic System—anatomy & histology.   2. Mouth—
embryology.   3. Odontogenesis—physiology. WU 101 A954e 2000]
RK280.A84 2000
611'.018931—dc21
DNLM/DLC   99-25601

01   02   03   /   9   8   7   6   5   4   3   2

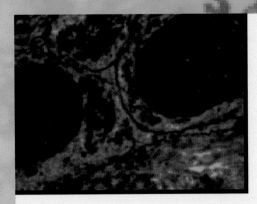

Preface

This textbook's purpose is to familiarize dental professionals with the parts of oral histology and embryology that are pertinent to clinical dental hygiene and dental practice. Developmental and structural microscopic anatomy are significant sciences for the practitioner. In acquiring an understanding of how cells, tissues, and organs develop and function, one gains a clearer perspective of these structures as a basis for their treatment.

Oral histology and embryology are the sciences most relevant to the understanding of clinical oral manifestations. Therefore this textbook has been designed to encompass histologic and embryologic information with specific consideration of clinical connotations. The text has been written especially for dental and dental hygiene students, practitioners, educators, and other co-associated professionals.

Several special features are found in this text. Numerous color photographs enhance visual learning. A concerted effort has been made to place all illustrative material as close as possible to the explanatory text. Each chapter has an overview to give a perspective of the chapter content, followed by more detailed descriptions of basic principles of oral histology and embryology and their relationship to clinical practice. This emphasis enables formation of both a practical and a theoretical approach to these essential sciences. Diagrams throughout the text facilitate further comprehension. Also included are low-magnification light microscopic and high-magnification electron microscopic photographs to assist with learning and to clarify concepts. A glossary has been included to augment learning.

Professional competence connotes more than technical ability. Therefore an effort has been made to indicate those aspects of basic sciences that complement the technical procedures. Clinical Comments appear throughout the text. Also, a new feature in this edition is the Consider the Patient case studies. These help the reader apply knowledge to possible clinical situations. Dental professionals must understand and appreciate these concepts involving clinical practice.

Pauline F. Steele

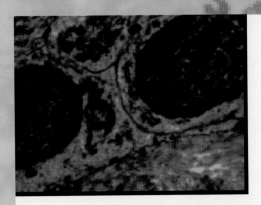

Acknowledgments

This text has been compiled during 40 years of interaction with students in histology lecture and laboratory instruction. I am grateful for the many questions and suggestions gained from these interactions. Initially, classroom guides were produced to facilitate instruction. These guides were gradually improved over the years until they approached textbook quality. Dr. Thomas Greene was especially helpful in the preparation of the guides. Also, a number of colleagues lectured in the histology course and then contributed chapters to a text, *Oral Development and Histology.* Many of their ideas and descriptions are included in this text. Individual colleagues' contributions have been recognized in the respective chapters where they appear.

One concept on which students and staff agreed was the placement of a figure as close as possible to the text that describes it. We have tried to adhere to this means of presenting descriptions in text that relate to illustrations. Another feature that staff and students liked was the **Clinical Comments.** This has been a popular addition. A feature that was added in this edition is the case-based **Consider the Patient** questions suggested by the reviewers. We are also grateful for the suggestion of chapter outlines and the introductory overview that begins each chapter. Again we are grateful for the suggestion of a glossary to introduce and explain new terms found throughout the book.

We are most appreciative of Dr. Alayne Evans for the artwork she produced throughout this text. She created many of these drawings while a student of dentistry at the University of Michigan. Mr. Chris Jung created additional artwork for this text. This book is also enhanced by Dr. Donald Strachan's expertise in scientific data presentation and analyses. I also thank Dr. Daniel Chiego Jr., a colleague who made many helpful suggestions during the preparation of this text. Finally, I wish to thank those authors who prepared chapters in the text *Oral Development and Histology* because information from some of those chapters was used in preparation of this book. All these contributions added immeasurably to the text we see today.

James K. Avery

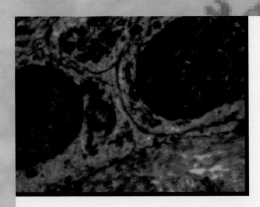

Contents

Essentials of
Oral Histology
and Embryology

A Clinical Approach

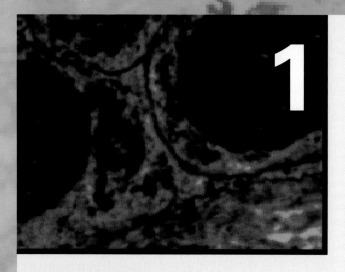

1 Development and Structure of Cells and Tissues

OVERVIEW

The smallest unit of structure in the human body is the cell, composed of a nucleus and cytoplasm. The nucleus contains **deoxyribonucleic acid (DNA)** and **ribonucleic acid (RNA)**, the fundamental structures of life. The cytoplasm functions in absorption and cell duplication, in which organelles perform specific actions. The cell cycle is the time required for the DNA to duplicate before mitosis. This chapter discusses the four stages of mitosis: prophase, metaphase, anaphase, and telophase. Also described are the three periods of prenatal development: proliferative, embryonic, and fetal. The fertilization of the ovum in the distal uterine tube, zygote migration, and the zygote's implantation in the uterine wall are discussed. In addition, the origin of human tissues—ectoderm, mesoderm, and endoderm—is presented, followed by the differentiation of tissue types, such as those of ectodermal origin, epithelium and skin with its derivatives, and the central and peripheral nervous systems. Next the chapter delineates development of the mesodermal components involving connective tissues of the body, such as fibrous tissue, three types of cartilage, two types of bone, three kinds of muscles, and the cardiovascular system. This chapter should help the reader better comprehend the origin, development, organization, and structure of the various cells and tissues of the human body.

CELL STRUCTURE AND FUNCTION

The human body is composed of cells, intercellular substance (the products of these cells), and fluid that bathes these tissues. Cells are the smallest living units capable of independent existence. They carry out the vital processes of **absorption, assimilation, respiration, irritability, conductivity, growth, reproduction,** and **excretion.** Cells vary in size, shape, structure, and function. Regardless of function, each cell has a number of characteristics in common with other cells, such as **cytoplasm** and a **nucleus,** which contains a **nucleolus.** However, some cell characteristics are related to function. A cell on the surface of the skin, for example, serves best as a thin, flattened disk, whereas a respiratory cell functions best as a cuboidal or columnar cell to facilitate adsorption with mobile cilia to move fluid from the lung to the oropharynx. Surrounding each cell is the **intercellular material** that provides the cell with nutrition, takes up waste products, and provides the body with form. It may be as soft as loose connective tissue or as hard as bone cartilage or teeth. **Fluid,** the third component of the body, is the blood and lymph that travel throughout the body in vessels or the tissue fluid that bathes each cell and fiber of the body.

Cell Nucleus

A nucleus is found in all cells except mature red blood cells and blood platelets. The nucleus is usually round to ovoid, depending on the cell's shape. Ordinarily a cell has a single nucleus; however, it may be binucleate, as are cardiac muscle cells or parenchymal liver cells, or multinucleate, as are osteoclasts and skeletal muscle cells. The nucleus is important in the production of deoxyribonucleic acid (DNA) and ribonucleic acid (RNA). DNA contains the genetic information in the cell, and the RNA carries information from the DNA to sites of actual protein synthesis, which are located in the cell cytoplasm. The nucleus is bound by a membrane, the **nuclear envelope,** which has openings at the **nuclear pores.** This envelope is composed of two phospholipid layers similar to the plasma membrane of the cell. The pores are associated with the endoplasmic reticulum that forms at the end of each cell division. The nucleus contains from one to four nucleoli, which are round, dense bodies constituting the RNA contained in the nucleus. Nucleoli have no limiting membrane (Fig. 1-1).

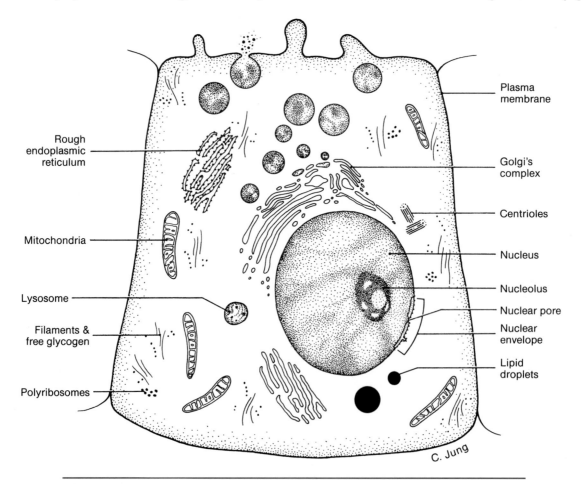

FIG. 1-1 Schematic diagram of cell structure illustrating components, such as nucleus, rough endoplasmic reticulum, mitochondria, Golgi's complex, and centrioles, as viewed by electron microscopy.

Cell Cytoplasm

Cytoplasm contains structures necessary for adsorption and for creation of cell products. The **cytosol** is the part of the cytoplasm that contains the organelles and solutes. The cytosol uses the raw materials brought into the cell to produce energy. It also functions in the excretion of waste products. These functions are carried out by the **endoplasmic reticulum (ER),** parallel membrane-bound cavities in the cytoplasm that contain newly acquired and synthesized protein. Two types of ER, smooth surfaced and granular or rough surfaced, can be found in the same cell. Rough-surfaced ER is caused by ribosomes on the surface of the reticulum and is the site at which protein production is initiated. Proteins are vital to the cell's metabolic processes, and each type of protein is composed of a number of different amino acids linked in a specific sequence. Amino acids form protein-containing groups, which in turn form acids or bases.

Ribosomes are particles that translate genetic codes for proteins and activate mechanisms for their production. They can be found as separate particles in the cytoplasm, clustered, or attached to the ER membranes. Ribosomes are nonspecific as to what type of protein they synthesize. The type is dependent on the messenger RNA (mRNA), which carries the message directly from the DNA of the nucleus to the RNA in the ER. This molecule attaches to the ribosomes and gives orders about the formation of the amino acids.

The ER transports substances in the cytoplasm. The ER is connected to Golgi's apparatus via small vesicles. **Golgi's apparatus** or **complex** helps sort, condense, package, and deliver proteins arriving from the ER. Golgi's apparatus is composed of cisternae (flat plates) or saccules, small vesicles, and large vacuoles. From here the secretory vesicles move or flow to the cell surface, where they fuse with the cell membrane and the plasmalemma and release their contents by exocytosis.

Lysosomes are small, membrane-bound bodies that contain a variety of acid hydrolase and digestive enzymes to help break down substances both inside and outside the cell. They are in all cells except red blood cells but are prominent in macrophages and leukocytes.

Mitochondria are membrane-bound organelles that lie free in the cytoplasm and are present in all cells. They are important in generating energy, are a major source of adenosine triphosphate (ATP), and therefore are the site of many metabolic reactions. These organelles appear as spheres, rods, ovoids, or threadlike bodies. Usually the inner layer of their trilaminar bounding membrane inflects to form transverse-appearing plates, the cristae (Fig. 1-1). Mitochondria lie adjacent to the area that requires their energy production.

Microtubules are small tubular structures in the cytoplasm that are composed of the protein tubulin. These structures may appear as singles, as doublets, or as triplets. They probably function as structural and force-generating elements and relate to cilia (motile cell processes) and to centrioles in relation to mitosis. They have cytoskeletal functions in maintaining cell shape. **Centrioles** are short cylinders appearing near the nucleus. Their walls are composed of nine triplets of microtubules. Centrioles are microtubule-generating centers and are important in mitosis, self-replicating before mitosis begins.

Surrounding the cell is the **plasma membrane** or plasmalemma, which envelops the cell and provides a selective barrier that regulates transport of substances into and out of the cell. All membranes are composed mainly of lipids and proteins with a small amount of carbohydrates. The plasma membrane also receives signals from hormones and neurotransmitters. In addition, cells contain proteins, lipids, or fatty substances that provide energy in the cell and are important components of cell membranes and permeability. Carbohydrates are also important in cells as the most available energy component in the body. These carbohydrates may exist as polysaccharide-protein complexes, glycoprotein complexes, glycoproteins, and glycolipids. Carbohydrate compounds are important in cell function and for development of cell products, such as supportive tissues and body lubricants.

Genetic mechanisms help a cell to develop and maintain a high degree of order. The ability is dependent on the genetic information that is expressed within the cell. The basic genetic processes in the cell are RNA and protein synthesis, DNA repair, and replication and genetic recombination. These processes produce type proteins and nucleic acids of a cell. These genetic events are relatively simple compared to other cell processes.

CELL DIVISION

Cell Cycle

Cell division is a continuous series of discrete steps by which the cell component divides. This function is related to the need for growth or replacement of tissues and is partly dependent on the length of the cell's life. Continually renewing cells line the gastrointestinal tract and compose the epidermis and the bone marrow. A second type of cell is part of an expanding population—the cells of the kidney, liver, and some glands. The third type of cell does not undergo cell division or DNA synthesis. An example is the neurons of the adult nervous system. For a somatic cell to undergo cell division, it must pass through a **cell cycle,** which ensures time for DNA genetic material in the daughter cells to duplicate that of the parent cell. However, in a sex cell, ovum, or spermatozoon, the process of meiosis occurs, in which a reduction division of chromosomes in the daughter cell takes place. The result is that half as many chromosomes are in the

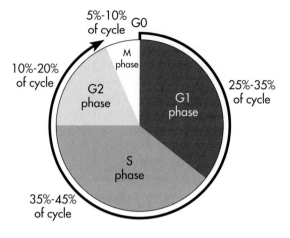

FIG. 1-2   Periods of cell cycle indicate relative time needed for each phase. G1 is the preduplication phase, or resting phase, which takes about 6 to 8 hours. In the S phase, DNA duplication takes place in 8 to 10 hours. The G2 phase is postduplication phase, which takes about 4 to 6 hours. In the M phase, mitosis takes about 35 to 40 minutes. These figures are for cultured mammalian cells. The total is 18 to 24 hours for the four stages of cytokinesis.

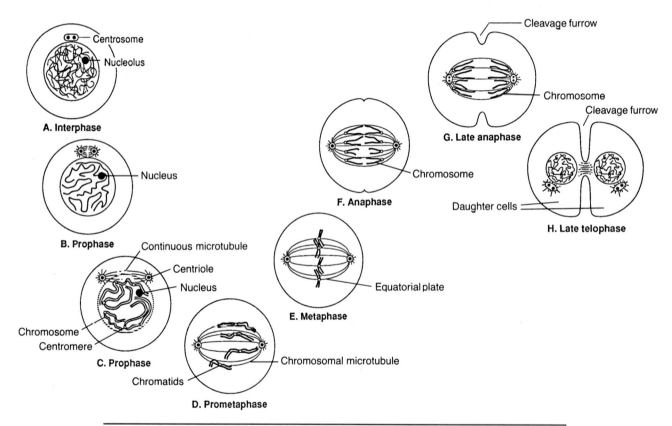

FIG. 1-3   Mitosis of somatic cell. The continuous process of cell division is shown. Mitosis is replication of parent chromosomes and distribution of two sets of chromosomes into two separate and equal nuclei. Stages are as follows: **A,** Interphase, resting cell. **B** and **C,** During prophase, chromatin thread shortens and thickens and becomes chromosomes, which then split into pairs of chromatids. Nuclear membrane disappears, and centrioles appear and begin migration to opposite poles of cell. **D,** In prometaphase, or early metaphase, chromatid pairs attach to centromere and line up in equatorial plate of cell. **E,** Metaphase occurs when centromeres and chromatids line up in middle of cell. Centrioles are at opposite ends of cell and attach to chromosomes by mitotic spindles. **F,** Anaphase is a division and movement of completed identical sets of chromatids (chromosomes) to opposite ends of cells. **G,** In late anaphase, identical sets of chromosomes have reached opposite ends of the cells as cleavage begins. **H,** In telophase a nuclear membrane reappears, nucleoli appear, and chromosomes lengthen and form chromatin thread. Mitotic spindles disappear, and centrioles duplicate so that each cell has completely identical properties.

daughter cell as are in the parent cell. Through meiosis, after fertilization of the ovum by the male chromosomes, the original (diploid) number of chromosomes is regained. The duration of the cell cycle in somatic cells is known now (Fig. 1-2). After mitosis the cells enter the reduplication or **G1 stage** of the interphase, the initial resting stage. This is followed by the **S phase,** in which DNA synthesis is completed. Next the cell enters the **G2 stage** or quiescent phase of the post-DNA duplication and proceeds into the mitotic stages of prophase, metaphase, anaphase, and telophase (Fig. 1-3). The cell then reenters and remains in the interphase stage until duplication resumes the mitotic process of developing two daughter cells identical to the parent cells.

Mitosis

Before mitosis the cell exists in the interphase, as seen in Fig. 1-3, *A.* The first step of mitosis is **prophase,** in which four structural changes occur (Fig. 1-3, *B*). The chromatin thread of the nucleus thickens into rodlike structures called **chromosomes.** Each chromosome then splits, forming two **chromatids.** These chromatids line up along the central area of the cell, called the **equatorial plate.** Each chromatid pair is attached to a spherical body called a **centromere.** The centriole pair duplicates, and the chromatids accompany the centrioles' migration to the opposite ends of the cell. Those fibers not formed between the migrating centrioles are **spindle fibers,** and those that form around the centrioles are **astral rays** or **asters** (Fig. 1-3, *C*). At this time the nucleolus disappears and its components become attached to the chromatids. Finally, the nuclear envelope breaks down and changes into granular elements, such as the ER (Fig. 1-3, *D*).

Chromatids have moved to the cell center by the **metaphase** stage. They are arranged along an equatorial plate at right angles to the long axis of the spindle (Fig. 1-3, *E*). The two chromatids of each chromosome become attached centrally at the equatorial plate to a centromere. These chromatids then split at the centromere into two sets of chromosomes.

In **anaphase** the daughter chromosomes move to the opposite poles of the cell with the full complement of 46 at each end (Fig. 1-3, *F* and *G*). This is thought to occur by movement of the chromosomal microtubules that attract the chromatids toward the poles. A constriction begins to appear around the midbody of the cell (Fig. 1-3, *G*).

In **telophase** the chromosomes detach from the chromosomal microtubules and the microtubules disintegrate. The chromosomes next elongate and disperse, losing their identity and regaining the chromatin thread appearance. Both the nucleoli within the nucleus and the nuclear envelope then reappear. As each nucleus matures, the cleavage furrow deepens in the midcell until the two daughter cells separate (Fig. 1-3, *H*).

CLINICAL COMMENT

All cells have a limited lifetime. For example, the life span of a white blood cell is only a few hours to a few days. Red blood cells live approximately 120 days before they are ingested by macrophages. Surface-covering cells—such as those of the skin, hair, or nails—renew as they are replaced as do cells lining the respiratory, urinary, and gastrointestinal tracts. Other cells in the body—such as those of the liver, kidneys, and thyroid gland—do not normally renew after maturity unless they are injured.

ORIGIN OF HUMAN TISSUE

Periods of Prenatal Development

Implantation and enlargement of the blastocyst, which contains the embryonic tissue, occur rapidly in the **proliferative period,** which lasts for 2 weeks. During this time, fertilization, implantation, and formation of the embryonic disk take place. After the second week this mass of cells begins to take the form of an embryo, so the period of 2 to 8 weeks is termed the **embryonic period.** During this period the different types of tissue develop and organize to form organ systems. The heart forms and begins to beat by the fourth week, and the face and oral structures develop during weeks 4 to 7. The embryo takes on a more human appearance in the eighth week and moves into the **fetal period,** which extends until birth (Fig. 1-4). During this period the tissues that developed in the embryonic stage enlarge, differentiate, and become capable of function.

CONSIDER THE PATIENT . . .

An expectant mother has reason for concern about the health of her baby. She asks whether tests are available to find out if her baby is healthy. She wants to know what the tests would reveal and if any risks are involved. (See discussion at end of chapter.)

Ovarian Cycle, Fertilization, Implantation, and Development of the Embryonic Disk

The origin of tissue begins with fertilization of the egg, or ovum, which occurs when sperm contact the egg in the distal part of the uterine tube (Fig. 1-5). The fertilized

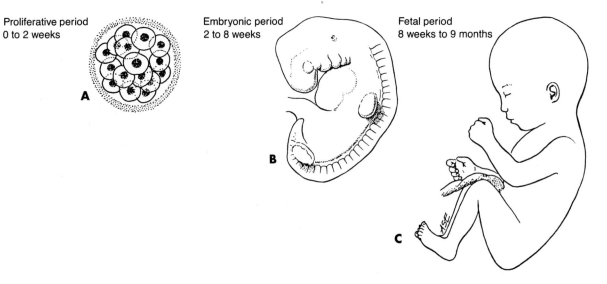

Proliferative period
0 to 2 weeks

Embryonic period
2 to 8 weeks

Fetal period
8 weeks to 9 months

FIG. 1-4   The developing human passes through three periods: **A,** Proliferative period, first 2 weeks, during which cell division is prevalent. **B,** Embryonic period, from second to eighth week. **C,** Fetal period, from eighth week to birth.

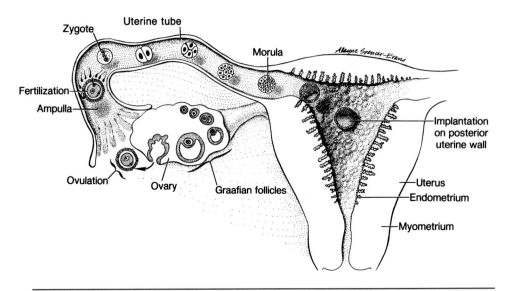

FIG. 1-5   Schematic diagram of uterus and uterine tubes shows path of sperm to distal tube, in which fertilization of newly appearing ovum from adjacent ovary occurs. Resultant zygote travels to uterus while undergoing cleavage, and implantation occurs on seventh day after conception.

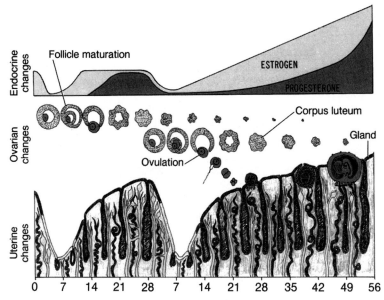

FIG. 1-6 Cyclical events of ovulatory cycle. *Top,* Endocrine changes: ovulation is controlled by estrogen and progesterone. *Center,* Ovarian changes: ovum matures, is expelled from ovary on fourteenth day, and if fertilized, becomes implanted in uterine wall 7 days later. *Bottom,* Uterine changes: uterine wall thickens and prepares for implantation each month. If implantation does not occur, uterine wall erodes with loss of blood vessels and gland ducts (menstruation).

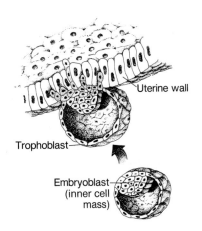

FIG. 1-7 Implantation of a fertilized ovum (zygote) in wall of uterus. Outer cells of trophoblast digest uterine cells to implant. Embryoblast develops within cell mass. As mass expands, a surrounding cavity is formed.

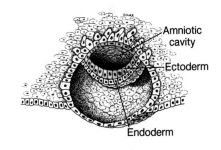

FIG. 1-8 Second small cavity lined with ectoderm develops (amniotic cavity). Other cavity (yolk sac) is lined with endoderm. The two cell layers contact in the center to form an area of ectoderm and endoderm for embryonic disk.

egg then grows and is termed the **zygote.** The cell mass produces a ball of cells (the **morula**) in the uterine tube. The morula grows and begins migration medially to the uterus, which it reaches at the end of the first week. The uterine cavity meanwhile prepares for the arrival of the fertilized ovum. The uterine lining **(endometrium)** thickens, and capillaries and glands develop to nourish the ovum. Estrogen and progesterone control this cyclical event (Fig. 1-6). The morula increases in size and is termed a **blastocyst.** As the blastocyst swells, it becomes hollow and develops a small inner cell mass. When this blastocyst or zygote reaches the uterine cavity, it attaches to the sticky wall of the uterus and becomes embedded in its surface. The cells of the zygote digest the uterine

endometrium, permitting deeper penetration. This process is known as **implantation** (Figs. 1-5 to 1-7). If no fertilized ovum reaches the uterine cavity, the development of capillaries and glands is terminated by menstruation (Fig. 1-6).

Two small cavities develop on either side of the inner cell mass. They reach each other in the center, where a small disk (the **embryonic disk**) is formed (Fig. 1-8). The embryonic disk becomes the embryo, composed of the common walls of the two adjacent sacs. One sac is lined with **ectodermal** cells, which will form the outer body covering **(epithelium).** The other sac is lined with **endodermal** cells. On the dorsal surface of the embryonic disk, the ectoderm forms the **neural plate,** whose

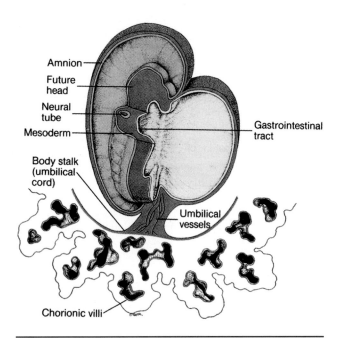

FIG. 1-9 A 3-week human embryo, viewed from the ventral-lateral aspect, illustrating an elongating gastrointestinal tube and dorsally located neural tube.

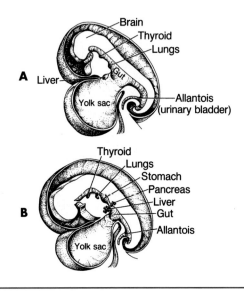

FIG. 1-10 Further development of the gastrointestinal tract at 4½ weeks **(A)** and at 5 weeks **(B)**. Outpouchings of the tube will form gastrointestinal organs.

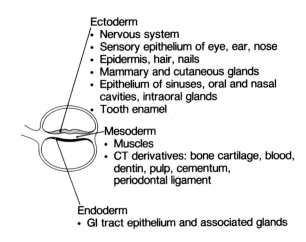

Ectoderm
• Nervous system
• Sensory epithelium of eye, ear, nose
• Epidermis, hair, nails
• Mammary and cutaneous glands
• Epithelium of sinuses, oral and nasal cavities, intraoral glands
• Tooth enamel

Mesoderm
• Muscles
• CT derivatives: bone cartilage, blood, dentin, pulp, cementum, periodontal ligament

Endoderm
• GI tract epithelium and associated glands

FIG. 1-11 Derivatives of ectoderm, mesoderm, and endoderm germ layers.

lateral boundaries elevate to form a **neural tube** that will become the brain and spinal cord (Fig. 1-9). The endodermal cells also form a tube, which will become the **gastrointestinal tract.** As this tube elongates, it anteriorly develops outpouchings that form the pharyngeal pouches, lung buds, liver, gallbladder, pancreas, and urinary bladder (Fig. 1-10).

Next, cells develop between the ectodermal and endodermal layers in the embryonic disk. This area becomes the **mesodermal** layer. These cells will develop into the muscles, skeleton, and blood cells of the embryo (Fig. 1-11). Mesodermal cells also accompany the elongating digestive tube and support its walls with muscle growth. This enables function and assists in the forming of organs arising from the developing gastrointestinal tube. From these three layers—ectoderm, mesoderm, and endoderm—develop all tissues of the body, as well as the complex organs (Fig. 1-11).

DEVELOPMENT OF HUMAN TISSUES

Epithelial Structures and Derivatives

The skin is a dual organ that has an **epidermis,** a surface cell layer that develops from the surface of ectodermal cells, and a **dermis,** which arises from the underlying mesoderm. The dermis originates in the **somites,** the masses of mesoderm that lie on either side of the neural tube (Fig. 1-12). From this mesoderm come both the dermis of the epithelium and the visceral mesoderm that covers the yolk sac and later becomes the gastrointestinal tract (Fig. 1-12). Therefore all the muscles functioning in peristalsis of the intestines arise from this mesoderm.

Initially the embryo is covered with a single layer of ectodermal cells (Fig. 1-13, *A*). By 11 to 12 weeks, this ectodermal layer of epithelium thickens into four layers. From the basal layer of cells come the more superficial cells of the epithelium (Fig. 1-13, *B*). Later **melanocytes** invade and pigment the skin. At birth the skin may show varying degrees of keratinization. Hair, teeth, nails, and mammary, sebaceous, and salivary glands all develop

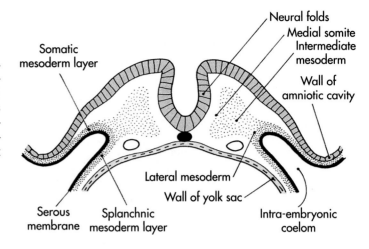

FIG. 1-12 Neural folds and somites in transverse section at approximately 20 days after conception. Medial somite (mesoderm) forms axial skeleton that surrounds neural tube. Intermediate mesoderm forms striated muscle of body, and lateral mesoderm forms dermis of the epithelium of body wall (somatic) and gastrointestinal tract (splanchnic).

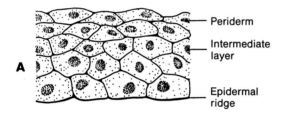

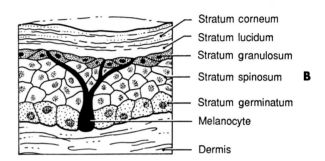

FIG. 1-13 Development of the skin at 4 weeks **(A)** and at 36 weeks **(B)**. Initial layer of epithelial cells thickens into multiple layers, and underlying connective tissue becomes dermis. Dermis and epithelium combine to become skin.

from a combination of epidermal and dermal cells. This development occurs when epithelial cells proliferate, invade the underlying dermis, and finally differentiate into glands or teeth, with both the epidermis and dermis contributing to each of these structures.

CLINICAL COMMENT

Environmental teratogens may affect the development of normal cells, tissues, organs, or organ systems. A defect in the development of a group of cells is considerably less damaging than a defect in an organ or organ system. The smaller and less complex the development, the less extensive the problem created. Development is also related to timing. Tissues are most susceptible to defective development when they begin to differentiate in the embryonic period (4 to 8 weeks).

NERVOUS SYSTEM

The neural folds appear during the third prenatal week. The lateral edges of the neural plate begin to elevate as folds arising dorsally (Fig. 1-9). These folds represent the first change in shape of the embryo's body from the flat sheet of cells (Fig. 1-8). These folds reach the midline, first in the cervical region, and then the neural tube closes both anteriorly and posteriorly (Fig. 1-14). When the anterior tube closes, it shows three dilations that form the primary brain vesicles, the **forebrain, midbrain,** and **hindbrain** (Fig. 1-15, *A*). The neural tube bends forward just behind the midbrain and backward behind the hindbrain (Fig. 1-15, *C* and *D*). The **cerebral hemispheres** develop from the forebrain vesicles. The midbrain is a pathway from the cerebral cortex to centers in the **pons** and **cerebellum** of the hindbrain. The fifth cranial nerve develops in the midbrain (Fig. 1-15, *B* to *D*). The cerebral hemispheres of the forebrain develop into the **frontal, temporal,** and **occipital** lobes.

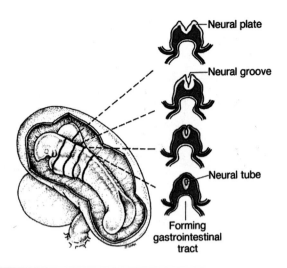

FIG. 1-14   *Left,* Dorsal view of closing neural tube of 3-week human embryo. Closure occurs initially in dorsal area, then anteriorly and posteriorly. *Right,* Transverse sections of neural folds appear anteriorly, and those of closed neural tube are in midbrain region.

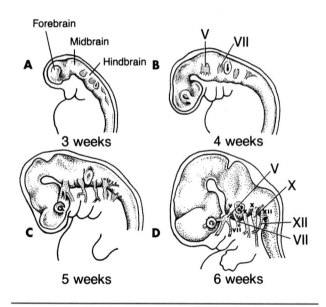

FIG. 1-15   Development of cranial nerves: **A,** 3 weeks; **B,** 4 weeks; **C,** 5 weeks; **D,** 6 weeks. At 3 weeks, forebrain has enlarged and sensory vesicles are laterally located. At 4 and 5 weeks, forebrain has bent forward and cranial nerves have grown into tissues they innervate. At 6 weeks, anterior brain has enlarged and bent back on posteriorly located cerebellum.

The ventricles of the brain are continuous and connect posteriorly with the spinal cord. The walls of the neural tube are lined with neuroepithelium. As these cells proliferate, they differentiate into **neuroblasts** and become the white and gray matter of the spinal cord. Neuroblasts are primitive nerve cells that develop into adult nerve cells called the **neurons.** These cells do not

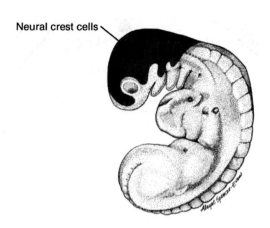

FIG. 1-16   Migration pathway of neural crest cells from neural folds to the developing face.

divide further. Along the surface of the developing brain and spinal cord, neural crest cells form the sensory system of the dorsal root ganglia of the cranial and spinal nerves (Fig. 1-16). The neural crest cells also contribute to tissues of the face, such as cartilage, muscles, teeth, and ligaments.

Connective Tissue
Connective Tissue Proper
Connective tissue develops from the somites as fibroblasts migrating from either side of the neural tube (Fig. 1-12). Early in formation, the ventromedial part of the somite differentiates into the **sclerotome,** the dorsolateral part becomes the **dermatome,** and a third division becomes the intermediate mesoderm or **myotome.** The medial sclerotome differentiates into **mesenchymal cells,** which become **osteoblasts, chondroblasts,** and **fibroblasts.** A large part of the embryonic skeleton develops from these cells. Dermatome cells form the dermis, the subcutaneous tissue, and the **visceral mesoderm,** which supports the endoderm of the gastrointestinal tract, as well as a system of mesenteries that stabilize and support the gastrointestinal tract (Fig. 1-17). Also, connective tissue arises from the somites, providing supporting connective tissues, bones, cartilage, tendons, and ligaments. The tendons connect the muscles to the skeleton as they develop. Connective tissue also functions as capsules of glands and the supporting tissues within them.

Cartilage and Bone
The initial skeletal component in the embryo is **cartilage.** Cartilage cells arise from the sclerotome and migrate to surround the notochord and spinal cord, which form the spinal column (Fig. 1-17, *C*). The skeleton de-

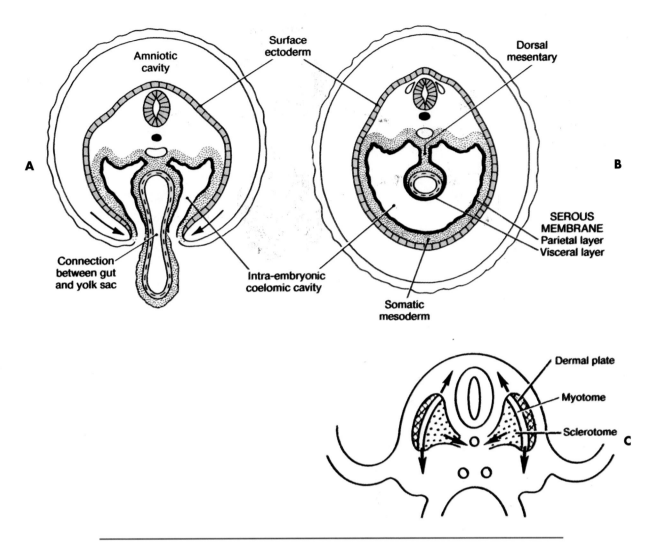

FIG. 1-17 **A** and **B,** Cross sections of embryo illustrating the yolk sac's role in development of gastrointestinal tube. Developing body wall is growing ventrally, closing ventral opening. **C,** Contributions of somite to skin, muscles, and cartilage. Cartilage forms a support for spinal column (sclerotome), which surrounds neural tube. Contribution of somitic mesoderm (dermal plate) to the body wall seen in **B.** Muscles arise from intermediate mesoderm (myotome).

velops in the same segmental pattern as the muscles do (Figs. 1-18 and 1-19). Chondroblasts also form cartilage in the appendages, the cranium, and the face, which first appear in the fifth prenatal week. Cartilage cells undergo both **appositional** (exogenous) and **interstitial** (endogenous) growth (Fig. 1-18, *B*).

Apposition of new layers of cartilage occurs on the surface of cartilage, and interstitial growth involves the proliferation and expansion of the cells within the matrix (Fig. 1-18, *B*). A supportive cartilage skeleton is produced rapidly to support the soft tissues of the growing embryo. Later most of this same cartilage skeleton is replaced by bone, which offers more rigidity and strength as muscles attach to it, making movement possible (Fig. 1-18, *C*). Most cartilage appears clear and

glasslike and is called **hyaline cartilage.** Cartilage may also contain elastic fibers and be termed **elastic** or **fibrous cartilage.** The intervertebral disks, for example, are fibrous cartilage, but the external ear contains elastic cartilage. Cartilage combines the properties of elasticity and strength.

Bone replaces cartilage by a process termed **endochondral bone development** (Fig. 1-20). In this case a small blood vessel enters the cartilage shaft (diaphysis), the cartilage calcifies and disintegrates in the center, and a marrow space is formed (Fig. 1-20, *B*). New bone develops on the surface of cartilage spicules that border the marrow space (Fig. 1-20, *C*). Small blood vessels enter the head of the long bones, and secondary ossification centers appear, repeating the process that took place in

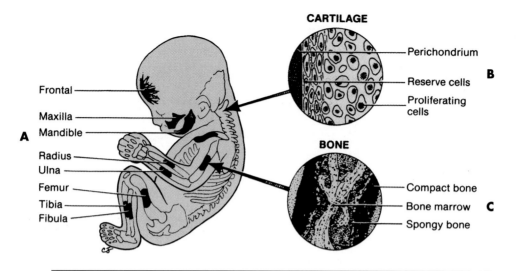

FIG. 1-18 **A,** Embryo's skeleton illustrating development of cartilage and bones. **B,** Cartilage development by both surface apposition and internal interstitial growth. **C,** Endochondral bone development in shaft of long bone.

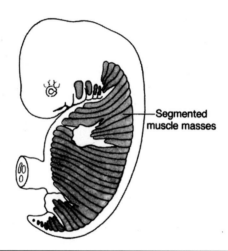

FIG. 1-19 Schematic diagram of primitive myotome in skeletal muscle formation in embryo.

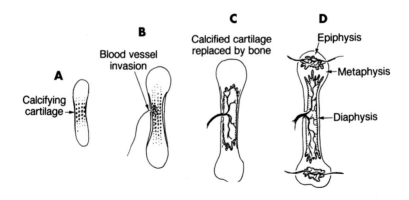

FIG. 1-20 Schematic diagram of endochondral ossification as seen in developing long bones of body. **A,** Original hyaline cartilage is calcified in center of diaphysis. **B,** A blood vessel invades center of shaft. **C,** Marrow space appears in center of shaft, and bone forms around the diaphysis. **D,** Bone formation continues in shaft, and secondary ossification sites appear in heads (epiphysis) of the bones. A disk of cartilage remains between bone forming in head and shaft (epiphyseal line).

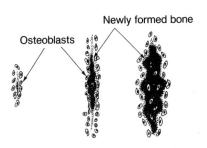

FIG. 1-21 Membranous bone formation that takes place in connective tissue. Initial membranous sites grow by apposition of new bone on their surfaces.

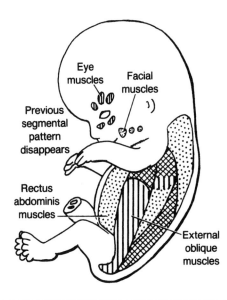

FIG. 1-22 Differentiation of skeletal muscle by enlargement of fibers and attachment to bony skeleton to become functional units. Previous segmental pattern disappears.

the shaft of the long bone (Fig. 1-20, *D*). During the growth period a developing cartilage disk remains in the neck of each long bone and bone forms on either side. This disk is known as the **epiphyseal line** and will remain as long as the bone is forming. The wider part of the diaphysis adjacent to the epiphyseal line is known as the **metaphysis** (Fig. 1-20, *D*). Cartilage develops and expands by **interstitial growth,** which is growth within the cartilage matrix by each cartilage cell enlarging and forming matrix around each cell. New bone forms along the cartilage margins of the epiphyseal line. After bone replaces the epiphysis, cartilage is limited to covering the heads of long bones, the nasal septum, the ears, and a few other sites.

Direct transformation of connective tissue into bone may also take place. In this case, collagen fibers of connective tissue organize into closely knit meshwork and this matrix gradually calcifies into bone by a process termed **intramembranous bone formation** or membranous bone formation (Fig. 1-21). It is much simpler for bone cells to organize in this manner and to form spicules of bone through coalescence with neighboring spicules until a bony plate is formed. The bones of the face and cranium develop in this manner.

DNA transcription is an example of **gene expression.** Transcription generates mRNAs that carry information for protein synthesis, as well as transferring ribosomal and other RNA molecules that have structural and catalytic functions. RNA molecules synthesize RNA polymerase enzymes, which make an RNA copy of a DNA sequence.

Muscle

By the tenth prenatal week, muscle cells (myoblasts) have begun migrating from the myotome, following a segmental pattern similar to that of the bony skeleton (Figs. 1-18 and 1-19). They gradually differentiate into elongated, multinucleated muscle fibers, which are specialized cells with the property of contractility. In this manner, muscle is able to provide motion on the basis of structural and functional characteristics.

Muscle is divided into three types: skeletal, smooth, and cardiac. Later these skeletal muscles lose their segmental pattern of development as they acquire insertion on skeletal elements. These muscle fibers become the **striated voluntary muscles,** which divide into groups that supply the dorsal and ventral parts of the limbs and provide both the deep and superficial muscle fibers (Fig. 1-22). These muscles are called striated because they have lines across them that are the contraction sites that cause the muscles to function.

Muscle cells also migrate to the gastrointestinal tract and support the trachea, bronchi, urogenital tract, and larger blood vessels. These muscle cells develop and become oriented in the direction in which their contractility will be exerted. They are termed **smooth muscle cells** and are under the control of the autonomic nervous system, not under conscious control as are skeletal muscles. The blood vessels that develop in the head region, limbs, and body wall gain their muscular coat from local mesenchyme.

Cardiovascular System

The cardiovascular system originates from cells termed **angioblasts,** which arise from **angiogenic clusters** from the visceral mesoderm located in the walls of the yolk sac during the third week of prenatal life (Fig. 1-23). As these cells separate into clusters, the outer cells organize into a series of elongating tubes and the inner cells become blood cells (Fig. 1-24). For the first few weeks nutrition moves from the yolk sac to the embryo through the developing **vitelline vascular system** (Fig. 1-25). The entire blood vascular system within the embryo is created

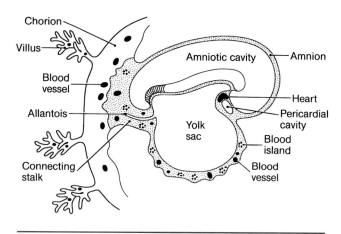

FIG. 1-23 Origin of blood cells and blood vessels in walls of yolk sac, placenta, and body stalk in 2½-week-old embryo.

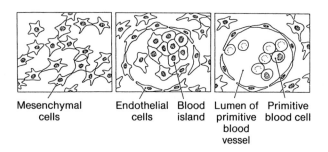

FIG. 1-24 Appearance of blood islands from mesenchymal cells in location noted in Fig. 1-23. The more peripheral cells form capillary walls, and the inner cells form red blood cells. The tubes or capillaries then lengthen.

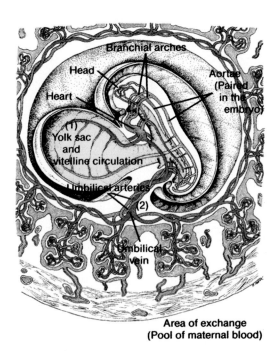

FIG. 1-25 Development of blood vascular system in embryo. *1,* In yolk sac, vitelline circulation develops, persisting for only a few weeks until this nutritional source is exhausted. *2,* Umbilical system develops in umbilical cord, supplying embryo and fetus with oxygen and nutrients until birth.

in the same manner with longitudinal growth of vessels and the appearance of blood cells within them. As vessels begin to develop in the embryo, they in turn form a vascular network connected to the placenta. Because it traverses the umbilical cord, this network is termed the **umbilical system** (Fig. 1-25). Through this umbilical system, nutrition and oxygen are conducted to the embryo and carbon dioxide and wastes to the placenta. By the fourth week the heart begins to beat. This vascular system takes over the functions as the vitelline system expires because the yolk sac has nothing more to contribute (Fig. 1-25).

Other mesenchyme cells migrate into the pericardial area to function in the development of heart tubes, and these cells later differentiate into cardiac muscle. Two angiogenic cell clusters initially form the straight bilateral endocardial heart tubes, which fuse during the third week. They then enlarge and bend back upon themselves (Fig. 1-26). As the great vessels that bring blood to the heart enlarge and become more extensive, the heart grows and internal partitioning begins. An opening persists between the right and left atria **(foramen ovale)** until birth. As the heart tube enlarges and twists during de-

velopment, strands of muscle take on the arrangement of parallel fibers. Like striated muscle, these fibers develop transverse markings termed **intercalated disks.** The myofibrils on either side of these disks exert contraction through the interaction of these many cells. Cardiac muscle is thus not under conscious control and begins to beat during the fourth week. Umbilical circulation then becomes active in transporting oxygen and nutrition from the placenta.

 CLINICAL COMMENT

The human placenta is often considered in terms of its function in exchanging fetal oxygen and carbon dioxide. It also exchanges nutrients and electrolytes, such as proteins and carbohydrates. The placenta produces hormones, such as progesterone and estrogen, which can help maintain pregnancy. It also produces a lactogenic hormone that gives the fetus first priority on circulating maternal blood glucose.

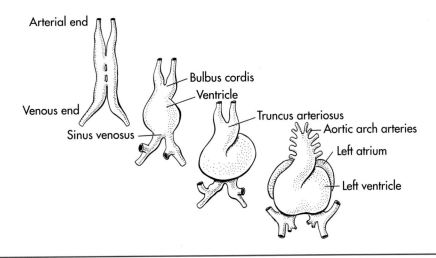

FIG. 1-26   Development of four-chamber heart from fusion of two lateral endocardiac heart tubes. Tubes fold laterally into single tube, which is next divided by internal septa into four-chamber heart.

SELF-EVALUATION QUESTIONS

1. What is the smallest unit of structure, and what are its eight functions in the body?
2. Name the structures found in cell cytoplasm, and describe their functions.
3. Name the cells that do not undergo division.
4. Describe changes in the embryonic disk during the third and fourth prenatal weeks.
5. Define the cell cycle and describe the activities that occur in the G1 and G2 phases.
6. What is the significance of the angiogenic clusters found in the vitelline and umbilical vascular systems?
7. What develops from the gastrointestinal tract?
8. Describe the characteristics of the three prenatal periods.
9. Name three types of cartilage, and describe where they are in the human body.
10. Name and describe three types of muscle fibers.

    CONSIDER THE PATIENT . . .

Discussion: Two diagnostic tests are available. Amniocentesis is the withdrawal of a small amount of amniotic fluid; it reveals genetic disorders and age of the fetus. Fetal ultrasound reflects body tissues to the video monitor; it reveals abnormal or normal development, vitality, sex, and fetal age. Neither test causes tissue damage. Ultrasound would be the choice in this case.

SUGGESTED READING

Avery JK, editor: *Oral development and histology,* New York, 1992, Thieme Medical.

Moore KL: *The developing human,* ed 6, Philadelphia, 1998, WB Saunders.

Sadler T, editor: *Langman's medical embryology,* ed 5, Baltimore, 1985, Williams & Wilkins.

Sperber GH: *Craniofacial embryology,* ed 4, Boston, 1989, Wright.

Tortora GJ: *Principles of human anatomy,* ed 7, New York, 1995, Harper Collins College.

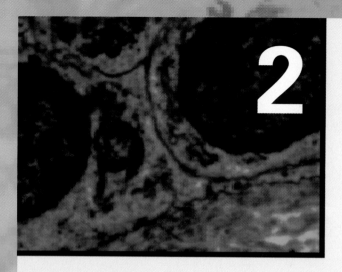

2 Structure and Function of Cells, Tissues, and Organs

OVERVIEW

This chapter describes the structure and function of the body's primary tissues: epithelial, neural, connective, and muscle. Chapter 1 presents information about the development of these tissues. This chapter continues with a description of the tissues and of how they function in organs and organ systems. The chapter first describes epithelial tissue as to cell type, structure, location, and function in the body. Simple squamous epithelium lines the blood vascular and respiratory systems, the kidney, most glands, and the intestine. Stratified squamous epithelium, on the other hand, is limited to the lining of the mouth, pharynx, larynx, vagina, and part of the urinary bladder.

Neural tissue is the next type considered. Both the central nervous system, which is composed of the brain and spinal cord, and the nerves and ganglia of the peripheral nervous system are discussed. The basic structural unit of the nervous system is the neuron. Along with the supporting neuroglia cells, this tissue forms a communication network. The two properties of a neuron are irritability and conductivity, both of which enable neurons to react and respond to stimuli.

The third tissue type discussed is connective tissue, characterized by its abundant matrix and composed of fibers and amorphous substance. This tissue is classified according to associated cells, fibers, location, and function. Connective tissue proper consists of loose and dense connective tissue and loose connective tissue with special properties. Two other specialized types of connective tissue are cartilage and bone. Three types of cartilage are described—hyaline, elastic, and fibrous—followed by both cancellous (spongy) and compact (dense) bone. A fourth type of connective tissue is blood and lymph.

The three types of muscle—striated voluntary and smooth and cardiac involuntary—are described according to cell shape, matrix, and their functions in the body.

Organ systems are then described to illustrate how tissues combine to carry out specialized functions in the human body. These organ systems are integumentary, digestive, respiratory, vascular, lymphatic, endocrine, urinary, reproductive, and special senses. Correlative tables help explain this information.

EPITHELIAL TISSUE

Epithelial tissue is composed of different layers. One is a superficial layer of closely packed sheets of cells covering the external surface of the body. Another, the dermis, is the connective tissue layer of the skin underlying the epithelial tissue. A much thinner layer of epithelial tissue also lines the internal cavities of the body and the tubes that drain glands and carry blood throughout the body. The **epidermis** and **dermis** constitute the skin. The epidermis, a form of epithelium, rests on a basement membrane that separates it from the dermis. The epithelial cells form membranes that are composed of closely associated cells with an intercellular substance between them. Most epithelium has the capability of cell renewal by mitosis of the basal cells, and the rate of renewal is dependent on the location of the epithelium in the body. For example, human buccal mucosa renews in 10 to 14 days, whereas the junctional epithelium of the gingiva renews in 4 to 6 days (Fig. 2-1). The dermis is closely associated with the epidermis and has an interdigitating relationship in some areas. Because epithelium does not contain blood vessels, the skin depends on vessels located in the connective tissue of the dermis.

The vessels are in close proximity, nourishing the skin and playing an important part in its function of thermal regulation. Nerves also exist in the dermis, and some penetrate the epithelial cells to function as receptors. Sweat glands, hair follicles and their associated sebaceous glands, and erector pili muscles are located in the dermis and subcutaneous tissue. Ectoderm is the source of the epithelial lining of some internal organs, but not of all epithelial-lined surfaces. For example, the epithelial lining of the alimentary canal is of endodermal origin. The epithelial lining of the peritoneal cavity and the endothelial lining of blood vessels are from mesoderm.

Epithelium is described according to cell shape and cell arrangement in one or more layers. Some cells form a single layer known as **simple epithelium.** Epithelium with all cells in contact with the basal lamina, but not with the surface, is known as **pseudostratified.** The type consisting of several cell layers with only the basal cell layer in contact with the basal lamina is known as **stratified epithelium** (Fig. 2-1). Further modifications are based on cell shape.

Epithelial membranes function in one or more of the absorptive processes: contractility, digestion, secretion, excretion, protection, and sensation. Table 2-1 shows the

Table 2-1

Classification of Epithelia

Cell Type	Cell Shape	Cell Modifications	Characteristics	Location
Simple				
1. Squamous				
a. Endothelial	Spindle			Lines heart, blood, and lymph vessels
b. Mesothelial	Oval to polygonal			Lines pleural, pericardial, and peritoneal cavities
2. Cuboidal	Cube		Cilia may appear	Kidney, glands, respiratory passages
3. Columnar	Rodlike		Microvilli, cilia may appear	Most glands, small intestines, respiratory passages
4. Pseudostratified	Rodlike with thin section		Cilia, stereocilia	Respiratory passages, male reproductive organs
Stratified				
1. Squamous	Polyhedral		Intercellular bridges	Covering of the body, mouth, pharynx, vagina
2. Columnar	Columnar cells on cuboidal or columnar on columnar			Oropharynx, larynx
3. Transitional	Cube to pear		Distension causes cell flattening	Urinary passages, bladder

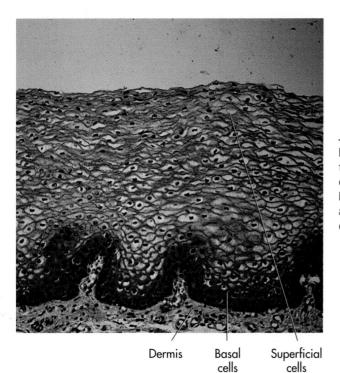

FIG. 2-1 Stratified squamous nonkeratinized epithelium from the oral cavity. Darker stained cells are basal cells, which are dividing to form more superficial layers. As cells develop in the basal layer, they gradually migrate to the surface and are lost by attrition. Dermis contains the blood vessels that nourish the epithelium.

Dermis   Basal   Superficial
           cells   cells

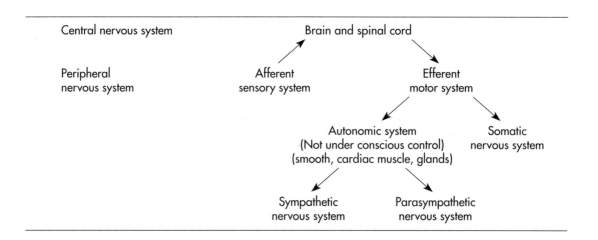

FIG. 2-2 Components of the nervous system.

classification of epithelia by cell type, cell shape, cell modifications, characteristics, and location.

NEURAL TISSUE

Neural tissue is a second type of tissue. It constitutes the central and peripheral nervous systems. The **central nervous system** (CNS) is the control center of the nervous system and is composed of the brain and spinal cord. The brain is located in the cranium and is connected to the peripheral tissues by cranial nerves and to the spinal cord by spinal nerves. All sensation received anywhere in the body is relayed to the brain and spinal cord, which act on the sensation. Nerve tissue is made from neuroepithelial cells, which are highly organized areas for reception and correlation. Nerve processes that carry information and convey it from the peripheral nervous system in muscles and glands to the CNS are called the **afferent (sensory) system.** Other neurons that convey responses from the CNS to muscles and glands are located in the **efferent (motor) system.** These two systems are further divided into **somatic** and **autonomic** nervous systems. The nervous system is closely associated with

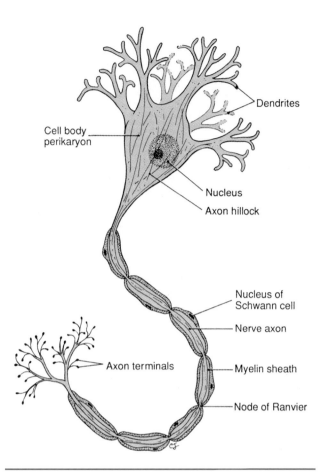

Cell body
perikaryon

Dendrites

Nucleus

Axon hillock

Nucleus of
Schwann cell

Nerve axon

Axon terminals

Myelin sheath

Node of Ranvier

FIG. 2-3 Diagram of a nerve cell and its processes. Myelin insulates the nerve axon and is produced by Schwann's cells. Impulses are received by the dendrites and travel to the cell body and then the axon terminals, where they may contact dendrites of an adjacent nerve cell.

the endocrine system, which is dependent on neural stimuli to function.

The somatic nervous system carries impulses to the voluntary muscles, such as the skeletal muscles, which are under conscious control. On the other hand, the efferent autonomic system carries impulses from the CNS to involuntary muscles, such as the smooth and cardiac muscles, and to all the glands. The viscera receive most of their impulses from this system.

The autonomic system produces responses involuntarily and is further divided into the **sympathetic** and **parasympathetic** divisions. These two divisions modify each other: the sympathetic causes increased activity, and the parasympathetic modifies or decreases activity. Fig. 2-2 outlines the nervous system.

The nervous system carries out numerous functions with only two principal types of cells, which are **neuron** and **neuroglia.** Neurons are the nerve cells that receive and conduct impulses and regulate muscle and gland activity. Neuroglia cells are the supporting cells of the nervous system. Each neuron consists of three parts. The first

part is the **cell body** or **perikaryon,** which contains the nucleus and the **cytoplasm.** The cytoplasm contains a chromatophilic substance or rough endoplasmic reticulum (RER). The function of the RER, as in other cells, is protein synthesis. Proteins travel from the perikaryon into the second part of the neuron, the **axon,** which is a long, thin singular process that varies in length from a few millimeters to several feet or more. The axon conducts nerve impulses away from the nerve cell body. It terminates by branching into **axon terminals** or synaptic end bulbs (Fig. 2-3). Axons outside the CNS are protected and insulated by a myelin sheath, which is a multilayer of phospholipid produced by the neurilemma (Schwann's cells). The third component of the neuron is the **dendrite,** usually multiple, which receives impulses and conducts them to the cell body (Fig. 2-3).

Neuroglia cells carry out the functions of support. These are 5 to 50 times more numerous than neurons. Neuroglia cells protect and support nerve cells, and some are even phagocytic, ingesting bacteria.

The brain continues into the spinal cord, which is within the vertebral canal. This canal is a cylindrical space extending from the brain to the lumbar vertebrae. It is composed of 31 segments with spinal nerves coming from each. The spinal cord conveys impulses from the peripheral nervous system to the brain and from the brain to the peripheral tissues.

CONNECTIVE TISSUE

Connective tissue varies in its proportion of cells, fibers, and intercellular substance and its location in the body. **Connective tissue proper** is classified as **loose, dense,** or **loose connective tissue with special properties.** Two other types of connective tissue are the skeletal tissues, **cartilage** and **bone.** Bone is classified as **compact** (dense) or **cancellous** (spongy) (Figs. 2-4 to 2-6). The three types of cartilage are **hyaline** (Fig. 2-7), **elastic,** and **fibrous** (Fig. 2-8). Other forms of connective tissue are **blood** and **lymph,** which are fluid connective tissues (Fig. 2-9).

Blood conducts oxygen to the cells, returns carbon dioxide from the cells to the lungs, clots to prevent blood loss, and regulates pH through a buffer system. It also

 CONSIDER THE PATIENT . . .

Case 1: An older patient appears with a fractured arm after minimal trauma. He asks if the fracture may have been caused by something other than the initial trauma.

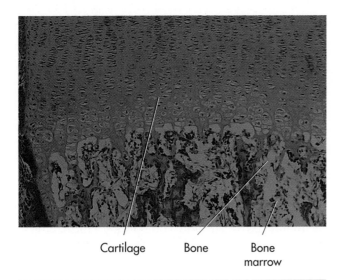

Cartilage   Bone   Bone
marrow

FIG. 2-4   Developing endochondral bone matrix. At the junction, below which are bone spicules and above which is cartilage, is an area of transition of cartilage into bone. The hyaline cartilage above becomes calcified and undergoes breakdown at the junction. Bone spicules form in the center of the long bone, called the bone marrow. New cartilage also forms as shown in the area at the top of the micrograph. This area maintains the cartilage until growth is completed.

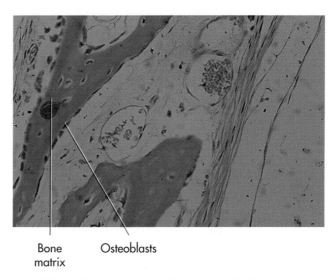

Bone   Osteoblasts
matrix

FIG. 2-5   Appearance of cancellous bone. If this were newly forming intramembranous bone, numerous osteoblasts would be on the surface of the trabeculae. A few elongated and flattened osteoblasts can be seen on the bone surface. Several thin-walled veins, which contain red blood cells, and scattered connective tissue cells can be seen in the field.

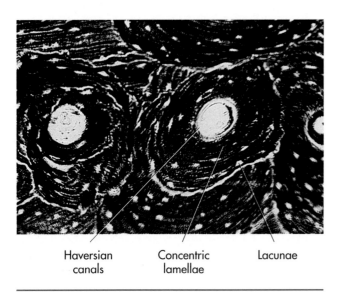

Haversian   Concentric   Lacunae
canals   lamellae

FIG. 2-6   Compact bone in transverse section illustrating haversian vascular channels. These haversian canals are surrounded by concentric lamellae and lacunae (white) appearing along the lamellae. This pattern indicates the deposition pattern of the bone. Between the haversian systems are some interstitial lamellae. In living bone, osteocytes would appear as live cells within the lacunae.

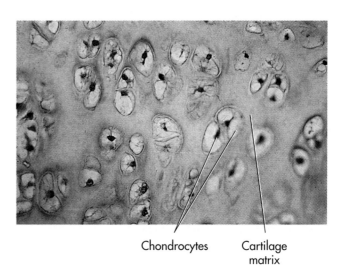

Chondrocytes   Cartilage
matrix

FIG. 2-7   Section of hyaline cartilage found in thyroid or tracheal cartilages. Large cells (chondrocytes) are surrounded by a homogenous-appearing cartilage matrix. Only darkstained nucleoli can be seen because cytoplasm of the cells is faintly stained. Cells exist in lacunae, which are open spaces in the matrix. Some cells have divided, and two cells appear in the same or adjacent lacunae.

Table 2-2
Formed Elements of the Blood

Element		Number	Function
Erythrocytes		Male: 5.4 million/ml^3 Female: 4.8 million/ml^3	Oxygen and carbon dioxide pickup and transport
Leukocytes		5000-9000/ml^3	
Granular	Neutrophils	55%-65%	Phagocytic to infectious agents
	Eosinophils	1%-3%	Helminthic parasitic diseases
	Basophils	0%-0.7%	Histamine, serotonin, heparin
Nongranular	Lymphocytes	20%-35%	Immunologic response, B, T, and NK cells
	Monocytes	3%-7%	Phagocytic, contribute osteoclasts
Platelets		5000-9000/ml^3	Function in clot formation, stimulate cell division

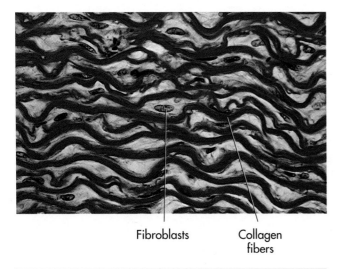

Fibroblasts   Collagen fibers

FIG. 2-8   Appearance of dense, irregular connective tissue. Large bundles of collagen fibers appear in longitudinal section with a few pale-stained fibroblasts interspersed between them. The faint banding of these collagen fibers cannot be seen at this magnification.

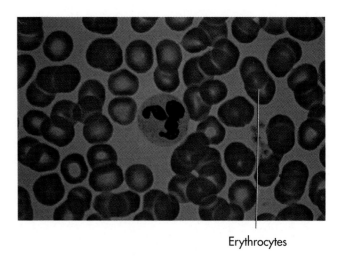

Erythrocytes

FIG. 2-9   Another type of connective tissue is the circulating blood. In the field are numerous red blood cells (erythrocytes) and white blood cells (neutrophils). The white blood cells are slightly larger than the red, and the red are nonnucleated. The red cells appear white in the center because they are biconcave disks and are very thin in this area. Whole blood consists of 55% plasma, which has no cells, and 45% cells and cell fragments.

regulates body temperature and provides protection from bacteria through its phagocytic and antigenic properties. Plasma is the fluid part of the blood in which the cells and particulate substance are suspended. Men have about 5 liters of blood, and women have about 4.5 liters, which is about 7% of body weight. The erythrocytes (red blood cells) are not true cells because they have no nucleus or other organelles. However, these cells do have the ability to take oxygen from the lungs, transport it to the tissues, and return carbon dioxide from the tissues to the lungs. Leukocytes (white blood cells) are of two types, granular and nongranular.

The lymphoid organs are part of the immune system and consist of lymph nodes, thymus, and spleen. Other aggregates of lymphatic tissue and lymphocytes are in the bone marrow, bloodstream, tonsils, Peyer's patches, and other locations of the alimentary canal. A characteristic of the immune system is its ability to recognize and react specifically to macromolecules that are foreign to the body.

Details of cellular and other elements of blood are noted in Table 2-2. Each type of connective tissue has specific associated cells and fibers with special functions and locations in the body (Table 2-3).

Table 2-3

Classification of Connective Tissue

Tissue Type	Associated Cells	Fibers		Location and Function

I. Connective tissue proper
  A. Loose connective
    tissue
	Fibroblasts, macro-
	phages, mast cells
		Yellow elastic
		White collagen
				Fascia, superficial and
				deep; organ framework
				support

B. Dense connective tissue 1. Dense regular	Fibroblasts, macrophages	White fibrous		Tendons, ligaments; muscle to bone attachment
2. Dense irregular	Fibroblasts, macrophages	Mostly white fibrous, elastic and reticular fibers		Sheets, dermis, some sternum, capsules; support of organs

C. Loose connective tissue
    with special properties
    1. Mucous connective
      tissue
	Stellate fibroblasts	Collagenous		Umbilical and vocal cords;
				support

2. Elastic tissue	Fibroblasts	Yellow elastic		Ligamenta nuchae, vocal cords; support
3. Reticular tissue	Reticular cells	Fine reticular		Framework of lymph node and spleen
4. Adipose tissue	Fat cells	None		Scattered in all loose connective tissue and in deposits
5. Pigment tissue	Melanoblasts	None		Corium of dark skin Choroid and iris of eye
II. Cartilage A. Hyaline cartilage	Chondrocytes	Fine collagenous		Articular and nasal cartilages, trachea, bronchi; support
B. Elastic cartilage	Chondrocytes	Elastic, collagenous		External ear, eustachian tube, epiglottis; support
C. Fibrous cartilage	Chondrocytes	Collagenous (dense)		Intervertebral disks; support
III. Bone A. Spongy or cancellous	Osteocytes, osteoblasts, osteoclasts	Collagenous		Center of long bones
B. Compact or dense	Osteocytes, osteoclasts, osteoblasts	Collagenous		Outer shaft of bones
IV. Blood and lymph	Erythrocytes, leukocytes			Blood vascular and lymphatic systems

MUSCLE TISSUE

The reaction to stimulus is motion, and the basis of motion in a muscle cell is the change from chemical to mechanical energy by enzymatic cleavage of adenosine triphosphate (ATP). This is a result of the action of two proteins, **actin** and **myosin,** which are arranged in the direction of contraction. Muscle is located throughout the body and consists of three types: **skeletal** or **voluntary** (Fig. 2-10), **smooth** (Fig. 2-11), and **cardiac** (Fig. 2-12). Skeletal muscle allows movement under voluntary control. The **involuntary** muscle (smooth muscle) of the alimentary canal assists with digestion and movement of food through the alimentary tract. The involuntary (car-

diac) muscle of the heart pumps blood through some 50,000 miles of blood vessels. Therefore the three muscle types in the body have specific characteristics permitting individualized functions. However, some features of muscle are common to all types. For example, each muscle fiber is covered with **perimysium,** and the entire muscle is covered with **epimysium.** Each muscle type contains actin and myosin, which cause the contraction so vital to muscle function. Table 2-4 shows the muscles' locations and the cells that function within each.

ORGAN SYSTEMS

Organ systems comprise the tissues in the body that are functionally integrated and specifically designed to perform designated functions. Cells, the basic structural and functional units of the body, may aggregate and form tissues or groups of tissues, which are organized together to form organs. These organs form for a specific function and relate to other organs to form organ systems. Fig. 2-13 shows most of the body's organ systems, which are described as follows.

Integumentary or Skin System

The largest organ in the body (skin) has numerous functions. One is the excretion of waste products, such as carbon dioxide, water, small amounts of salts, and urea. The skin also eliminates heat, serves as a protection against invasion of foreign materials, and receives stimulation from nerves. These varying functions are possible because of the skin's multicellular layers of epithelium and layers of connective tissue that carry blood vessels, muscles, and nerves. Epithelium has five cell-type layers: a basal or germinating layer, a spinous layer called stratum spinosum, a layer of cells with keratohyalin granules called the granular layer, a clear layer called the stratum lucidum, and the covering layer of keratinocytes that protects all the deeper layers. The dermis has two layers: a superficial papillary layer and a deep reticular layer. The skin also has hair follicles and sweat glands and sebaceous glands, which assist in the multifunctional nature of the skin.

Table 2-4

Classification of Muscle

Type	Cell Shape	Diagrams	Location
A. Skeletal Skeletal wall, voluntary	Very long multinucleated fiber with cross-striations composed of actin (thin) and myosin (thick) components.		Bony skeleton or fascia, limbs and body, pharynx, upper esophagus
B. Smooth Visceral, involuntary	Spindle-shaped fibers with a single elongated nucleus and myofilaments. Nuclei located in center of fiber.		Hollow organs, wall of intestines, ducts of glands, blood vessels
C. Cardiac muscle Striated, involuntary	Long cross-striated fibers that branch and contain intercalated discs (junctional complexes). Some muscle fibers are specialized to conduct impulses: Purkinje's fibers. Nuclei in center of fiber.		Wall of heart, major veins opening into the heart

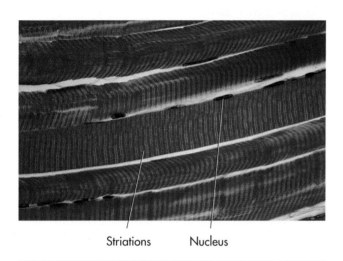

Striations   Nucleus

FIG. 2-10   Skeletal muscle fibers in longitudinal section. Cross striations are seen as alternating light and dark bands, indicating fiber contraction sites. Each large fiber contains a number of nuclei on the periphery. These are muscle fibers of the arms, legs, and body wall and are controlled voluntarily.

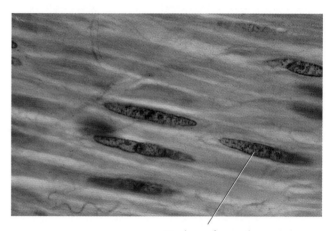

Nucleus of smooth
muscle cell

FIG. 2-11   Smooth muscle fibers in longitudinal section can be compared to skeletal muscle. Smooth muscle fibers are spindle shaped with the large, longitudinal nucleus in the center of the fiber. Small amounts of connective tissue surround the fibers. This muscle surrounds the gastrointestinal tract and muscular blood vessels. It is controlled involuntarily.

Digestive System

Functions of the digestive system's alimentary canal are to absorb, transform, and extract needed components from food ingested and to excrete all unused solid waste. In addition, carbon dioxide, water, and heat are lost. A long tube (approximately 26 feet) composed of the pharynx and esophagus conducts food to the stomach, a mixing and digestive chamber where food is reduced to liquid chyme. Further digestion takes place in the small intestine, which adds glandular secretions from the liver, pancreas, and spleen. The large intestine, which absorbs nutrition, also dehydrates food and compresses it into solid waste. Digestion takes place throughout the tract through function of salivary glands in the oral cavity,

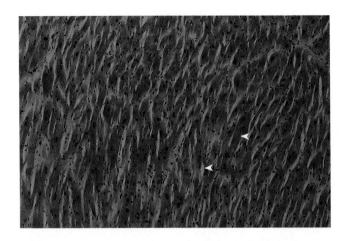

FIG. 2-12 Section of cardiac muscle found in the heart wall. Muscle fibers appear striated and are similar to skeletal muscle fibers except that some of the fibers branch *(arrowheads)*. The nuclei of these fibers are located centrally, as seen in smooth muscle, and the areas at the ends of the nuclei are pale staining.

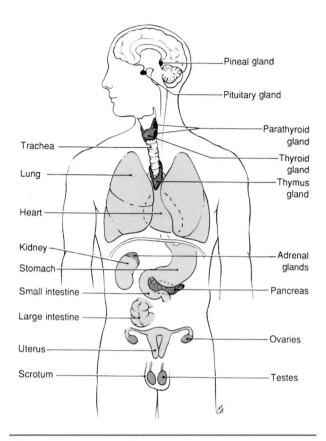

FIG. 2-13 Diagram of the human body with glands listed on the right side and organs listed on the left.

gastric glands in the stomach, and liver, gallbladder, pancreas, and spleen in the small intestine. The walls of the tract are composed of functional layers: lining epithelium, connective tissue layers, and layers of muscle. Muscle aids in peristaltic movement of food through the tract (Figs. 2-14 and 2-15).

Respiratory System

The function of the respiratory system is primarily to exchange gases in several phases. The process includes both inflow (inspiration) of oxygen and outflow (expiration) of carbon dioxide. The blood cells exchange oxygen and carbon dioxide with other cells in the body and with the pulmonary air sacs. The respiratory system includes the nasal chambers, in which the air is warmed by blood flowing close to the surface and which becomes moist through the mucus secreted by goblet cells. These also trap dust particles. Cilia of the lining cells of the respiratory tract move these particulate substances to the pharynx and out of the respiratory system. In addition, the system includes the pharynx, trachea, and bronchi, which function as conduction chambers, and the lungs proper, which function in respiration (Fig. 2-16).

Vascular System

The vascular system includes the heart, large elastic arteries, smaller muscular arteries, and miles of capillaries, as well as veins that carry blood from the capillaries back to the heart. The heart, which is the size of an adult's clenched fist, pumps an estimated 5 to 6 liters of blood approximately 60 times a minute. The function of the bloodstream is to carry oxygen to the cells in all areas of the body and to return carbon dioxide from these cells to the lungs. The blood vascular system provides nutrition from the walls of the alimentary canal and other organs. Blood also carries waste products to the kidneys, the gastrointestinal tract, and other organs of excretion, such as the skin. Arteries function in conduction and distribution, capillaries in oxygen exchange and nutrition of the extracellular spaces, and veins in the return of blood to the heart. The blood vascular system additionally functions in blood clotting, and some white blood cells function in phagocytosis. Blood also conducts various hormones to their sites of action through the activities of the neuroendocrine system. Table 2-2 shows cellular and other elements of the blood.

Lymphatic System

The lymph system consists of lymphatic tissue throughout the body, such as lymph nodes, thymus, spleen, and tonsils (palatine, lingual, and pharyngeal). Aggregations of lymphatic tissue appear in the lower intestine, such as Peyer's patches and the appendix. Circulating lymphocytes in the bloodstream and the lymphatic vessels must also be included. Lymphocytes have the ability to recog-

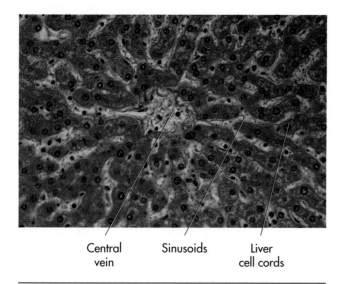

Central   Sinusoids   Liver
vein   cell cords

FIG. 2-14 Section of liver tissue illustrating liver cell cords radiating from a central vein. Blood filters from periphery of each liver (hepatic) lobule. This organ filters the blood and provides a storage area. Spaces between the cell cords are termed sinusoids. Also, large oval nuclei of liver cells can be seen.

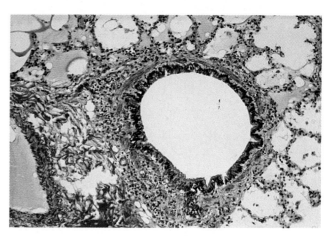

FIG. 2-16 A lung section showing a bronchiole in the center of the field and air sacs in the upper right. The bronchiole is lined with simple columnar ciliated epithelium, and signs of inflammation are seen in the cells surrounding the bronchiole.

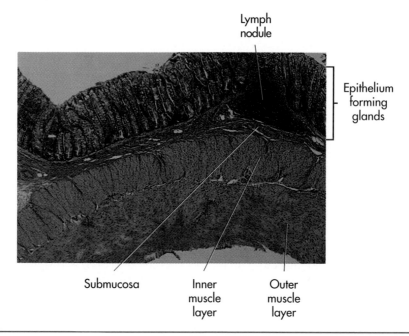

Lymph
nodule

Epithelium
forming
glands

Submucosa   Inner   Outer
              muscle   muscle
              layer   layer

FIG. 2-15 Section of a colon illustrating epithelium-forming deep glands in the mucosa. Supported by connective tissue, lymph nodules are seen as dense aggregations of lymphocytes in this layer of glands. Beneath this is the submucosa, made up of connective tissue containing arteries, veins, capillaries, and nerves. Below this zone are the muscular layers; the inner layer is longitudinal and the outer is circular. On the surface of the intestine is thin connective tissue, the serosal layer.

nize macromolecules that are foreign to the body. B, T, and NK cells are among the lymphocyte types recognized today.

Endocrine System

The endocrine system includes the thyroid, parathyroid, and pituitary glands, ovaries, testes, pancreas, and adrenal medulla. A basic function of these glands is to secrete hormones into the vascular circulation, which then circulates and acts only on target cells through the second messenger, cyclic adenosine monophosphate (cAMP). Although 50 or more hormones traverse the bloodstream, each acts only on specific receptor cells. Hormones help regulate metabolism energy balance and aid in regulation of involuntary smooth and cardiac muscle fibers. Hormones vary body activities, regulate centers of the immune system, play a role in growth and development, contribute to the process of reproduction, and regulate volume and composition of the extracellular environment. Some organs have endocrine function but also have other functions. Examples of these organs are the pancreas, testes, ovaries, thymus, hypothalamus, stomach, intestine, liver, kidneys, heart, and skin. The hypothalamus is the major neural coordinating system between the nervous and endocrine systems.

Urinary System

The urinary system includes the kidneys, ureters, bladder, and urinary tract. The system filters toxic and unnecessary substances from the bloodstream and concentrates them before excretion. Kidneys excrete not only water, but also nitrogenous wastes and bacterial toxins. The major function of the urinary system is to control blood volume and pressure and composition of the urine. Also, this system restores water to the blood. In this manner, renin helps regulate blood pressure. Urine is stored in the urinary bladder until excreted.

Reproductive System

The male reproductive system includes the testes, prostate, and seminal vesicles, and the female system includes the ovaries, uterus, and vagina. The female produces eggs, and the male produces sperm along with secretions of the accessory glands that produce semen. The sperm and the egg each have half the chromosome complement that enables fertilization of the egg, which produces a zygote. The uterus then provides an environment in which the embryo can develop. The testes secrete the hormone testosterone, and the female system produces estrogen and progesterone to ensure development of the embryo.

Special Senses

The special senses system permits the detection of changes in the surrounding environment. This system includes vision, hearing, equilibrium, smell, and taste.

The eye focuses a distortion-free image on the retina. The retina responds to various colors and intensities and encodes spatial and temporal parameters for transmission to the brain.

The ear is composed of three parts. The external ear receives sound waves; the middle ear translates these waves into mechanical vibrations; and the internal ear receives the vibrations and changes them into specific impulses that are transmitted by the acoustic nerve to the brain.

Equilibrium is controlled by the vestibular organs, which are located in the internal ear.

The olfaction organ is located in the olfactory epithelium, which is a pseudostratified, ciliated columnar epithelium located in the roof of the nasal cavity. The olfactory cells are bipolar nerve cells, and their axons transmit to nerve trunks in the connective tissue underlying the olfactory epithelium. From there olfactory impulses are transmitted to the brain.

The taste modality is located in cells of the taste buds, which are in the circumvallate papillae on the tongue's posterior dorsal surface. Taste is discussed in Chapter 14.

CLINICAL COMMENT

Oral infections can cause pain, tenderness, swelling, and enlarged lymph nodes. Pain is due to the response of a nerve receptor and its transmission to the brain, with corresponding efferent response to both autonomic and somatic systems. This results in a change in vascular tone, causing swelling. Lymph nodes enlarge as defense cells proliferate and become active, filtering and destroying the bacteria and their products in the local lymph nodes.

CLINICAL COMMENT

The heart, which weighs less than a pound and is the size of a clenched fist, pumps 1899 gallons of blood a day or 1.3 million gallons a year. This figure is for a person who is resting; it increases considerably with exercise.

SELF-EVALUATION QUESTIONS

1. Describe four types of loose connective tissue that have special properties.
2. Describe two types of connective tissue proper.
3. Describe three types of cartilage and their locations in the body.
4. Describe cancellous and compact bone and the location of both types.
5. Describe two types of muscle that have involuntary movement and their functions.
6. What are the nonstratified epithelial cell types, and where are they located in the body?
7. Describe the location of stratified squamous and columnar epithelium.
8. Discuss the function of the autonomic nervous system.
9. Describe how the sympathetic and parasympathetic nervous systems work together.
10. Name and briefly describe each of the nine organ systems.

CONSIDER THE PATIENT . . .

Discussion 1: Osteoporosis, caused generally by lack of sex hormones, is a probable cause. Osteoporosis affects older men and women who lose calcium from their skeletons. Women lose calcium earlier (after age 40 to 45) than men (after age 60). Another possible cause of bone loss among older clients is lack of protein (collagen) production, which results in brittle bones and loss of bone matrix.

Discussion 2: Given her symptoms, you should suspect hypothyroidism, which requires evaluation of the level of thyroid hormone in the blood.

SUGGESTED READING

Alberts B et al: *The molecular biology of the cell,* ed 2, New York, 1989, Garland.

Fawcett DW: *The cell,* ed 2, Philadelphia, 1981, WB Saunders.

Geneser F: *Textbook of histology,* Copenhagen, 1986, Munksgaard.

Ross MH, Reith E: *Histology, a text and atlas,* New York, 1985, Harper & Row.

Tortora GJ: *Principles of human anatomy,* ed 7, New York, 1995, HarperCollins College.

Weiss L: *Cell and tissue histology,* ed 5, New York, 1983, Elsevier.

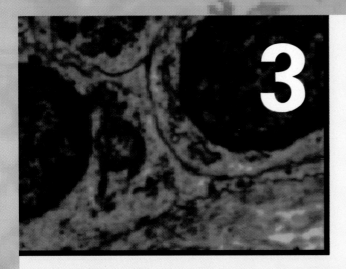

3

Development of the Oral Facial Region

OVERVIEW

This chapter concerns development and orientation of the tissues that form the human face and neck. During the fourth week of development, the human embryo consists of a flat disk that bends down at its anterior extremity as the overlying brain expands and enlarges. This action pushes the heart beneath the brain. A pit develops in the midline between the brain and the heart and becomes the oral cavity or stomodeum (Fig. 3-1). Beneath this pit the first **branchial arch,** termed the **mandibular arch,** forms. The **maxillary tissues** that form the cheeks grow from this first arch. Below the mandibular arch four other branchial arches or bars appear during the fourth to seventh prenatal week. The second arch is called the **hyoid** (Fig. 3-2). These parallel arches are important in the development of the face and neck, and each contains blood vessels, muscles, nerves, and skeletal elements. Aortic arch blood vessels, which course through each branchial arch from the heart below to the brain above, are important to craniofacial development.

The first, second, and fifth of these vessels soon disappear. The third arch vessel quickly assumes the role of supplying nutrients to the tissues of the first and second arches. This third arch vessel also shifts the blood supply to the face from the internal carotid vessels to the external carotid. Muscles arise in each of the branchial arches: the mandibular arch muscles become the masticatory muscles; the second arch muscles become the facial expression muscles; and the muscles of the third and fourth arches become the constrictor muscles of the throat. Cranial nerves enter each of these muscle masses as they arise. The fifth nerve enters the mandibular arch to innervate the muscles of mastication. The seventh innervates the second arch muscle mass, and other cranial nerves innervate the muscles of the neck. Cartilage also appears in each arch: **Meckel's cartilage bar** in the first, the **superior hyoid** in the second, the **inferior hyoid** in the third, and the **laryngeal cartilages** in the fourth. The **cranial base cartilages** arise to support the brain and from them come the auditory and olfactory sense capsules. All the creative events described in this chapter take place from the fourth to seventh prenatal week, the short time required for facial organization.

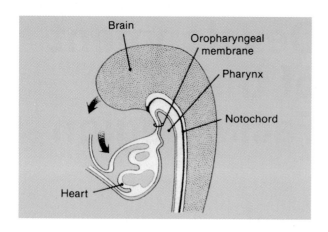

FIG. 3-1 The embryo bends anteriorly with the growth and expansion of the developing brain. This pushes the heart ventrally, and the oral pit (stomodeum) develops between the brain and the heart.

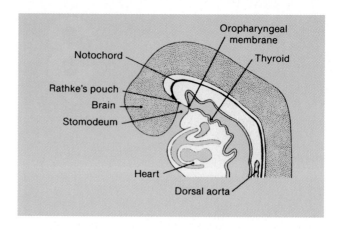

FIG. 3-3 Internal view of oral pit at 3½ weeks. Oropharyngeal membrane separates the oral (stomodeum) and pharyngeal cavities. This membrane will soon rupture, allowing the cavities to join.

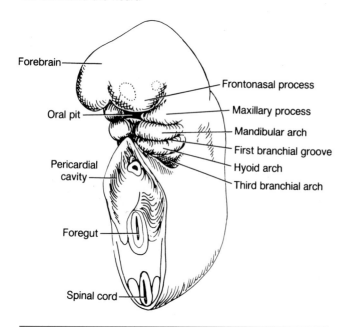

FIG. 3-2 Facial development in the fourth prenatal week. The oral pit is surrounded by facial primordia, which are the frontonasal process, the maxillary process, and the mandibular arch. Branchial arches are defined by grooves. The heart develops in the thorax, which is within the pericardial cavity.

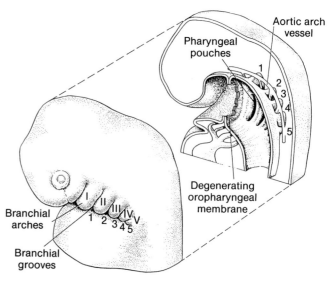

FIG. 3-4 Sagittal view of branchial arches with corresponding grooves between each arch. The pharyngeal pouches are seen in the wall of the pharynx. The aortic arch vasculature leads from the heart dorsally through the arches to the face.

DEVELOPMENT OF THE OROPHARYNX

The oropharynx is composed of the primitive oral cavity and the area of foregut called the pharynx. The oral pit first appears in the fourth week of development, when the neural plate bends ventrally as the neural folds develop to form the forebrain (Fig. 3-1). This cephalocaudal bend pushes the heart ventrally, and the yolk sac becomes enclosed to form an elongating tube known as the foregut (Fig. 3-1).

The deepening oral pocket then appears between the forebrain and the heart and eventually becomes the oral cavity (Fig. 3-2). At its deepest extent is the **oropharyngeal membrane,** which ruptures in the fifth week, opens the oral cavity to the tubular foregut, and soon becomes the **oropharynx** (Figs. 3-3 and 3-4). The mandibular arch will grow laterally to the oral pit, developing the maxillary process, which forms the cheeks.

The enlarging heart now becomes positioned below the mandibular arch in the thorax and begins beating at the end of the fourth week (Fig. 3-3). Blood is forced through the vessels in the branchial arches supplying the

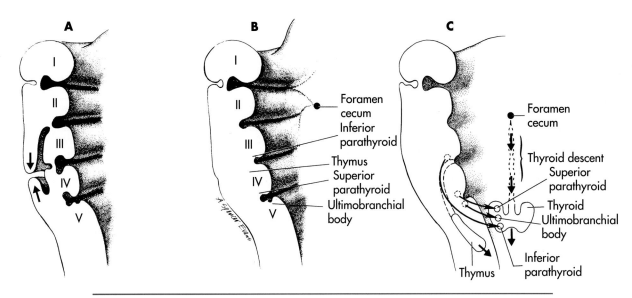

FIG. 3-5 **A,** Tissue from arch II and V growing toward each other *(arrows)* to make branchial arches and grooves disappear. **B,** Resulting appearance following overgrowth. **C,** Contribution of each pharyngeal pouch.

face, neck, and brain. The forming face now grows away from the forebrain and presses against the chest and heart.

DEVELOPMENT OF THE BRANCHIAL ARCHES

The **branchial** arches are so termed because they bend around the sides of the pharynx as bars of tissue. Each arch is separated by vertical grooves on the lateral sides of the neck at the fifth week. Within the pharynx, grooves called **pharyngeal pouches** separate each arch. These pouches match the branchial clefts on the external aspects of the neck (Fig. 3-4).

 CONSIDER THE PATIENT . . .

A patient appears with a swelling in the lateral area of the neck and states that the swelling subsides from time to time but then resumes. He asks you what you think the cause may be.

The five arches with their clefts resemble the embryonic gill slits of fish and amphibians. This is one of many similarities between human embryos and other embryos during early development. The first arch is termed the mandibular arch because it will later form the bony mandible and the associated muscles of mastication, nerves, and blood supply. The second, or hyoid, arch forms the facial muscles, vessels, and hyoid bone. The third, fourth, and fifth arches consist of paired right and

left bars that are divided before they reach the midline by the presence of the bulging heart (Fig. 3-2). The arches become progressively smaller anterior to posterior. The outer surface of each arch is covered with ectoderm as are the inner surface of the first arch and the covering of the anterior surface of the second. This ectoderm is the epithelial lining of the oral cavity. The pharyngeal surface of the remaining four arches is, however, lined by endoderm, which is the same as the lining of the gastrointestinal tract (Fig. 3-4). The cores of the arches—the blood vessels, muscles, nerves, cartilages, and bones—will differentiate and are important in the development of the adult human face.

 CLINICAL COMMENT

The face develops during the short span from the fourth to seventh prenatal weeks. Environmental factors can cause a facial or branchial arch defect, which would probably affect these tissues before the fourth week. This is the time to be especially careful of irradiation and chemical, hormonal, dietary, or stress-related factors.

Branchial Grooves and Pharyngeal Pouches

The first branchial groove deepens to become the **external auditory canal** leading to the middle ear. The membrane at the depth of this tube becomes the **tympanic membrane.** The **middle ear** and **eustachian tube** develop from the corresponding first pharyngeal pouch. Af-

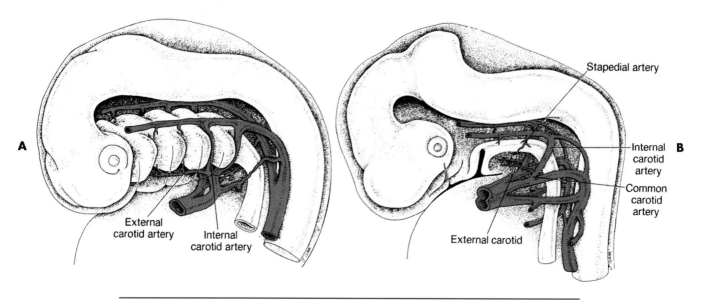

FIG. 3-6 Aortic vasculature development. **A,** At 4 weeks the anterior aortic vessels have passed through each branchial arch tissue and have disappeared. The pouches project laterally between each arch. **B,** At 5 weeks the third branchial arch vessel becomes the common carotid, which supplies the face by means of the internal carotid and stapedial arteries.

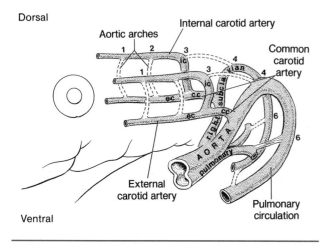

FIG. 3-7 Details of the aortic arch changes during early development. Aortic arch vessels numbers 1, 2, and 5 disappear. Arch 3 becomes the common carotid artery. Arch 4 becomes the dorsal aorta and enlarges so that the common carotid arises from the aorta. Arch 6 becomes the right and left pulmonary arteries.

ter the fifth week no other branchial grooves are seen externally as the tissue of the second and fifth arch grow over the other arches and grooves and make contact with each other (Fig. 3-5, *A*). This overgrowth obscures the tissue of both the arches and the grooves externally, although their internal structures are unaffected and provide an important role in facial and body development (Fig. 3-5, *A* and *B*).

The endodermal lining of the pharyngeal pouches differentiates into several important organs. The second pharyngeal pouch becomes the **palatine tonsils;** the third becomes the **inferior parathyroids** and **thymus;** the fourth becomes the **superior parathyroids;** and the fifth becomes the **ultimobranchial body** (Fig. 3-5, *C*).

The palatine tonsils function in the development of lymphocytes, which are important in the immunology of the body. The parathyroid glands regulate calcium balance throughout life. The thymus, located behind the sternum and between the lungs, is large at birth and continues to grow until puberty, during which it begins to atrophy but continues to function. Although its full importance is unknown, the thymus produces **T cells** that destroy invading microbes and are therefore important to the body's immune system. The ultimobranchial body fuses with the thyroid and contributes parafollicular cells to the thyroid. The function of the ultimobranchial body remains unknown (Fig. 3-5, *B* and *C*).

Vascular Development

Each of the five branchial arches contains a **right** and a **left aortic arch vessel** that leads from the heart through the arches to the face, brain, and posterior regions of the body (Fig. 3-4). Not all of these paired aortic arches are present at the same time, however. The first and second begin to develop in the fourth week and disappear in the fifth week (Fig. 3-6). The third arch vessels then become prominent, taking over the facial area of the first two. As the fourth and fifth arch vessels arise, the fourth becomes prominent and the fifth disappears (Fig. 3-7). Next the sixth arch vessels appear and become dominant along with those of the third and fourth.

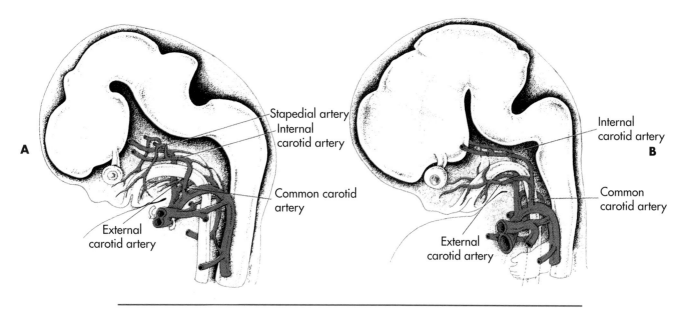

FIG. 3-8   Shift in the vascular supply to the face. **A,** Face and brain are supplied first by the internal carotid artery. **B,** Facial vessels detach from the internal carotid artery and attach to the external carotid.

The third arch vessels become the **common carotid arteries,** which supply the neck, face, and brain. The fourth arch vessels become the dorsal aorta, which supplies blood to the remainder of the body, and the vessels of the sixth arch supply the lungs with **pulmonary circulation** (Fig. 3-7).

An important feature of the common carotid arteries is the supply of blood to the face, neck, and brain from the **internal carotid** artery. However, after 7 weeks the circulation to the face and neck shifts from the internal to the **external carotid** (Fig. 3-8). The internal carotid continues to supply the growing brain.

Muscular and Neural Development

Muscle cells in the first arch become apparent during the fifth week and begin to spread within the mandibular arch into each muscle site's origin in the sixth and seventh week (Fig. 3-9). By the tenth week the muscles of the second arch have formed a thin sheet that extends over the face and posterior to the ear (Fig. 3-10). As these muscles grow over the face, they develop into the various groups of muscles that attach to the newly ossifying bones of the facial skeleton. The muscle masses of the mandibular arch, on the other hand, remain in the first arch and become easily recognized muscles of mastication (Fig. 3-9, *A*). These are the **masseter, medial,** and **lateral pterygoid** and **temporalis muscle.** They all relate to the developing mandible (Fig. 3-11).

The masseter and medial pterygoid form a vertical sling that inserts into the angle of the mandible. The temporalis muscle spreads into the infratemporal fossa

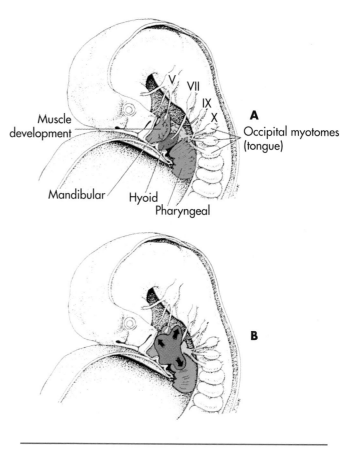

FIG. 3-9   Development of muscles and nerves of the branchial arches. **A,** Mandibular arch muscle mass expands to form the muscles of mastication. **B,** At 7 weeks the muscles of the second arch grow upward to form the muscles of the face.

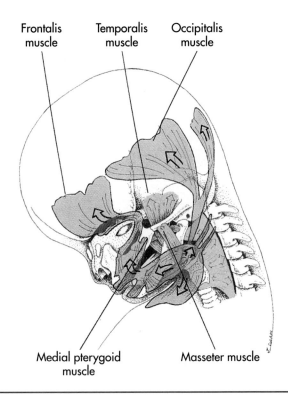

FIG. 3-10   Facial muscles grow from the second branchial arch to cover the face, scalp, and posterior to the ear. These all become muscles of facial expression.

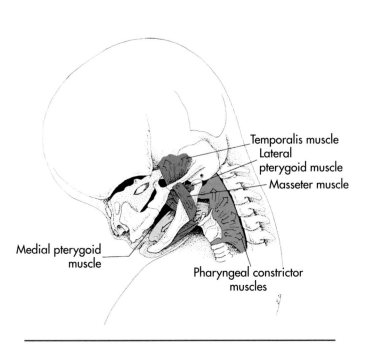

FIG. 3-11   Masticatory muscles of the mandibular arch. The medial pterygoid and masseter muscles attach as a sling to the angle of the mandible. Temporalis muscle grows from the coronoid process into the infratemporal fossa, and lateral pterygoid extends from the head of the condyle anteriorly to the sphenoid bone and the pterygoid bone in the infratemporal fossa.

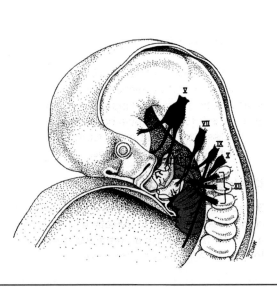

FIG. 3-12   Cranial nerves growing into branchial arches. Nerve V grows to the mandibular arch, and nerve VII to the hyoid arch. Nerves IV, VI, IX, and X contribute to tongue muscles, which are developing anteriorly.

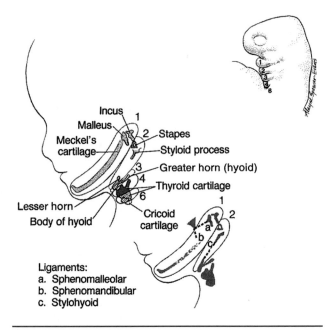

FIG. 3-13   Cartilages derived from branchial arches. Meckel's cartilage and incus come from arch 1; stapes, styloid, and lesser hyoid from arch 2; greater hyoid from arch 3; and thyroid and laryngeal cartilages from arches 4 and 5.

that inserts into the developing coronoid process of the mandible. The lateral pterygoid extends horizontally from the neck of the condyle, and some fibers insert into the temporomandibular disk (see Chapter 13). The pharyngeal constrictor muscles in the fourth arch have differentiated in the neck and function to enclose the pharynx (Fig. 3-11).

Nerves develop in conjunction with the developing muscle fibers. By the end of the seventh week the fibers of the fifth nerve have entered the mandibular muscle mass as has the seventh nerve in the facial muscle mass in the second arch (Fig. 3-12). As these muscle masses develop, the nerves are present and follow or lead them as they migrate to their position of differentiation, maturation, and function. The seventh nerve supplies the stylohyoid and stapedius muscles and the posterior belly of the digastric muscle. The ninth (glossopharyngeal) nerve enters the third arch and supplies the stylopharyngeal and upper pharyngeal constrictor muscles. The tenth (vagus) nerve innervates muscles of the fourth arch, which are the inferior constrictors and laryngeal muscles. The tongue, which is primarily muscle, relates to the branches of the ninth nerve, which are the receptors of taste for the posterior third of the tongue, and to the seventh nerve, which is the taste receptor for the anterior two thirds. The fifth nerve is the sensory nerve to the same area of the anterior tongue (Fig. 3-12). The tongue is a good example of muscle cell migration because it originates in the occipital myotome and migrates anteriorly into the floor of the mouth. During migration the nerves mentioned enter the muscle mass and later carry out their functions (Fig. 3-13).

Cartilaginous Skeletal Development

The initial skeleton of the branchial arches develops as cartilaginous bars. In the first arch, **Meckel's cartilages** appear bilaterally (Fig. 3-13). The anterior aspects of these two cartilages approach each other near the midline but do not coalesce. Posteriorly each terminates in an enlarged bulbous structure called the **malleus**. The malleus lies adjacent to a small cartilage called the **incus**. Farther posterior is a third body of cartilage, the **stapes** (Fig. 3-13). These three bilateral cartilages later transform into bone and function in the middle ear as hearing bones.

Substantial evidence shows that the contact point of the malleus and incus is the articulation of the lower jaw for the first 20 weeks of prenatal life. Then the second temporomandibular joint, which is the articulation of the condyle and the temporal fossae, becomes functional (Fig. 3-14). Chapter 13 has further information about the temporomandibular joint.

The rod-shaped cartilage of the second or hyoid arch is known as Reichert's cartilage. The stapes, styloid process, lesser horn, and upper body of the hyoid arise from this arch (Fig. 3-13). The third arch cartilage forms

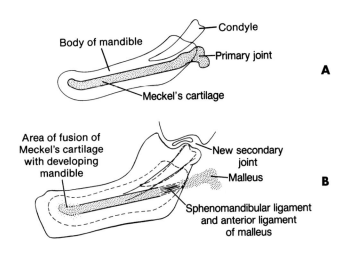

FIG. 3-14 Relationship between primary and secondary jaws. **A,** Meckel's cartilage with its posterior malleus-incus joint functions in jaw movement during the first 4 months of prenatal life. **B,** A shift to the condylar-temporal articulation occurs. Incus, malleus, and stapes transform into bones for hearing.

the greater horn and the lower part of the hyoid body. The fourth arch contributes to the hyoid cartilage, which then supports the gland. The fifth arch has no adult cartilage derivatives, and the sixth arch cartilage forms the laryngeal cartilage (Fig. 3-13).

DEVELOPMENT OF THE CRANIOFACIAL SKELETON

Cartilages of the Face

The earliest formed skeletal elements in the craniofacial area are the cartilaginous nasal capsule **(ethmoid),** the **sphenoid,** the **auditory capsules,** and the **basioccipital cartilages.** All these cartilages initially arise as a single cartilaginous continuum in the midline underlying the brain (Fig. 3-15). Anteriorly the nasal capsule contains the organ of smell. Laterally the auditory capsules protect the organs of hearing (Fig. 3-15). The sphenoid cartilage is posterior to the ethmoid. It later forms wings of bone that spread out under the brain laterally (Fig. 3-16). Behind the sphenoid is the occipital cartilage. Although the ethmoid capsule, sphenoid, and basioccipital cartilages are formed as a single cartilaginous unit initially, they separate later to form individual bones. These cartilages underlie and support the brain and are known as the **cranial base.** The cranial base is determined by drawing a line from the nasal bone **(nasion)** to **sella turcica** of the sphenoid to **basion** as seen in Fig. 3-17. These cartilages are transformed into bone by endochondral bone formation.

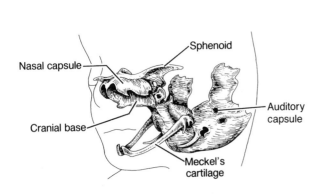

FIG. 3-15 Cartilages of the face and skull. Note that the cranial base cartilage supports the maxillary area of the face and Meckel's cartilages of the mandibular arch. The locations of the sphenoid and auditory capsules are shown.

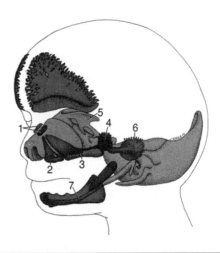

FIG. 3-18 Relationship of cartilage to membrane bone growth of the lateral face at 8 weeks. The facial bones are numbered: *1*, nasal; *2*, premaxilla; *3*, maxilla; *4*, zygomatic; *5*, sphenoid; *6*, temporal; and *7*, mandible.

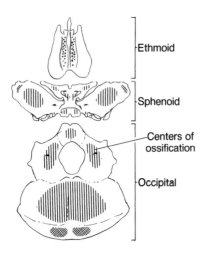

FIG. 3-16 Development of the cranial base as viewed from the inferior surface of the brain. Initiating cartilage centers *(lined areas)* are shown in the center of each site with bony growth extending outward.

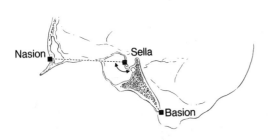

FIG. 3-17 Lateral view of the cranial base. A line from nasion to sella to basion is a cranial base landmark used to evaluate facial growth.

Bones of the Face

The protective covering of the brain is formed by membrane bones. These bones are termed **frontal, parietal,** and squamous portions of the **temporal** and **interoccipital** bones (Fig. 3-18). Membrane bones form directly from connective tissue and do not initially form from cartilage.

CLINICAL COMMENT

Branchial arch syndromes are seen clinically as combinations of such defects as underdevelopment of the mandible, retracted tongue, large tongue, small mouth, malformed ears, and cleft palate. A rare disorder, Treacher Collins syndrome, is directly attributable to branchial arch deficiencies.

The facial bones, which also form in membrane bone, complete the facial skeleton. They develop overlying the nasal capsule and are called the **premaxillary, maxillary, zygomatic,** and **petrous portions** of the temporal bone (Fig. 3-18). These bones initially appear as tiny ossification centers in the face and then increase in diameter, spreading anteriorly, posteriorly, and upward into the tissues surrounding the orbit (Fig. 3-19).

The maxillary bones also grow medially into the palate to support the palatine shelf tissue (Fig. 3-20). The bones of the maxilla grow as the facial tissues continue to develop. The height of the maxilla is due partially to the growth in length of the roots of the teeth.

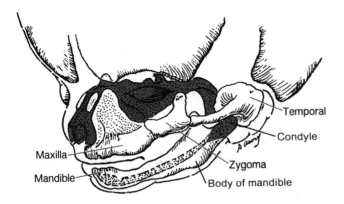

FIG. 3-19   The facial skeleton at the twelfth prenatal week illustrating the positional relationships of the maxillary, zygomatic, and temporal bones, the membrane bone of the body, and cartilaginous condyle of the mandible.

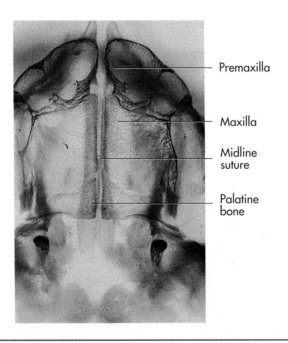

FIG. 3-20   Cleared human specimen. Ossification of the human palate in eighth prenatal month. Sutures are shown in the midline and between each of these bones anteroposteriorly. These provide for further growth of the palate. The developing teeth are enclosed in premaxillary, maxillary, and palatine alveolar tooth crypts.

The bony mandible grows laterally to the first arch cartilage as well as posteriorly to join the bony body with the cartilaginous condyle. Together, the body of the mandible and the cartilaginous condyle replace Meckel's cartilage (Fig. 3-19).

The mandible develops as several units: a **condylar** unit forms the articulation, allowing movement of the mandible; the **body** is the center of all growth and function of the mandible; the **angular process** responds to the lateral pterygoid and masseter masticatory muscles;

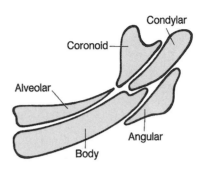

FIG. 3-21   Developing areas of the mandible that respond to different influences. The body, condyle, and alveolar, angular, and coronoid processes all unify as the mandible in common function.

the **coronoid process** responds to the temporalis muscle development and attachment; the **alveolar process** responds to development of the teeth (Fig. 3-21). This development produces the mature mandible (Fig. 3-22).

CLINICAL COMMENT

Many facial defects are due to lack of transformation of the branchial arches to their adult derivatives. Branchial cysts and fistulas may appear along the sides of the neck because the epithelial-lined pockets remain as a result of the overgrowth of the arches. These defects may also open in the pharynx. Cysts and fistulas may result in swelling or draining of mucus from an opening on the side of the neck.

Sutures of the Face

A system of articulations develops between each of the major bones of the face to facilitate growth. These articulations are positioned in the direction of facial growth, which is forward, away from the brain, and downward to facilitate lengthening of the face. The articulations are termed **sutures** and are defined as fibrous joints in which the opposing surfaces are closely united. A suture develops between the **zygomatic, maxillary, frontal,** and **temporal facial bones.** Sutures are named for the two or more bones with which they articulate. Facial sutures are named **zygomaticomaxillary, frontomaxillary,** and **zygomaticotemporal** (Fig. 3-23).

These articulations are growth sites that allow the associated bones to expand and to maintain orientation at their junctions by means of the fibrous attachment that controls their relationship with the adjacent bones. Such

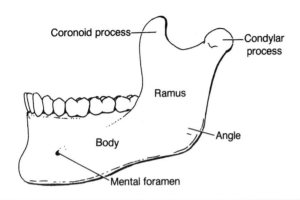

FIG. 3-22   Adult mandible. The bilateral halves fuse in the midline to form a single mandibular bone.

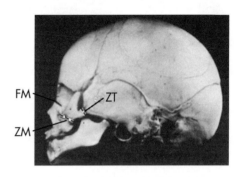

FIG. 3-23   Sutures of the developing skull of the newborn: *FM,* frontomaxillary; *ZM,* zygomaticomaxillary; and *ZT,* zygomaticotemporal. The pterygopalatine suture is not present at this age but is present in the adult (Fig. 3-28).

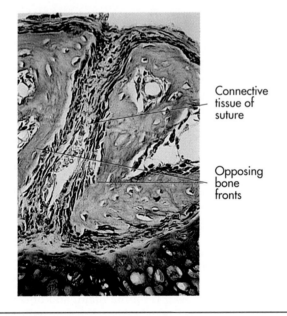

FIG. 3-24   Histology of a simple suture illustrating opposing bony fronts to the right and left with connective tissue between them. Osteoblasts form bone on opposing bone fronts, causing growth. The connective tissue band maintains space between the fronts, allowing the bone surfaces to grow.

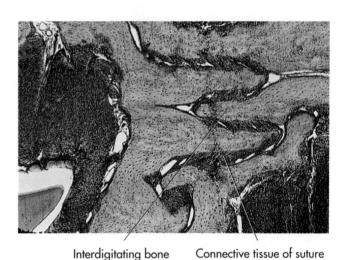

FIG. 3-25   Histology of serrated suture of skull. Interposing (interdigitating) fingers of bone are shown with connective tissue between each of these projections.

Bone   Connective tissue

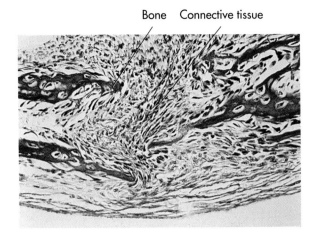

FIG. 3-26 Histology of a developing squamous suture of the parietal and temporal bones. The bones of the suture overlap and have connective tissue between them.

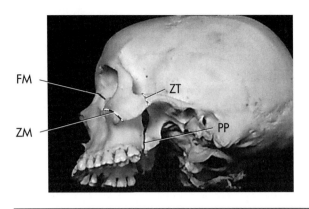

FIG. 3-27 Sutures of the adult human skull: *FM*, frontomaxillary; *ZM*, zygomaticomaxillary; *ZT*, zygomaticotemporal; and *PP*, pterygopalatine. The positions are different from those in the skull of the newborn (Fig. 3-23).

articulations may consist of a band of connective tissue termed **syndesmosis** (Fig. 3-24). In the center of this band are osteogenic cells, which along the periphery provide for new bone growth. The sutures of the face are of three types: **simple,** which is an uncomplicated band of tissue between bony fronts (Fig. 3-24); **serrated,** which is an **interdigitating** type of suture (Fig. 3-25); and **squamosal,** which has a beveled or overlapping type junction (Fig. 3-26). Each connective tissue suture consists of a central zone of proliferating connective tissue cells with osteogenic cells along the peripheral bony fronts. Each suture is surrounded by a fibrous connective tissue (Figs. 3-24 to 3-26). When the position of these sutures in the fetal skull is compared with the position of the sutures in the adult skull, the relationship of these articulations appears similar, although adult bones are larger (compare Fig. 3-23 to Fig. 3-27). When facial growth is complete, all of these sutures will become inactive, although the interface of the apposing bones remains and defines the boundary of the facial bones.

In contrast to the sutures of the external face, those in the midline consist of an interposing band of cartilage. This type of suture is termed **synchondrosis** and is located in the midline (Fig. 3-28). Synchondrosis sutures grow by forming new cartilage in the center of the suture as cartilage transforms to bone at the periphery of the suture (Fig. 3-28). These cartilage sutures are of only one type and exist between the ethmoid and sphenoid bones

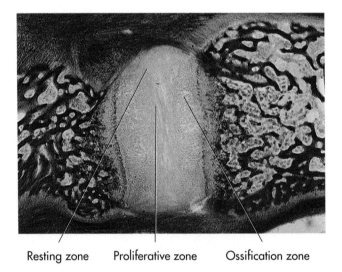

Resting zone   Proliferative zone   Ossification zone

FIG. 3-28 Histology of synchondrosis. This band of cartilage is in the midline between the ethmoid and sphenoid bones. Cartilage cells differentiate in the center of the suture as cartilage is replaced by bone peripherally along the bony fronts.

in the midline during facial growth. They become known as the **ethmosphenoid suture.** Fig. 3-29 presents a summary of all structures that develop from the branchial arches, branchial grooves, and pharyngeal pouches.

BRANCHIAL GROOVES — Adult Derivative	Arch No.	Cranial Nerve	Branchiomeric Muscles	Skeletal Derivative	Aortic Arch	PHARYNGEAL POUCHES — Adult Derivative
Ext. Auditory Meatus	I Mandibular	V Trigeminal	Muscles of mastication, anterior belly of digastric, mylohyoid, tensor tympani, tensor palatini	Malleus, incus, sphenomandibular ligament, sphenomalleolar ligament (Meckel's cartilage)	I	1 Middle ear / Eustachian tube
	II Hyoid	VII Facial	Muscles of facial expression, stapedius, stylohyoid, posterior belly of digastric	Stapes, styloid process, stylohyoid ligament, lesser cornu of hyoid, upper part of body of hyoid	II	2 Palatine tonsil
	III	IX Glossopharyngeal	Stylopharyngeus	Greater cornu of hyoid, lower part of body of hyoid	III	3 Thymus, inferior parathyroid
	IV	X Vagus	Laryngeal musculature, pharyngeal constrictors	Laryngeal cartilages	IV	4 Superior parathyroid
Cervical Fistula	V	XI Spinal accessory	Sternocleidomastoid / Trapezius		VI	5 Ultimobranchial body

BRANCHIAL ARCH STRUCTURES

FIG. 3-29 Summary of structures that develop from branchial arches, branchial grooves, and pharyngeal pouches.

SELF-EVALUATION QUESTIONS

1. Define a branchial arch and a pharyngeal arch.
2. Describe several important events that occur in the second branchial arch during the fourth and seventh prenatal weeks.
3. Discuss the origin and growth of the facial muscles.
4. Discuss the origin and growth of the tongue muscles.
5. What are the contributions of pharyngeal pouches number one, two, three, and four?
6. Describe the origin and growth of the masticatory muscles.
7. Discuss the origin, descent, and function of the thyroid gland.
8. Discuss the origin and time of the shift in the facial blood supply.
9. Describe the cartilages of the early facial skeleton and the bones that they replace.
10. Name, locate, and describe the connective tissue sutures of the face.

CONSIDER THE PATIENT . . .

Discussion: The symptoms suggest a branchial cleft and related cyst. Surgery would be recommended to correct this condition.

SUGGESTED READING

Avery JK: *Oral development and histology,* New York, 1994, Thieme Medical.

Enlow DH: *Handbook of facial growth,* Philadelphia, 1982, WB Saunders.

Hall BK: *Developmental and cellular skeletal biology,* New York, 1978, Academic Press.

Sadler TW: *Langman's medical embryology,* ed 7, Baltimore, 1995, Williams & Wilkins.

Snyder, GB et al: *Your cleft lip and palate child,* Gainesville, Fla, 1972, Florida Cleft Palate Association and Mead Johnson Laboratories.

Sperber GH: *Craniofacial embryology,* ed 4, Boston, 1989, Wright.

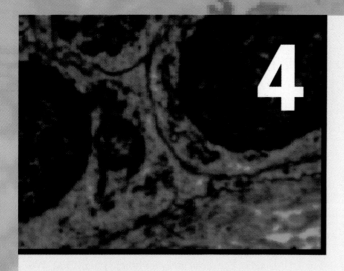

4

Development of the Face and Palate

OVERVIEW

This chapter describes the development of the human face and the palatine defects that may occur. An understanding of this subject is important to the dental health professional for two reasons. First, the professional must understand the variability that can occur in facial form and, second, must be aware that the human face and palate are among the areas most susceptible to malformations.

The human face develops early in gestation, during the fifth through seventh weeks, and the palatal processes begin to close during the eighth week. These two structures are closely related in time of development and sometimes have related malformations. The face develops from the tissues immediately surrounding the oral pit, but the forehead develops from the frontal area that lies above the pit (Fig. 4-1). The nose later develops from this area as well, so the name changes from frontal area to frontonasal area (Fig. 4-2). Below the oral pit is the mandibular arch, from which the mandible arises and articulates with the temporal bone. Lateral to the oral pit are the right and left maxillary processes, which develop from the mandibular arch. Cheek tissues come from these processes. Intraorally, the palate forms the mouth's roof, which separates the oral and nasal cavities. First the medial palatal segment forms as part of the medial nasal segment. This segment provides the first separation of the oral and nasal cavities. Next, two lateral palatine shelves arise from the maxillary processes and grow horizontally to close the palate posterior to the pharynx. At the same time the tongue develops in the floor of the oral cavity but grows rapidly and expands into the nasal cavity. The tongue functions in palatine shelf closure because the shelves must override it before closure can be accomplished.

Many environmental factors can cause clefts of the face, palate, or both. These defects of the lip or palate may be unilateral or bilateral and also incomplete or complete.

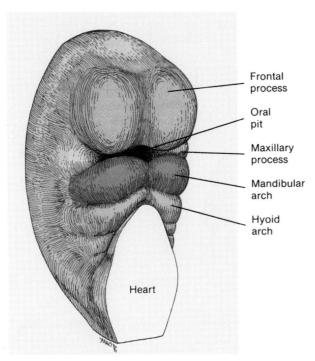

FIG. 4-1 Human face during fourth prenatal week. Frontal and maxillary processes and mandibular arch, although seemingly unrelated tissue masses, are grouped around oral pit. Below mandibular arch is hyoid arch. Heart is below face.

FIG. 4-2 Human face during fifth prenatal week. Nasal pits are located on the sides of face during this week. Frontal process changes to the frontonasal process.

FACIAL DEVELOPMENT: WEEKS 4 TO 7

Tissue Organization

The face develops primarily from tissues surrounding the oral pit. Above the oral pit is the covering of the brain termed the **frontal process,** from which develops the **forehead.** Lateral to the oral pit are the right and left **maxillary processes,** from which develop the **cheeks,** and below the oral pit is the **mandibular arch,** from which forms the **lower jaw.** In the fourth week, when the facial tissues have just begun to organize, they measure only a few millimeters in height and width and are only as thick as a sheet of paper. Further growth of the face from this minute assembly of tissue sites is anterior to the brain. Lying inferior to the mandibular arch is the second branchial or **hyoid** arch, and its muscles expand into and contribute to the face. The hyoid arch also forms part of the external and middle ear.

Development of the human face is most easily described in terms of the changes that occur at weekly intervals from the fourth to the seventh prenatal weeks.

Fourth Week

At 4 weeks the oral pit is surrounded by several masses of tissue. Branchial arches are also evident below the pit and on the sides of the neck. The frontal processes of the brain bulge forward and laterally to dominate the facial area. Below the frontal processes are two small wedge-shaped tissues, termed the maxillary processes, that lie lateral to the oral pit. Beneath the maxillary processes is the mandibular arch, which appears divided or constricted in the midline (Fig. 4-1). The heart lies immediately below the face and is one of the fastest growing organs. During the fourth week the heart begins to pump blood throughout the body.

Fifth Week

During the fifth week the bilateral nasal placodes, or thickened areas of epithelium, appear in the upper border of the lip. They develop into nostrils as the tissues around these placodes grow, resulting in two slits opening into the oral pit. At this point the frontal area becomes known as the **frontonasal process.** The nostrils deepen as the tissues around them continue to grow, and the **internasal area,** the distance between the nostrils, represents the width of the face (Fig. 4-2). Gradually the frontal prominence diminishes and the face broadens. The eyes become prominent on the sides of the head (Fig. 4-2). Throughout the fifth week the mandibular arch loses its midline constriction (Fig. 4-2).

Sixth Week

At the beginning of the sixth week the lateral parts of the face expand, broadening the face. This is also due to a lateral growth of the brain. The eyes and maxillary processes, which were located on the sides of the face in

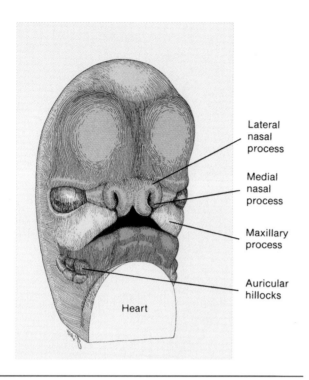

FIG. 4-3 Human face during sixth prenatal week. Nasal pits appear more centrally located in medial nasal process. Growth in lateral area of face causes eyes to approach front of face. Nasal slits may be sites of cleft lips. Auricular hillocks bordering ear canal have merged.

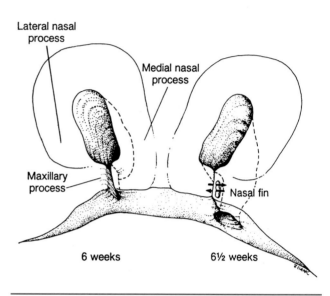

FIG. 4-4 Fusion of nostrils' floor. At left, epithelial coverings of medial nasal and maxillary processes are separated. At right, the processes are in contact and fused and the epithelial layers form a fin. As soon as the fin forms, it is penetrated by mesenchymal cells, which grow through the epithelium to bind lip crevice together.

the fifth week, come to the front of the face. The mouth slit widens to the point at which the maxillary and mandibular tissues merge. The nasal processes are limited to the middle of the upper lip, which results in the face's appearing more human. The upper lip is now composed of a medial nasal process and two lateral maxillary segments (Fig. 4-3). The medial nasal process is called the **philtrum.** A ridge of tissue surrounds each nasal pit. The tissue lateral to the pits is the **lateral nasal process,** and the tissue medial to the pits is the **medial nasal process.**

The medial nasal process is in close contact with the medial aspect of the maxillary process, and the lateral nasal process is above the maxillary process. The border of the lip consists of two maxillary processes, and the medial third is the medial nasal. A lack of contact or fusion of the **medial nasal** and **maxillary processes** results in a **cleft lip,** either unilateral or bilateral. The epithelial coverings of the medial nasal and maxillary processes normally contact and create a zone of fusion termed the **nasal fin** (Fig. 4-4). This epithelial fin is soon penetrated by connective tissue growth, which binds together the two maxillary and medial nasal parts of the lip. If this penetration were not to occur, the lip could pull apart.

Soon the **orbicularis oris** muscle grows around the oral pit to provide support to the upper lip. The nasal pits continue behind the nasal fin to open into the roof of the mouth at 6½ weeks (Fig. 4-4). Extending from the nostrils to the eyes is an oblique groove, which is the **oro-naso-optic groove.** In the tissue beneath this groove the **nasolacrimal duct** develops. A modification of the first branchial groove into the ear canal or **auditory tube** also appears below the corners of the mouth. Six small hillocks of tissue, termed the **auricular hillocks,** are grouped around the external ear canal. Three of these come from the mandibular arch and three from the second or hyoid arch (Figs. 4-3 and 4-5).

 CLINICAL COMMENT

Environmental factors play a significant role in facial and palatal malformations. The period before the fifth week is the critical time during which these factors can affect facial development.

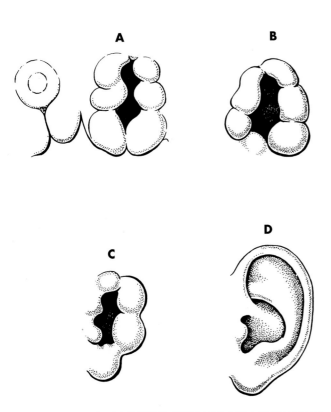

A

B

C

D

FIG. 4-5 Development of external ear (auricle). **A,** The three auricular hillocks on the left are from mandibular arch, and the three on the right are from hyoid arch. **B,** Auricular hillocks begin to merge around the first branchial groove. **C,** The hillocks merge. **D,** The ear is developed.

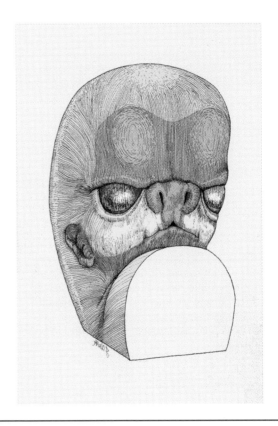

FIG. 4-6 Human face during seventh prenatal week. Median nasal and maxillary processes have merged. Eyes are closer to the front of face. Nose and eyes are on same horizontal plane, which will change with vertical growth of face. Auricles of ear have developed.

Seventh Week

By the seventh week the face has a more human appearance (Fig. 4-6). The eyes approach the front of the face, and the nose represents less of the face than it did at the fourth week. The lateral growth of the brain, resulting in facial expansion, causes the eyes to appear on the front of the face, which makes it more recognizable as a human face. A third of the face has been added lateral to each nostril (Fig. 4-6). The eyes are on the same horizontal plane as the nostrils, which will change after the bridge of the nose develops and lengthens. The upper lip has fused, producing a medially located philtrum. The mouth is limited in size with the change in facial pro-

CLINICAL COMMENT

Because much of the face arises from tissues on the surface of the brain, defects of the anterior brain may result in developmental alteration of facial form.

portions. The ear hillocks have fused and grown to form the ears (auricles). The ridges around the eyes will soon develop into eyelids (Figs. 4-5 and 4-6). The danger of a cleft lip has passed. In just 3 prenatal weeks, separate tissue masses have enlarged, fused, and merged into a recognizable human face.

PALATAL DEVELOPMENT: WEEKS 7 TO 9

Medial and Lateral Palatal Processes

The palate is the tissue that separates the oral and nasal cavities. This palate, although thin, is supported by bone, which provides rigidity. The palate develops from an anterior wedge-shaped medial part and two lateral palatine processes (Fig. 4-7, *A*). The medial part is also known as the **primary palate** because it develops first and is a floor to the nasal pits. Next, the **lateral palatine processes** develop from the maxillary tissues laterally and grow to the midline. This further limits the oral cavity from the nasal cavity posteriorly to the nasopharynx (Fig. 4-7, *B*). As the palatine shelves grow medially, they contact the tongue, which grew upward into the nasal cavity during the seventh week. When the palatine shelves contact the

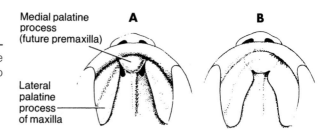

FIG. 4-7   Development of palate. **A,** Medial and lateral palatine processes develop. **B,** Lateral palatine process moves medially to midline.

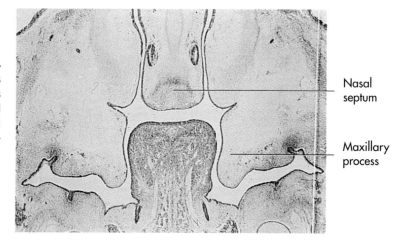

FIG. 4-8   Cross section of face showing tongue's growth upward into nasal cavity. Palatine shelves (maxillary processes) contact tongue during medial growth. Tongue then grows down beside the palatal shelves. During seventh week, tongue muscle begins differentiation.

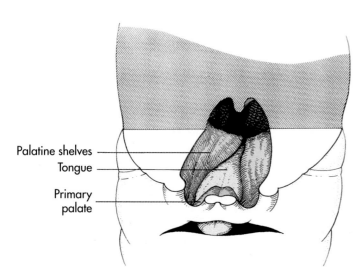
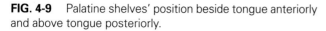

FIG. 4-9   Palatine shelves' position beside tongue anteriorly and above tongue posteriorly.

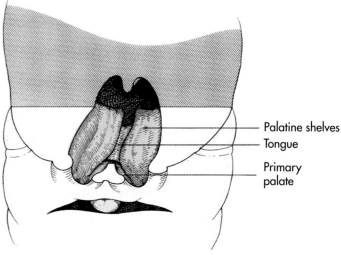

FIG. 4-10   Palatine shelves' elevation over tongue. Shown is tongue's position when palatine shelves move above it and also anteriorly during the elevation process.

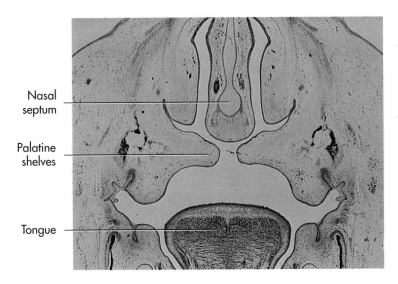

FIG. 4-11 Tongue with overlying palatine shelves. Shelves are in near midline position as well as near the overlying nasal septum.

Nasal septum

Palatine shelves

Tongue

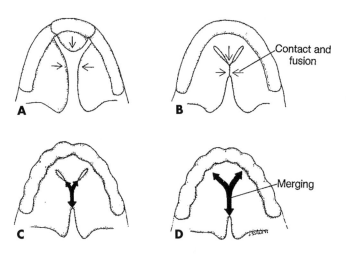

A

B   Contact and fusion

C

D   Merging

FIG. 4-12 **A,** Horizontal palatine shelf growth to attain contact in the midline. **B,** Initial contact behind medial palatal segment. **C** and **D,** Tissues merge anteriorly and posteriorly from point of initial contact.

tongue, they grow downward on either side of the tongue (Fig. 4-8).

Palatal Shelf Elevation and Closure

At its posterior limits the tongue is below the palatine shelves. This is because posteriorly the tongue is attached to the floor of the mouth and the posterior roof of the mouth is above the tongue. During the eighth prenatal week the posterior shelves push together, forcing the tongue forward and down (Fig. 4-9). This action causes the palatal shelves to slide over the tongue (Fig. 4-10). The process is known as **palatal shelf elevation** and is presumed to take place rapidly, about as fast as the act of swallowing. For this reason, palatal shelf elevation has never been precisely recorded.

As soon as the palatine shelves reach the resulting horizontal position, the tongue broadens and pushes upward against the shelves, which helps mold them together (Fig. 4-11). The shelves have a final growth surge until they con-

tact in the midline; this contact is known as **palatine shelf closure** or **fusion** (Fig. 4-12). The first site of contact is just posterior to the medial palatine process (Fig. 4-12). From this point of initial contact the shelves merge anteriorly and posteriorly (Fig. 4-12). The final step in fusion is the removal of the midline epithelial barrier between the right and left shelves. This occurs by enzymatic action of epithelial cells, which results in self-destruction. As soon as the epithelial cells begin to break down and disappear, connective tissue grows through the midline and completes the fusion of the palate. This is the same process as the one that occurred in lip fusion and is illustrated in Figs. 4-13 and 4-14. The fusion of the entire palate takes weeks while the palate grows in length. The palatal shelves also fuse with the overlying nasal septum in the midline of the face. This causes a complete separation of the oral and nasal cavities back to the nasopharynx. Then both the oral and nasal cavities open into the pharynx.

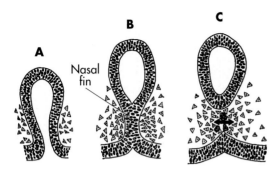

FIG. 4-13 **A,** Open floor of nasal cavity. **B,** Fusion of nasal cavity floor to form nasal fin. **C,** Arrows indicate growth of connective tissue through epithelial barrier as epithelial cells degenerate.

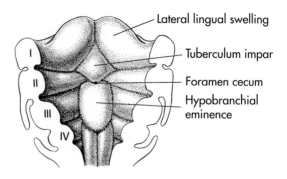

FIG. 4-15 Early tongue development. Tongue body develops from two lateral lingual swellings and a midline tuberculum impar. Tongue base develops from second and third branchial arches.

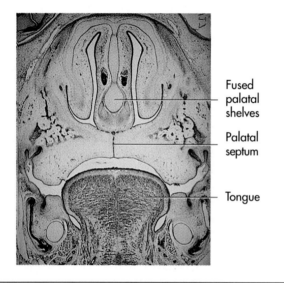

FIG. 4-14 Histologic cross section of palatine shelf fusion in the midline. On contact the epithelial seam breaks down between the shelves and the overlying septum.

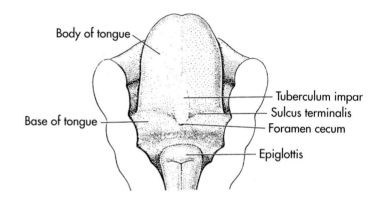

FIG. 4-16 Late tongue development illustrating body and base of tongue. Foramen cecum is the site of origin of tubular epithelial cord growth down the neck, and from it comes the thyroid gland.

Tongue Development

Body and Base

The tongue originates from the muscles of the occipital myotomes as described in Chapter 3 (see Figs. 3-9 to 3-11). From this posterior location the forming muscles migrate anteriorly into the floor of the mouth and are joined by other muscles of the first and second branchial arches. The tongue is innervated by the fifth, seventh, ninth, and tenth cranial nerves. This extensive innervation is due to the long distance the muscle cells migrate to reach the tongue. The muscles travel in the paths of these various nerves. The first branchial arch tissue forms the anterior (movable) body of the tongue. The second and third arches form the posterior, nonmovable base of the tongue. Tissues of the tongue have three parts, the central **tuberculum impar** and the **two lateral lingual swellings** (Fig. 4-15). The lateral parts rapidly enlarge

and merge, overgrowing the central tubercle. A U-shaped sulcus develops around the anterior part of the tongue, separating it from the jaw tissues and allowing freedom of movement (Fig. 4-16). Gradually the three parts of the anterior tongue merge to form a unified structure. The surface of the body and base of the tongue are separated by a V-shaped groove called the **terminal sulcus.** Posterior to the terminal sulcus the base of the tongue forms the **lingual tonsil** on the dorsal surface. The lingual tonsil forms part of the ring of tonsils (Waldeyer's ring) in the pharynx along with the **palatine** and **pharyngeal tonsils.** In later stages of development, several types of papillae differentiate on the oral mucosa of the tongue's dorsal body. The lingual tonsil differentiates on the surface of the tongue's base.

Thyroid Gland

The thyroid gland develops as an epithelial proliferation from the **foramen cecum** on the surface of the tongue at the junction of the body and base. Cells arise and mi-

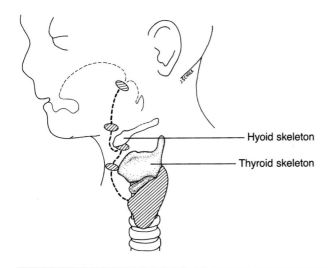

FIG. 4-17 Migratory path of gland tissue. Sometimes epithelial cysts and fistulae arise along this path of descent. Site can be in region of thyrohyoid skeleton.

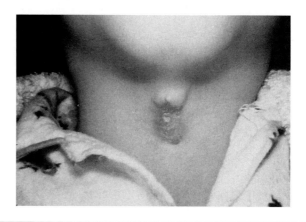

FIG. 4-18 Clinical view of thyroglossal fistulae appearing in the usual location, at midline of the neck in region of hyoid apparatus.

grate ventrally in the throat, creating the thyroid gland (Figs. 4-16 and 4-17). Then the cells from the foramen cecum rim descend in the midline floor of the pharynx past the hyoid cartilages to the level of the laryngeal cartilage. Finally, by the seventh week, the thyroid descends to the front of the trachea. During this long migration the thyroid gland remains attached to the tongue by an epithelial cord or duct termed the **thyroglossal duct,** which later becomes solid and eventually disappears (Fig. 4-17). Chapter 3 presents information about this process also (see Fig. 3-5, *B*).

Cysts and fistulas are along the route of descent of the thyroid tissue. A **thyroglossal cyst** is a blind pocket lined with thyroid epithelium. This cyst appears as a swelling and is commonly found in the area of the hyoid bone. A thyroglossal fistula appears as a swelling that has an opening on the surface of the neck (Fig. 4-18). The gland finally acquires two lateral lobes joined by a thin central isthmus of cells. By the end of the third month of prenatal life, the gland becomes functional.

MALFORMATIONS

Facial and palatal clefts usually occur because of a combination of environmental and genetic factors. An individual's susceptibility to stress is one factor that can have adverse effects.

Cleft lip is the most common facial malformation. Genetic factors play a role, as shown by the differences between racial groups. In the white American population the incidence of cleft lip is 1 in every 700 births. Proportionately, significantly fewer black Americans have clefts, the incidence being only 1 in 2000 newborns. In the

Asian population the incidence is 3 in 2000 births. Asians with one child born with a cleft palate have a 1 in 25 chance of a second child with the defect. The disparity is not surprising because congenital malformation affects races in different ratios. Evidence shows that a hereditary role exists along with various environmental susceptibility factors.

The incidence of clefts in males and females differs according to type of cleft. White males have nearly twice the number of cleft lips or cleft lips and palates as females. However, more white females have cleft palates, which occur at the rate of about 1 in every 2000 births. Overall, cleft palate is less frequent than cleft lip or a combination of cleft lip and palate.

Facial Clefts

Facial clefts are classified according to position and extent. A cleft may affect one or both sides of the lip (unilateral or bilateral) and can be either incomplete or complete (Figs. 4-19 to 4-21). An incomplete cleft lip ranges in size from a notch to a deep groove in the upper lip but does not involve an opening of the nostril into the oral cavity (Fig. 4-19). A true harelip is a midline cleft of the maxilla. The term harelip is used because a rabbit's upper lip develops with a midline cleft. The rabbit does not develop a medial nasal process, so the two maxillary processes meet in the midline. This condition, which is rare in humans, involves a notch in the medial nasal tissue that may be minute or may extend as a cleft into the nose (Fig. 4-22).

A cleft of the mandible may appear in the midline, although this also is rare (Fig. 4-23). A midline constriction in the mandible is observed during the fourth week. In this case the early constriction did not disappear and

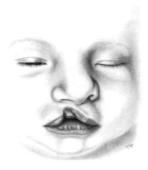

FIG. 4-19 Clinical view of unilateral incomplete cleft of the lip. This partial cleft is located in the line of fusion of medial nasal and maxillary processes.

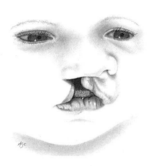

FIG. 4-20 Clinical view of unilateral complete cleft lip. In this case, maxillary and medial nasal processes did not fuse and then pulled farther apart during facial growth.

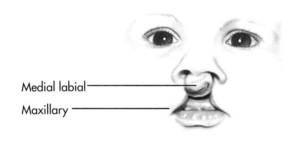

Medial labial

Maxillary

FIG. 4-21 Clinical view of bilateral complete cleft of the lip. The maxillary processes' contour results from a lack of contact and fusion. In this situation, anterior facial growth extruded the medial nasal and palatal tissues.

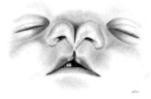

FIG. 4-22 Clinical view of midline cleft of the maxilla. This rare cleft occurs when the two parts of the medial nasal process fail to merge. The etiology of this condition can be seen in Fig. 4-3.

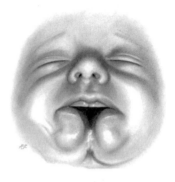

FIG. 4-23 Clinical example of a midline cleft of the mandible. The two parts of the first branchial arch, including the bony mandible, are separated at birth in this rare condition.

later resulted in a separation of the mandible's halves. This condition is believed to occur because of pressure from the adjacent enlarged heart, which begins beating before the mandible's midline fusion.

 CONSIDER THE PATIENT . . .

A patient tells you she heard that prenatal surgery has been developed in the past 10 years to correct life-threatening malformations. In this procedure, the fetus is removed from the uterus, corrections are made, and the fetus is returned to the uterus until proper delivery time. One advantage is a lack of scarring. She asks if any prenatal surgeries in the area of dentistry may be of interest.

Palatal Clefts

All the preceding facial clefts involve the lip, but some may extend into the palate as unilateral and bilateral cleft lip and palate defects (Fig. 4-24). Because the palatine shelves meet in the midline, both unilateral and bilateral clefts of the palate are in the midline clefts. Clefts must, however, extend around the medial palatal segment before they proceed in the midline (Fig. 4-24). Just as clefts of the lip can occur alone, clefts of the palate may occur as an isolated defect (Fig. 4-24, *B*). These palatal clefts can extend just a short distance into the posterior of the palate, can appear in the anterior, or can appear in both locations. However, the majority of cleft palates occur in combination with cleft lips (Figs. 4-25 and 4-26).

Other Defects

A number of other facial deformities appear clinically, some that are common and others that are rare. For ex-

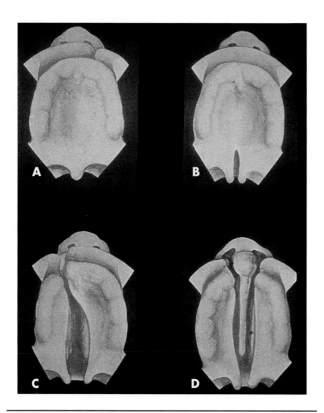

FIG. 4-24 Examples of cleft lip and palate. **A,** Cleft lip alone. **B,** Cleft palate alone. **C,** Unilateral cleft lip and palate. **D,** Bilateral cleft lip and palate.

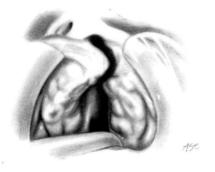

FIG. 4-25 Combined unilateral cleft of lip and palate. Clefts of the palate go lateral to the medial palatal segment and then posteriorly in the midline between the two palatal processes. Nasal tissue is distorted.

ample, Fig. 4-3 shows the origin of an oronasal optic cleft extending from the mouth to the eye. The most common defects are various malocclusions of the teeth. Midfacial hypoplasia—such as Apert's and Crouzon's syndrome—is a less common abnormality. Chapter 3 describes the developmental aspects of the first and second branchial arch syndromes.

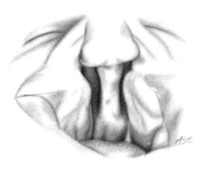

FIG. 4-26 Combined bilateral cleft of palate and lip. Cleft extends lateral to the medial processes and then down the midline.

CLINICAL COMMENT

Cleft lip and palate are among the most common congenital malformations. They appear in 1 of every 700 births in the white population and in 1 of 2000 births in the black population in the United States.

SELF-EVALUATION QUESTIONS

1. From what four embryonic processes does the face arise?
2. During which 3 prenatal weeks does the face develop human characteristics?
3. When do the palatine shelves elevate and begin closure?
4. Name the upper lip's three segments. When do they begin to coalesce into one unit?
5. From what structure does the nasal fin arise, and why is its disappearance important?
6. What is the origin of the auricles of the ear? From what branchial arches do they arise?
7. Define the primary and secondary palates, explain when each appears, and discuss their relative importance.
8. Describe the process of palatal elevation and the tissues that are believed to contribute to this event.
9. Compare the ratios of facial and palatal defects in the Asian, white, and black American populations.
10. From what three masses does the body of the tongue arise? What is the origin of the tongue base?

CONSIDER THE PATIENT . . .

Discussion: Prenatal surgery could correct cleft lip and cleft lip and palate without leaving scars.

SUGGESTED READING

Moore KL: *The developing human, clinically oriented embryology,* Philadelphia, 1998, Saunders.

Sadler TW: *Langman's medical embryology,* ed 7, Baltimore, 1995, Williams & Wilkins.

Snyder GB et al: *Your cleft lip and palate child,* Gainesville, Fla, 1972, Florida Cleft Palate Association and Mead Johnson Laboratories.

Sperber, GH: *Craniofacial embryology,* ed 4, Boston, 1989, Wright.

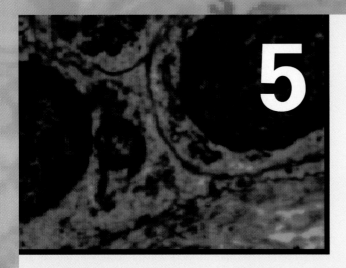

5 Development of Teeth

OVERVIEW

In the human, 20 primary and 32 permanent teeth develop from the interaction of the oral epithelial cells and the underlying mesenchymal cells. Each developing tooth grows as an anatomically distinct unit, but the basic developmental process is similar for all teeth.

Each tooth develops through successive bud, cap, and bell stages (Fig. 5-1, *A* to *C*). During these early stages the tooth germs grow and expand and the cells that are to form the hard tissues of the teeth differentiate. Differentiation takes place in the bell stage, setting the stage for enamel and dentin formation (Fig. 5-1, *D* and *E*). As the crowns are formed and mineralized, the roots of the teeth begin to form. After the roots calcify, the supporting tissues of the teeth—the cementum, periodontal ligament, and alveolar bone—begin to develop (Fig. 5-1, *F* and *G*). This formation occurs whether the tooth is an incisor with a single root, a premolar with several roots, or a molar with multiple roots. Subsequently, the completed tooth crown erupts into the oral cavity (Fig. 5-1, *G*). Root formation and cementogenesis continue until a functional tooth and its supporting structures are fully developed (Fig. 5-1, *G* and *H*).

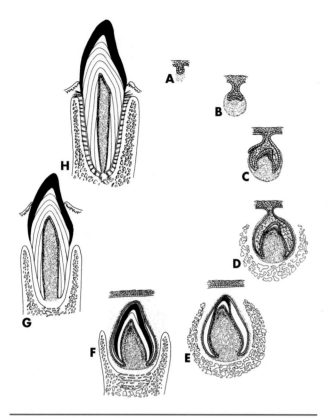

FIG. 5-1 Stages of tooth development. **A,** Bud. **B,** Cap. **C,** Bell. **D** and **E,** Dentinogenesis and amelogenesis. **F,** Crown formation. **G,** Root formation and eruption. **H,** Function.

INITIATION OF TOOTH DEVELOPMENT

Teeth develop from two types of cells: oral epithelial cells form the enamel organ, and mesenchymal cells form the dental papilla. Enamel develops from the enamel organ, and dentin forms from the dental papilla. The interaction of these epithelial and mesenchymal cells is vital to the initiation and formation of the teeth. In addition to these cells, the **neural crest cells** contribute to tooth development. The neural crest cells arise from the neural tissue at an early stage of development and migrate into the jaws, intermingling with mesenchymal cells. They function by integrating with the dental papillae and epithelial cells of the early enamel organ, which aids in the development of the teeth. The cells also function in the development of the salivary glands, bone, cartilage, nerves, and muscles of the face. Chapter 1 discusses neural crest cells and explains the cell's migration (see Fig. 1-16).

The first sign of tooth formation is the development of **dental lamina** rising from the oral epithelium. Dental lamina develops into a sheet of epithelial cells that pushes into the underlying mesenchyme around the perimeter of both the maxillary and mandibular jaws

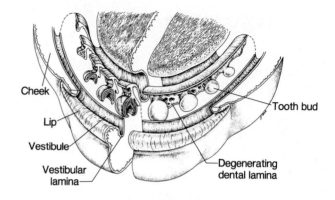

FIG. 5-2 Development of tooth buds in alveolar process. Anterior teeth are more advanced in development than posterior teeth. Anterior lamina has begun to degenerate as posterior lamina forms. When tooth buds have differentiated, lamina is no longer needed.

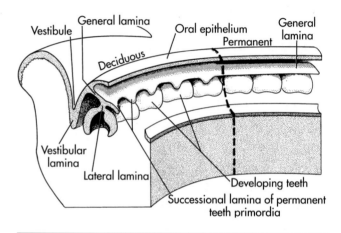

FIG. 5-3 Dental lamina system is shown in relation to general lamina. From successional lamina come permanent teeth, which replace primary teeth except in the posterior area of the arch.

(Fig. 5-2). At the leading edge of the lamina, 20 areas of enlargement appear, which form tooth buds for the 20 primary teeth (Fig. 5-2). At this early stage the tooth buds have already determined their crown morphology of an incisor or molar. This is due to gene expression. After primary teeth develop from the buds, the leading edge of the lamina continues to grow to develop the permanent teeth, which succeed the 20 primary teeth. This part of the lamina is thus called the **successional lamina** (Fig. 5-3). The lamina continues posteriorly into the elongating jaw and from it comes the posterior teeth, which form behind the primary teeth (Fig. 5-3). In this manner, 20 of the permanent teeth replace the 20 primary teeth and 12 posterior permanent molars develop behind the primary dentition (Fig. 5-3). The last teeth to develop are the third molars, which develop about 15 years after birth. Because the molars do not succeed the

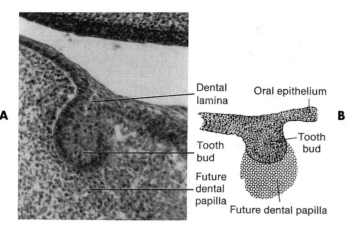

A

primary teeth, they do not form from the successional lamina but from the general lamina. The initiating dental lamina that forms both the successional and general lamina begins to function in the 6th prenatal week and continues to function until the 15th year, producing all 52 teeth. In general the teeth develop anteroposteriorly, which relates to the growing jaws. The posterior molars do not develop until space is available for them in the posterior jaw area. The second dentition does not develop until after the primary teeth are formed and functioning. Gradually the permanent teeth form under the primary crowns and later posteriorly to the primary molars.

CLINICAL COMMENT

Tooth development is dependent on the interaction of oral epithelial and underlying mesenchymal cells. Tooth formation can be affected by deficiencies of vitamin A, which is important in epithelial growth; vitamin C, which is important in connective tissue development; and vitamin D, which is essential in calcification. Other vitamins, minerals, and hormones also affect tooth development.

STAGES OF TOOTH DEVELOPMENT

Although tooth formation is a continuous process, it is characterized by a series of easily distinguishable stages known as the bud, cap, and bell stages. Each stage is defined according to the shape of the epithelial enamel organ, which is a part of the developing tooth. The initial stage, **bud stage,** is a rounded, localized growth of epithelial cells surrounded by proliferating mesenchymal cells (Fig. 5-4). Gradually, as the rounded epithelial bud enlarges, it gains a concave surface, which begins the **cap stage** (Fig. 5-5). The epithelial cells now become the

enamel organ and remain attached to the lamina. The mesenchyme forms the **dental papilla**, which becomes the dental pulp. The tissue surrounding these two structures is the **dental follicle.**

After further growth of the papilla and the enamel organ, the tooth reaches the morphodifferentiation and histodifferentiation stage, also known as the **bell stage** (Fig. 5-6). At this stage the inner enamel epithelial cells are characterized by the shape of the tooth they form (Fig. 5-6). Also, the cells of the enamel organ have differentiated into the **outer enamel epithelial cells,** which cover the enamel organ, and **inner enamel epithelial cells,** which become the **ameloblasts** that form the enamel of the tooth crown. Between these two cell layers are the **stellate reticulum cells,** which are star shaped with processes attached to each other. A fourth layer in the enamel organ is composed of **stratum intermedium cells.** These cells lie adjacent to the inner enamel epithelial cells. They assist the ameloblast in the formation of enamel. The function of the outer enamel epithelial cells is to organize a network of capillaries that will bring nutrition to the ameloblasts.

From the outer enamel epithelium, nutrients will percolate through the stellate reticulum to the **ameloblasts.** During the bell stage, cells in the periphery of the dental papilla become **odontoblasts.** These cells differentiate from mesenchymal cells. As the odontoblasts elongate and become columnar, they form a matrix of collagen fibers identified as **predentin.** After 24 hours this increment of matrix calcifies and becomes **dentin.** When several increments of dentin have formed, the differentiated ameloblasts deposit an enamel matrix. Dentinogenesis always precedes amelogenesis. After the enamel organ is differentiated, the dental lamina begins to degenerate by undergoing lysis. The dental lamina disappears in the anterior part of the mouth, although it remains active in the posterior region for many years (Figs. 5-2 and 5-3).

Cells interact through a system of effectors, modulators, and receptors called **cell signaling.** An example of

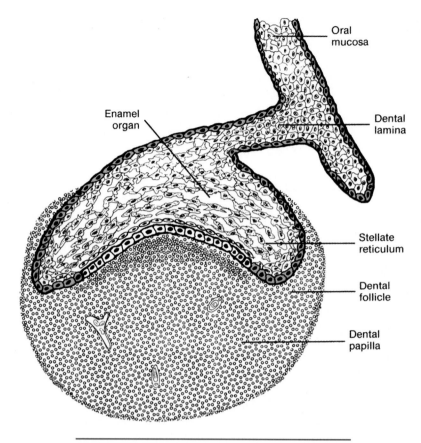

FIG. 5-5 Tooth development, diagram of cap stage.

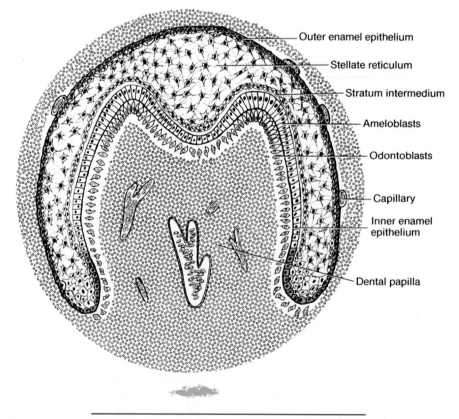

FIG. 5-6 Tooth development, diagram of bell stage.

such a system is epithelial-mesenchymal interaction in tooth development. The precursor cells, odontoblast and ameloblast, establish a positional relationship by means of effectors and receptors that are on the cell surface. The ameloblast differentiates first, causing the precursor odontoblast to locate itself adjacent. Then the odontoblast differentiates, establishing with the ameloblast a basement membrane that then forms a dentinal matrix. After this formation occurs, the ameloblast forms the enamel matrix. Thus it is not only cells, but also basal lamina and dentin matrix, that contain substances that cause cell changes and position.

DEVELOPMENT OF THE DENTAL PAPILLA

Densely packed cells characterize the dental papilla. This is evident even in the early bud stage, during which cells proliferate around the enlarging tooth buds at the leading edge of the dental lamina (Fig. 5-7). The papilla cells are believed to be significant in furthering enamel organ bud formation into the cap and bell stage. This cell density is maintained as the enamel organ grows. Cells of the dental papilla are found on close examination to be fibroblasts and appear to be in a delicate reticulum (Fig. 5-8). Blood vessels appear early in the dental papilla, ini-

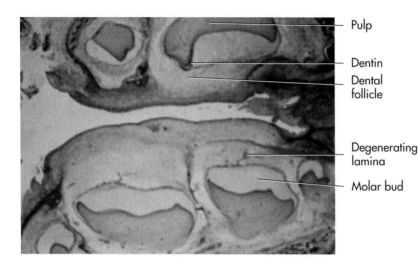

Pulp

Dentin

Dental follicle

Degenerating lamina

Molar bud

FIG. 5-7 Histology of tooth development with a sagittal view of the maxillary and mandibular human molar tooth buds.

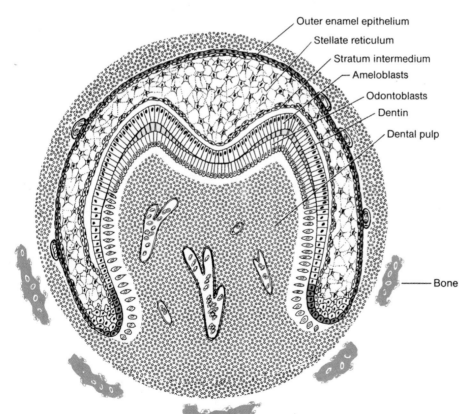

Outer enamel epithelium
Stellate reticulum
Stratum intermedium
Ameloblasts
Odontoblasts
Dentin
Dental pulp
Bone

FIG. 5-8 Tooth development, diagram of dentinogenesis.

tially in the central region along with nerve fibers associated with these vessels. The vessels bring nutrition to the rapidly growing organ. As the papilla grows, smaller vessels are also seen in the periphery of the area, bringing nutrition to the elongating odontoblasts (Fig. 5-6). Cellular changes result in formation of a hard shell around the central papilla. As this occurs, the papilla becomes known as the **dental pulp.**

DENTINOGENESIS

As the odontoblasts elongate, they gain the appearance of a protein-producing cell. A process develops at the proximal end of the cell, adjacent to the dentinoenamel junction. Gradually the cell moves pulpward, and the cell process, known as the **odontoblast process,** elongates (Fig. 5-9). The odontoblast becomes active in dentinal matrix formation similar to an osteoblast when it moves away from a spicule of bone. Increments of dentin are formed along the dentinoenamel junction. The dentinal matrix is first a meshwork of collagen fibers, but within 24 hours it becomes calcified. It is called **predentin** before calcification and **dentin** after calcification. At that time the dental papilla becomes the **dental pulp** as dentin begins to surround it. The odontoblasts maintain their elongating processes in dentinal tubules (Fig. 5-9).

When the odontoblasts are functioning, their nuclei occupy a more basal position in the cell and the or-ganelles become more evident in the cell cytoplasm. The appearance of granular endoplasmic reticulum, Golgi's complex, and mitochondria indicates the protein-producing nature of these cells (Fig. 5-10, *C* to *E*). The odontoblasts then secrete protein externally via vesicles at the apical part of the cell and along the cell processes (Fig. 5-10). The collagenous dentinal matrix is laid down in increments like bone or enamel, which is indicative of a daily rhythm for hard tissue formation. The site of initial formation is at the cusp tips (Fig. 5-8), and as further increments are formed, more odontoblasts are activated along the dentinoenamel junction (Fig. 5-9). As the odontoblastic process elongates, a tubule is maintained in the dentin and the matrix is formed around this tubule (Fig. 5-10, *C* and *D*).

Dentinogenesis takes place in two phases. First is the collagen matrix formation followed by the deposition of calcium phosphate (hydroxyapatite) crystals in the matrix. The initial calcification appears as crystals that are in small vesicles on the surface and within the collagen fibers (Fig. 5-11). The crystals grow, spread, and coalesce until the matrix is completely calcified. Only the newly formed band of dentinal matrix along the pulpal border is uncalcified (Fig. 5-12). Matrix formation and mineralization therefore are closely related. Mineralization proceeds by an increase in mineral density of the dentin. As each daily increment of predentin forms along the pulpal boundary, the adjacent peripheral increment of predentin formed the previous day calcifies and becomes dentin (Figs. 5-10, 5-12, and 5-13).

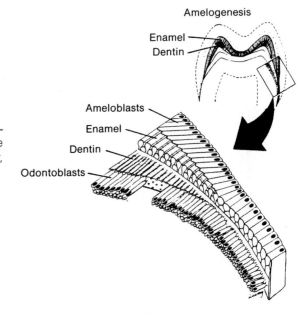

FIG. 5-9 Tooth development. Ameloblasts and odontoblasts move away from the dentinoenamel junction and away from each other, depositing enamel and dentin matrix.

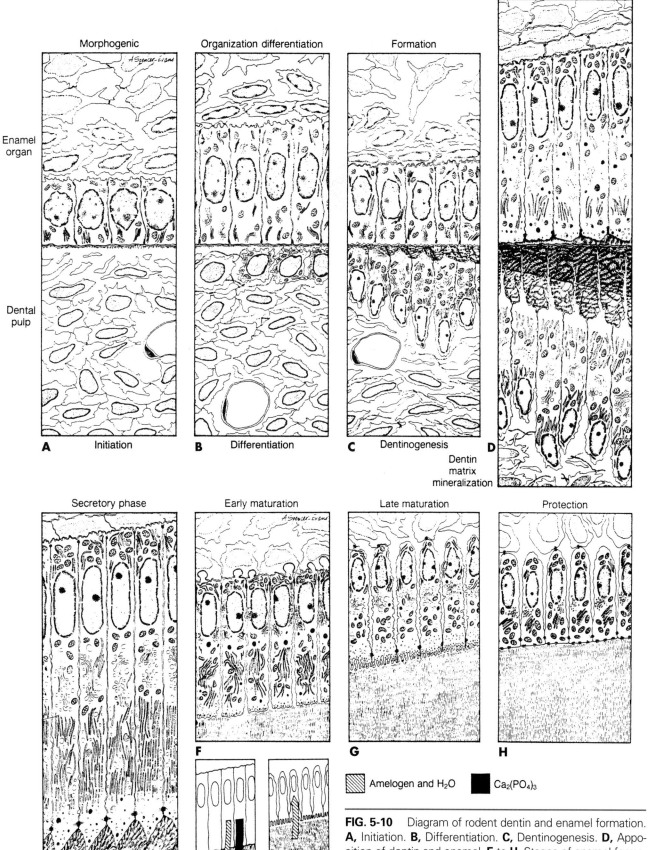

Apposition

Morphogenic

Organization differentiation

Formation

Enamel organ

Dental pulp

A Initiation

B Differentiation

C Dentinogenesis

Dentin matrix mineralization

D

Secretory phase

Early maturation

Late maturation

Protection

E

F

G

H

Amelogen and H$_2$O   Ca$_2$(PO$_4$)$_3$

FIG. 5-10   Diagram of rodent dentin and enamel formation. **A,** Initiation. **B,** Differentiation. **C,** Dentinogenesis. **D,** Apposition of dentin and enamel. **E** to **H,** Stages of enamel formation: **E,** secretory; **F,** early maturation; **G,** late maturation; and **H,** protective. During maturation of enamel an influx of mineral is accompanied by a loss of organic matter and water from the enamel matrix.

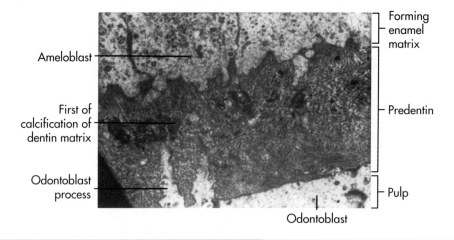

FIG. 5-11 Electron micrograph shows a band of predentin at the dentinoenamel junction. Ameloblasts are above, and odontoblastic cytoplasm is below. Calcification of predentin will spread from nucleation (first) sites within the predentin.

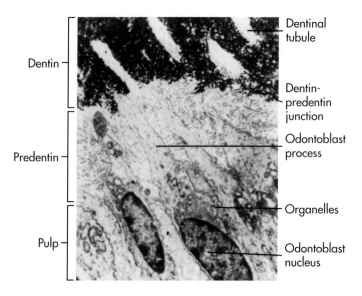

FIG. 5-12 Dentinogenesis. Calcified dentin seen above and predentin and odontoblasts below. Mineralization occurs along the dentin-predentin junction. (Electron micrograph.)

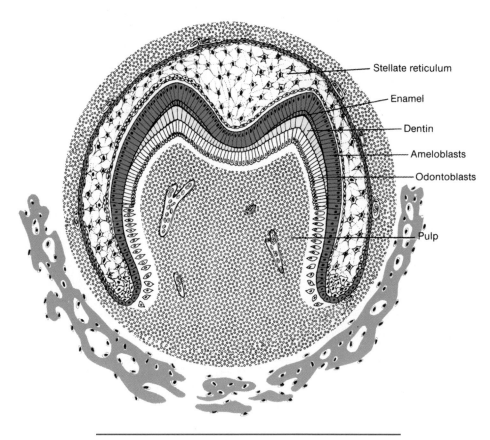

FIG. 5-13 Tooth development, diagram of amelogenesis.

AMELOGENESIS

Ameloblasts begin enamel deposition after a few micrometers of dentin have been deposited at the dentinoenamel junction (Fig. 5-14). At the bell stage, cells of the inner enamel epithelium differentiate. They elongate and are ready to become active secretory ameloblasts. The ameloblasts then exhibit changes as they differentiate and pass through five functional stages: (1) morphogenesis, (2) organization and differentiation, (3) secretion, (4) maturation, and (5) protection (Fig. 5-10). Golgi's apparatus appears centrally in the ameloblasts, and the amount of rough-surfaced endoplasmic reticulum (RER) increases in the apical area (Fig. 5-10, *D* and *E*). The row of ameloblasts maintains orientation by cell-to-cell attachments (desmosomes) at both the proximal and distal ends of the cell. This maintains the cells in a row as they move peripherally from the dentinoenamel junction depositing enamel matrix (Fig. 5-9).

Short conical processes **(Tomes' processes)** develop at the apical end of the ameloblasts during the secretory stage (Figs. 5-10, *E*, and 5-15). Junctional complexes called the **terminal bar apparatus** appear at the junction of the cell bodies and Tomes' processes and maintain contact between adjacent cells (Fig. 5-10, *E*). As the ameloblast differentiates, the matrix is synthesized within the RER, which then migrates to Golgi's apparatus, where it is condensed and packaged in membrane-bound granules. Vesicles migrate to the apical end of the cell, where their contents are exteriorized and deposited first along the junction of the enamel and dentin (Fig. 5-16). This first enamel deposited on the surface of the dentin establishes the dentinoenamel junction. Fig. 5-17 is an electron micrograph of young enamel matrix formed along the dentinoenamel junction. The Tomes' process of the ameloblast indents the surface of the enamel (Figs. 5-10, *E*, 5-15, and 5-16). This is because the center of the rod does not form at the same rate as the rod walls and can best be seen in Fig. 5-17. As the enamel matrix develops, it forms in continuous rods from the dentinoenamel junction to the surface of the enamel.

When ameloblasts begin secretion, the overlying cells of the stratum intermedium change in shape from spindle to pyramidal (Fig. 5-10, *B* to *F*). As amelogenesis proceeds, both of these cell layers, ameloblasts and stratum intermedium, are held together by cell junctional com-

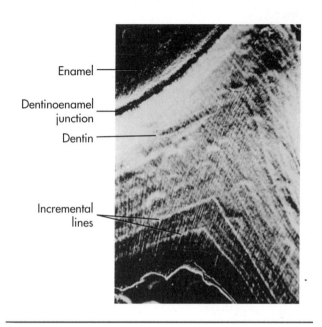

FIG. 5-14 Dentin microradiograph showing incremental lines in dentin.

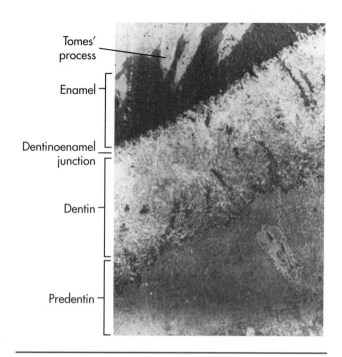

FIG. 5-16 Ultrastructure of early enamel and dentin matrix formation at dentinoenamel junction. Above is enamel, and below are dentin and predentin.

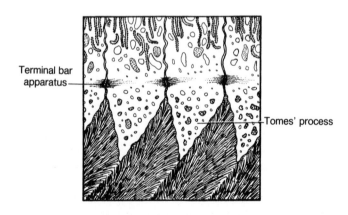

FIG. 5-15 Development of Tomes' process of ameloblast during amelogenesis.

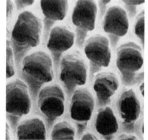

Human deciduous molar

Developing enamel surface

Height of field, 15–18 μm

FIG. 5-17 A scanning electron micrograph of ameloblast-enamel matrix interface during amelogenesis. Pits indicate where Tomes' process is present.

plexes termed **desmosomes,** with synthesis of enamel occurring in both cells. Substances needed for enamel production arrive via the blood vessels and pass through the stellate reticulum to the stratum intermedium and ameloblasts. In this manner the protein **amelogenin** is produced. Only a few ameloblasts at the tip of the cusps begin to function initially (Fig. 5-13). As the process proceeds, more ameloblasts become active and the increments of enamel matrix become more prominent.

Growth of individual cusps by incremental deposition continues until tooth eruption. This occurs in posterior multicuspid teeth as the ameloblasts continue to differentiate from the inner enamel epithelium and form enamel. Cusps then coalesce in the intercuspal region of the crown (Fig. 5-18). In radiographs, cusps initially appear separated and are joined together as growth progresses. The inner enamel epithelium forms the blueprint for the shape of the developing crown.

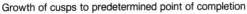
Growth of cusps to predetermined point of completion

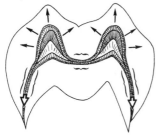

FIG. 5-18 Growth areas of developing crown. Growth at cusp tip, intercuspal region, and cervical region.

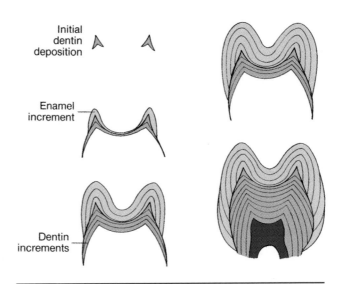
Initial dentin deposition

Enamel increment

Dentin increments

FIG. 5-19 Incremental pattern of dentin and enamel formation from initiation to completion. This begins in diagram at upper left and proceeds to completion at lower right.

CROWN MATURATION

As amelogenesis is completed and amelogenin is deposited, the matrix begins to mineralize (Fig. 5-10, *F* to *H*). As soon as the small crystals of mineral are deposited, they begin to grow in length and diameter. The initial deposition of mineral amounts to approximately 25% of the total enamel. The other 70% of mineral in enamel is a result of growth of the crystals (5% of enamel is water). The time between enamel matrix deposition and its mineralization is short. Therefore the pattern of mineralization closely follows the pattern of matrix deposition. The first matrix deposited is the first enamel mineralized, occurring along the dentinoenamel junction. Matrix formation and mineralization continue peripherally to the tips of the cusps and then laterally on the sides of the crowns, following the enamel incremental deposition pattern (Fig. 5-19). Finally, the cervical region of the crown mineralizes. During this process, protein of the enamel changes or matures and is termed **enamelin.**

The mineral content of enamel is approximately 95% as it rapidly surpasses that of dentin (69%) to become the most highly calcified tissue in the human body. Because of the high mineral content of enamel, almost all water and organic material are lost from it during maturation (Fig. 5-10, *E* to *H*).

As the ameloblast completes the matrix deposition phase, its terminal bar apparatus disappears and the surface enamel becomes smooth (Fig. 5-10, *F* and *G*). This phase is signaled by a change in the appearance of the cell as well as by a change in the function of the ameloblast. The apical end of this cell becomes ruffled along the enamel surface. The length of the ameloblast decreases, as does the number of organelles within it. The enamel has now reached the maturation phase, and the ameloblast becomes more active in absorption of the organic matrix and water from enamel, which allows mineralization to proceed (Fig. 5-10, *F* to *H*).

CLINICAL COMMENT

Functional enamel is the hardest tissue in the human body. To attain this status, the formative ameloblast cell must secrete protein during enamel formation as well as be active in absorbing water and protein from the matrix during its final mineralization process.

The increased mineral content in enamel is dependent on the loss of fluid and protein. This process of exchange occurs throughout much of enamel maturation and is not limited to the final stage of mineralization. Even after the teeth erupt, mineralization of enamel continues.

Finally, after the ameloblasts have completed their contributions to the mineralization phase, they secrete an organic cuticle on the surface of the enamel, which is known as the **developmental** or **primary cuticle.** The ameloblasts then attach themselves to this organic covering of the enamel by **hemidesmosomes** (Fig. 5-10, *H*). A hemidesmosome is half of a desmosome attachment plaque. Whereas a desmosome functions in attaching a cell to an adjacent cell, a hemidesmosome relates to the attachment of a cell to a surface membrane. The hemidesmosome attachment plaque is developed by the ameloblast, and this stage of plaque formation and attachment is known as the **protective stage** of ameloblast function. The ameloblasts shorten and contact the stratum intermedium and other enamel epithelium, which fuse together to form the **reduced enamel epithelium.**

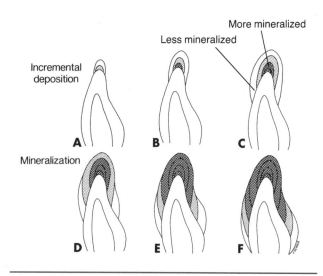

FIG. 5-20   Summary of enamel mineralization stages. **A,** Initial enamel is formed. **B,** Enamel is calcified, and more matrix is formed. **C,** More increments are formed. **D,** Matrix deposition and mineralization proceed. **E** and **F,** Matrix is formed at sides and cervical areas of the cusp.

FIG. 5-21   Histologic section of nearly mineralized enamel of crown. Enamel matrix is seen only at cervical region.

This cellular organic covering remains on the enamel surface until the tooth erupts into the oral cavity.

With mineralization of enamel complete and its thickness established, the crown of the tooth is formed (Fig. 5-20). The completed crown with the reduced enamel epithelium is seen in Fig. 5-21. Meanwhile dentin formation proceeds. The next stage of development will be root formation.

CONSIDER THE PATIENT . . .

A patient complains that white, chalky areas appear in the cervical enamel of some of his crowns. He asks what could cause this condition.

DEVELOPMENT OF THE TOOTH ROOT

Root Sheath

As the crown develops, cell proliferation continues at the cervical region or base of the enamel organ, where the inner and outer enamel epithelial cells join to form a root sheath (Fig. 5-22). When the crown is completed, the cells in this region of the enamel organ continue to grow, forming a double layer of cells termed the **epithelial root sheath,** or **Hertwig's root sheath** (Fig. 5-22, *A*). The inner cell layer of the root sheath forms from the inner enamel epithelium or ameloblasts in the crown, and enamel is produced. In the root, these cells induce odontoblasts of the dental papilla to differentiate and form dentin. The root sheath originates at the point that enamel deposits end (Fig. 5-22, *A*). As the root sheath lengthens, it becomes the architect of the root. The length, curvature, thickness, and number of roots are all dependent upon the inner root sheath cells (Fig. 5-22). As the formation of the root dentin takes place, cells of the outer root sheath function in the deposition of **intermediate cementum,** a thin layer of acellular cementum that covers the ends of the dentinal tubule and seals the root surface. Then the outer root sheath cells disperse into small clusters and move away from the root surface as **epithelial rests** (Fig. 5-22, *B*). At the proliferating end the root sheath bends at a near 45-degree angle. This area is termed the **epithelial diaphragm** (Fig. 5-22). The epithelial diaphragm encircles the apical opening of the dental pulp during root development. It is the proliferation of these cells that causes root growth to occur.

As the odontoblasts differentiate along the pulpal boundary, root dentinogenesis proceeds and the root lengthens. Dentin formation continues from the crown into the root (Fig. 5-23). The dentin tapers from the crown into the root to the apical epithelial diaphragm. In the pulp adjacent to the epithelial diaphragm, cellular proliferation occurs. This is known as the **pulp proliferation zone** (Fig. 5-22). It is believed that this area produces new cells needed for root lengthening. Dentinogenesis continues until the appropriate root length is developed. The root then thickens until the apical opening is restricted to approximately 1 to 3 mm, which is sufficient to allow neural and vascular communication between the pulp and the periodontium.

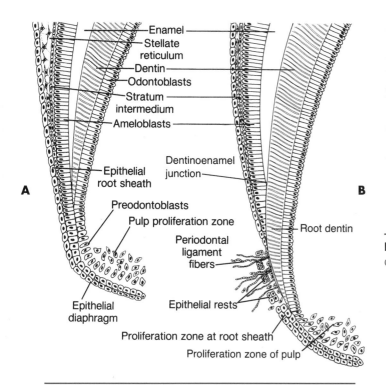

FIG. 5-22 Root sheath and epithelial diaphragm formation. **A,** Stage of initiation of root sheath at dentinoenamel junction. **B,** A later stage of root sheath development. Root dentin has formed below the cervical enamel.

With the increase in root length, the tooth begins eruptive movements, which provides space for further lengthening of the root. The root lengthens at the same rate as the tooth eruptive movements occur (Fig. 5-24).

 CLINICAL COMMENT

The root sheath determines whether a tooth has single or multiple roots, is short or long, or is curved or straight. However, roots conform to whatever area is available.

Single Root

The root sheath of a single-rooted tooth is a tubelike growth of epithelial cells that originates from the enamel organ, enclosing a tube of dentin and the developing pulp (Fig. 5-23). As soon as the root sheath cells deposit the **intermediate cementum,** the root sheath breaks up, forming **epithelial rests** (Figs. 5-22, *B,* and 5-25). The epithelial rests persist as they move away from the root surface into the follicular area. Mesenchymal cells from the tooth follicle move between the epithelial rests to contact the root surface. Here, they differentiate into cementoblasts and begin secretion of **cementoid** on the

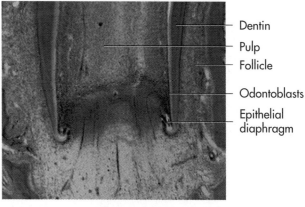

FIG. 5-23 Histology of root sheath and epithelial diaphragm. Root dentin and highly cellular pulp are shown.

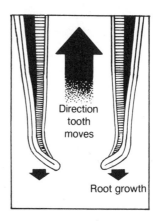

FIG. 5-24 Direction of root growth versus eruptive movements of tooth.

surface of the intermediate cementum. Cementoid is noncalcified cementum that soon calcifies into mature cementum (Fig. 5-26). The root sheath is never seen as a continuous structure because its cell layers break down rapidly once the root dentin forms. However, the area of the epithelial diaphragm is maintained until the root is complete; then it disappears.

Multiple Roots

The roots of multirooted teeth develop in a similar fashion to single-rooted teeth until the furcation zone begins to form (Fig. 5-27). Division of the roots then takes place through differential growth of the root sheath. The cells of the epithelial diaphragm grow excessively in two or more areas until they contact the opposing epithelial extensions (Fig. 5-27). These extensions fuse, and then the original single opening is divided into two or three openings. The epithelial diaphragm surrounding the opening to each root continues to grow at an equal rate. When a developing molar is sectioned through the cen-

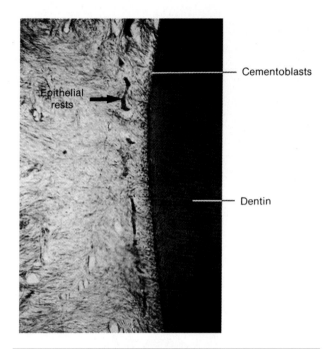

FIG. 5-25 Histologic micrograph of epithelial rests from root sheath along surface of root dentin.

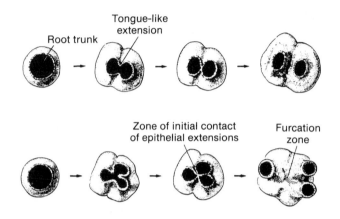

FIG. 5-27 Multiple-root development. Epithelial diaphragms extend as they make contact and fuse to divide a single root into two or three roots.

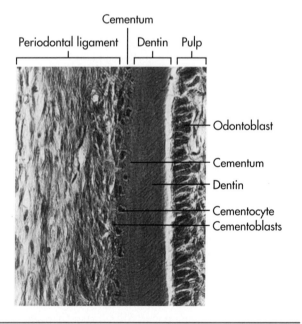

FIG. 5-26 Micrograph of cellular cementum on tooth surface. Cementocytes are in the cementum as well as on its surface. Periodontal cells are on left. Cementum contacts with tubular dentin. Odontoblasts and pulp cells are on right.

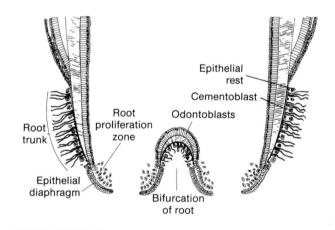

FIG. 5-28 Cell activity in multiple-root development. Bifurcation zone is shown. Root trunk is common root area from crown to site of root bifurcation.

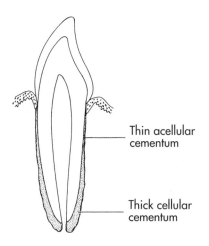

FIG. 5-29   Location of acellular cementum in cervical area and cellular cementum at root apex.

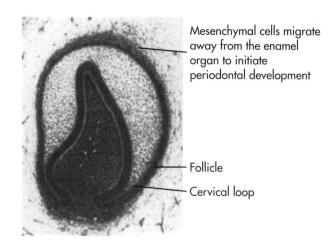

Mesenchymal cells migrate away from the enamel organ to initiate periodontal development

Follicle

Cervical loop

FIG. 5-30   Histology of enamel organ at bell stage of tooth development when cervical loop is present. Mesenchymal cells on surface of enamel organ migrate at this time peripherally and initiate development of future periodontium.

ter of its root, it would show the root sheath as an island of cells (Fig. 5-28).

As the multiple roots form, each one develops by the same pattern as a single-rooted tooth. After the root is complete and the sheath breaks up, the epithelial cells migrate away from the root surface as they do in a single-rooted tooth. Cementum then forms on the surface of the intermediate cemental surface. The cementum usually appears cellular, although the cementum near the cementoenamel junction is less cellular than that at the apices of the root (Fig. 5-29). Because the apical cementum is thicker, it is said to require more cells to maintain vitality. The primary function of this cementum involves the attachment of the principal periodontal ligament fibers.

CLINICAL COMMENT

Growth of the jaws is necessary for the change from the primary to permanent dentition. With the lengthening of the jaws, the permanent molars have space to develop, erupt, and function. The jaws protect each developing tooth with a shell-like enclosure of bone.

DEVELOPMENT OF SUPPORTING STRUCTURES

The mesenchymal cells surrounding the teeth are known as the **dental follicle** (Fig. 5-7). Some of these follicular cells, which lie immediately adjacent to the enamel organ, migrate during the cap and bell stages from the enamel organ peripherally into the follicle to develop the alveolar bone and the periodontal ligament (Fig. 5-30). These cells have been traced from this origin to the site where they differentiate into osteoblasts and form bone or fibroblasts, which form ligament fibers. After tooth eruption these tissues serve to support the teeth during function.

Periodontal Ligament

Cells of the dental follicle differentiate into collagen-forming cells of the ligament and form cementoblasts, which lay cementum on tooth roots. Some cells of the ligament invade the root sheath as it breaks apart. Other cells of the ligament area form delicate fibers, which appear along the forming roots near the cervical region of the crown. These are probably the stem cell fibroblasts that form more fiber groups, which appear as the roots elongate (Fig. 5-31). As these fibers become embedded in the cementum of the root surface, the other end attaches to the forming alveolar bone. Evidence suggests that these fibers turn over rapidly and are continually renewed as the location of origin is established. Collagen fiber turnover takes place throughout the ligament, although the highest turnover is in the apical area and the lowest is in the cervical region. Maturation of the ligament occurs when the teeth reach functional occlusion. At this time the density of fiber bundles increases notably.

Alveolar Process

As the teeth develop, so does the alveolar bone, which keeps pace with the lengthening roots. At first the alveolar process forms a labial and lingual bony trench in which the tooth organs develop. As the walls lining this trench increase in height, bony septa appear between the teeth to complete the crypts (Fig. 5-32). When the teeth

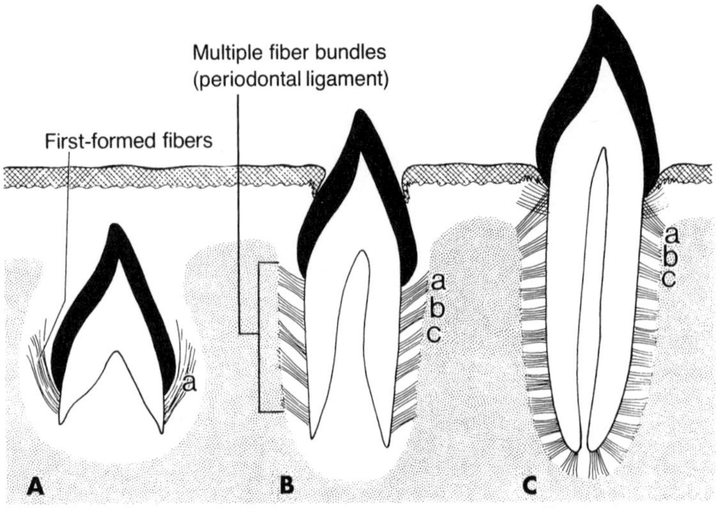

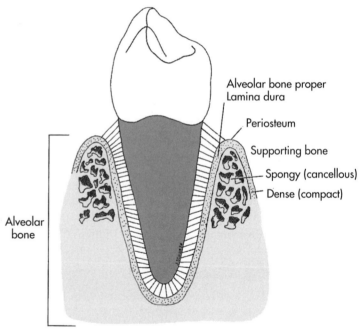

FIG. 5-31   Initial fiber bundle development of periodontal ligament. **A,** Initial fiber formation. **B,** Development of secondary fibers. **C,** Further fiber development. Initial fiber groups change in direction.

First-formed fibers

Multiple fiber bundles (periodontal ligament)

Tooth below alveolar crest

Tooth above alveolar crest

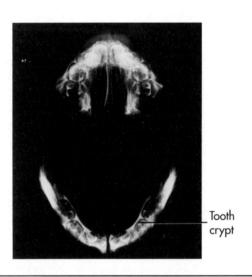

FIG. 5-32   Microradiograph of maxillary and mandibular arches, illustrating alveolar bone with tooth crypts enclosing developing teeth in embryo.

Tooth crypt

Alveolar bone proper
Lamina dura

Periosteum

Supporting bone

Spongy (cancellous)

Dense (compact)

Alveolar bone

FIG. 5-34   Tooth in alveolar bone. Alveolar bone is composed of alveolar bone proper, which lines the socket, and supporting bone. Supporting bone consists of spongy or cancellous bone and dense or compact bone.

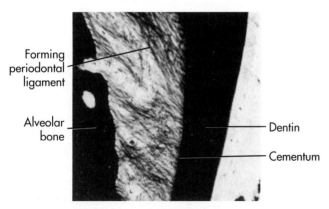

Forming periodontal ligament

Alveolar bone

Dentin

Cementum

FIG. 5-33   Appearance of periodontal ligament fibers during tooth eruption. Density of the fibers is similar to C in Fig. 5-31.

erupt, the alveolar process and intervening periodontal ligament mature to support the newly functioning teeth (Fig. 5-33). Bone that forms between the roots of the multirooted teeth is termed **interradicular** bone. In the mature form, alveolar bone is composed of **alveolar bone proper** and **supporting bone.** Alveolar bone proper lines the tooth socket, sustained by supporting bone, which is composed of both spongy and dense or

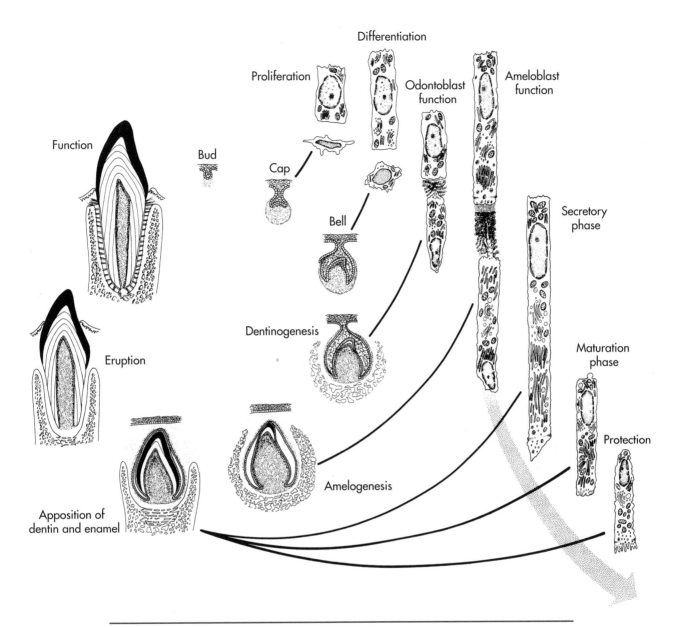

FIG. 5-35 Changes in formative cells of developing teeth are shown on right side of diagram and relate to the morphologic changes shown on left. Cell proliferation relates to the cap stage, and cell differentiation relates to the bell stage. Odontoblast function relates to dentinogenesis, and ameloblast function to amelogenesis. The labels secretory phase, maturation phase, and protection phase relate to the ameloblast function.

compact bone. Supporting bone forms the cortical plate, which covers the mandible (Fig. 5-34).

In summary, tooth development involves the interactive events of two types of tissues: epithelial and mesenchymal. These tissues develop through the soft tissue stages of bud, cap, and bell. This level is followed by the hard tissue formative stages of dentinogenesis and amelogenesis. Root formation logically follows crown development. Each developmental progression includes morphologic changes in shape and size, which are coordinated with microscopic changes in cell shape and function. Most of these relationships are seen in Fig. 5-35.

CLINICAL COMMENT

Accessory root canals may connect the pulp with the periodontal ligament at any point along the root, although it usually appears near the root apex. Pulp or periodontal infection can spread by means of this route to the adjacent tissue. A periodontal pocket that is resistant to treatment could be caused by this defect.

SELF-EVALUATION QUESTIONS

1. What two cell types interact in tooth development?
2. Describe two characteristics of the bell stage of tooth development.
3. List and describe each stage of tooth development.
4. Describe the dental papilla. When does it become the dental pulp organ?
5. Describe the differentiation of the odontoblast and the initiation of dentin formation.
6. Why is dentinogenesis called the two phases process?
7. What are the five phases of enamel production?
8. What structures enable the ameloblasts to move in a row rather than individually during enamel production?
9. What areas of enamel are first and last to calcify in the crown?
10. What two processes signal enamel completion?

 CONSIDER THE PATIENT . . .

Discussion: White, chalky areas in the cervical enamel of some crowns are caused by a lack of mineralization of the enamel. The chalkiness occurs in this location because this is the last area of the crown to calcify and sometimes the crown erupts before the cervical enamel has completely mineralized.

ACKNOWLEDGMENTS

Dr. Nicholas P. Piesco and Dr. N.M. ElNesr contributed to the production of chapters in Avery JK: *Oral Development and Histology,* ed 2, 1994, New York, Thieme Medical. Some of the figures in that text have been used in preparation of this chapter.

SUGGESTED READING

Kallenbach E, Piesco, NP: The changing morphology of the epithelium-mesenchyme interface in the differentiation of growing teeth of selected vertebrates and its relationship to possible mechanisms of differentiation, *J Biol Buccale* 6:229-240, 1978.

Marks SC et al: Tooth eruption, a synthesis of experimental observations. In Davidovich, Z, editor: *The biological mechanisms of tooth eruption and root resorption,* Birmingham, Ala, 1988, EBSCO Information Services, pp 161-169.

Robinson C, Kirkham J: Dynamics of amelogenesis as revealed by protein compositional studies. In *The chemistry and biology of mineralized tissues,* Birmingham, Ala, 1985, EBSCO Media, pp 248-263.

Thesleff I, Vaahtokari A: The role of growth factors in the determination of odontoblastic cell lineage, *Proc Finn Dent Soc* 88(SI):357-368, 1992.

Warshasky H et al: The development of enamel structure in the rat incisor as compared to the teeth of monkey and man, *Anat Rec* 299:371, 1981.

Wise GE, Marks SC Jr, Cahill DR: Ultrastructural features of the dental follicle associated with the eruption pathway in the dog, *J Oral Pathol* 14:15-26, 1985.

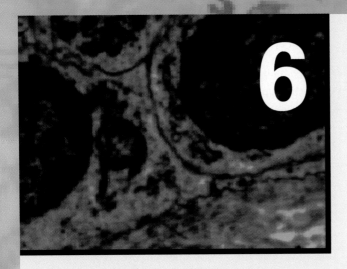

6 Eruption and Shedding of Teeth

OVERVIEW

Tooth eruption is the process by which developing teeth emerge through the soft tissue of the jaws and the overlying mucosa to enter the oral cavity, contact the teeth of the opposing arch, and function in mastication. The movements related to tooth eruption begin during crown formation and require adjustments relative to the forming bony crypt. This is the **preeruptive phase.** Tooth eruption is also involved in the initiation of root development and continues until the tooth's emergence into the oral cavity, which is the **prefunctional eruptive phase.** The teeth continue to erupt until they reach incisal or occlusal contact. Then they undergo functional eruptive movements, which include compensation for jaw growth and occlusal wear of the enamel. This stage is the **functional eruptive phase.** Eruption is actually a continuous process that ends only with the loss of the tooth. Each dentition, primary and permanent, has various problems during eruption and in the sequencing of eruption in the oral cavity. Teeth differ extensively in their eruptive schedules as well. This chapter describes these events. Finally, the process of tooth shedding or exfoliation of the primary dentition is discussed. Primary tooth loss results from three fundamental causes.

PREERUPTIVE PHASE

The preeruptive phase includes all movements of primary and permanent tooth crowns from the time of their early initiation and formation to the time of crown completion. Therefore this phase is finished with early initiation of root formation. The developing crowns move constantly in the jaws during the preeruptive phase. They respond to positional changes of the neighboring crowns and to changes in the mandible and maxilla as the face develops outward, forward, and downward away from the brain in its maturing growth path. During the lengthening of the jaws, primary and permanent teeth make mesial and distal movements. Eventually the permanent tooth crowns move within the jaws, adjusting their position to the resorptive roots of the primary dentition and the remodeling alveolar processes, especially during the mixed dentition period from 8 to 12 years of age.

Early in the preeruptive period the permanent anterior teeth begin developing lingual to the incisal level of the primary teeth (Figs. 6-1 and 6-2). Later, however, as the primary teeth erupt, the permanent successors are positioned lingual to the apical third of their roots. The permanent premolars shift from a location near the occlusal area of the primary molars to a location enclosed within the roots of the primary molars (Fig. 6-2). This change in relative position is due to the eruption of the primary teeth and an increase in height of the supporting structures. On the other hand, the permanent molars, which have no primary predecessors, develop without this type of relationship (Fig. 6-3). Maxillary molars develop within the tuberosities of the maxilla with their occlusal surfaces slanted distally. Mandibular molars develop in the mandibular rami with their occlusal surfaces slanting mesially (Fig. 6-3). This slant is due to the angle of eruption as the molars arise from the curvature of the condyle of the posterior mandible. All movements in the preeruptive phase occur within the crypts of the developing and growing crown before root formation begins.

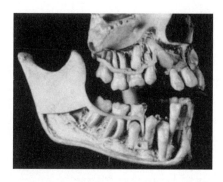

FIG. 6-3 Human jaws at 8 to 9 years of age, during mixed dentition period. Permanent teeth are replacing primary teeth, and positions of each are shown. Permanent mandibular molar has not emerged from coronoid process.

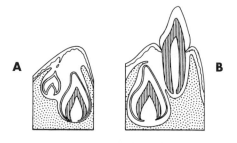

FIG. 6-1 Relative position of primary and permanent incisor teeth in, **A,** preeruptive and, **B,** prefunctional eruptive periods.

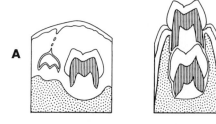

FIG. 6-2 Relative position of primary molar and permanent teeth in, **A,** preeruptive and, **B,** prefunctional eruptive periods.

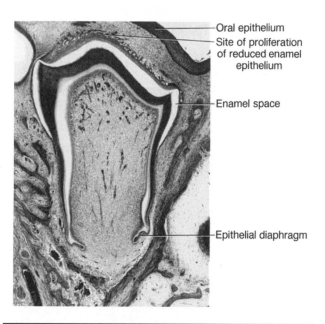

Oral epithelium
Site of proliferation of reduced enamel epithelium
Enamel space
Epithelial diaphragm

FIG. 6-4 Histology of prefunctional eruptive phase. Root develops, and reduced epithelium overlying crown approaches oral mucosa. Reduced enamel epithelium proliferates.

PREFUNCTIONAL ERUPTIVE PHASE

The prefunctional eruptive phase starts with the initiation of root formation and ends when the teeth reach occlusal contact. Four major events occur during this phase:

1. **Root formation** requires space for the elongation of the roots. The first step in root formation is proliferation of the epithelial root sheath, which in time causes initiation of root dentin and formation of the pulp tissues of the forming root. Root formation also causes an increase in the fibrous tissue of the surrounding dental follicle (Fig. 6-4).
2. **Movement** occurs incisally or occlusally through the bony crypt of the jaws to reach the oral mucosa. The movement is due to a need for space in which the enlarging roots can form. The reduced enamel epithelium next contacts and fuses with the oral epithelium (Fig. 6-5). Both of these epithelial layers proliferate toward each other, their cells intermingle, and a fusion occurs. A reduced epithelial layer overlying the erupting crown arises from the reduced enamel epithelium (Fig. 6-6).
3. **Penetration** of the tooth's crown tip through the fused epithelial layers allows entrance of the crown enamel into the oral cavity. Only the organic developmental cuticle (primary), secreted earlier by the ameloblasts, covers the enamel (Fig. 6-7).
4. **Intraoral occlusal** or **incisal movement** of the erupting tooth continues until clinical contact with the opposing crown occurs. The crown continues to move through the mucosa, causing gradual exposure of the crown surface, with an increasingly apical shift of the gingival attachment (Fig. 6-7). The exposed crown is the clinical crown, extending from the cusp tip to the area of the gingival attachment. In contrast, the anatomic crown is the entire crown, extending from the cusp tip to the cementoenamel junction.

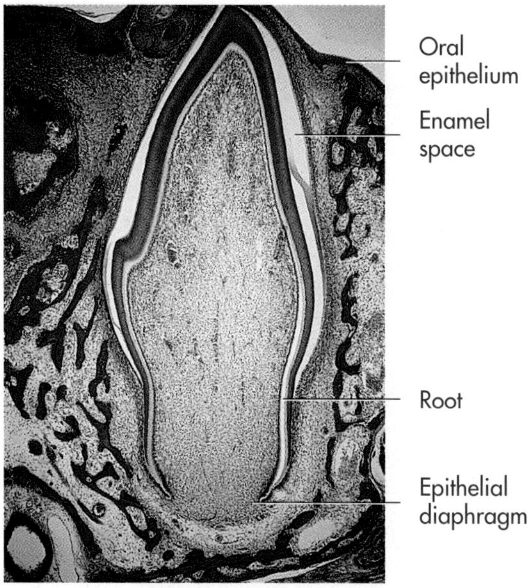

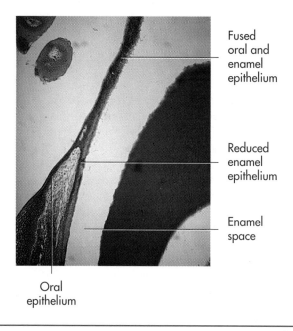

Fused oral and enamel epithelium

Reduced enamel epithelium

Enamel space

Oral epithelium

FIG. 6-6 Histology of erupting tooth. Fused enamel and oral epithelium are stretched over enamel of crown. (Enamel space occurs as enamel is dissolved in preparation of slide.)

Oral epithelium

Enamel space

Root

Epithelial diaphragm

FIG. 6-5 Histology of erupting cuspid tooth. Crown tip is contacting oral epithelium.

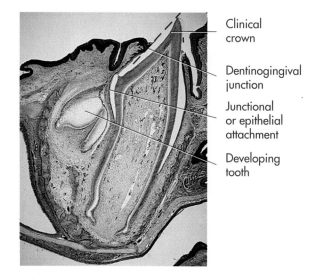

Clinical crown

Dentinogingival junction

Junctional or epithelial attachment

Developing tooth

FIG. 6-7 Histology of erupting primary tooth and appearance of clinical crown in mouth. Permanent tooth's position is shown on left. Dotted line indicates cuticle overlying enamel surface of erupting tooth.

CLINICAL COMMENT

Hypereruption occurs in the loss of an apposing tooth. This condition allows the tooth or teeth to erupt farther than normal into the space.

Changes in Tissues

The prefunctional eruptive phase is characterized by significant changes in the tissues **overlying, surrounding,** and **underlying** the erupting teeth.

Overlying the Teeth

The dental follicle changes and forms a pathway for the erupting teeth. A zone of degenerating connective tissue fibers and cells immediately overlying the teeth appears first (Figs. 6-8 and 6-9). During the process the blood vessels decrease in number and nerve fibers break up into pieces and degenerate. The altered tissue area overlying the teeth becomes visible as an inverted triangular area known as the **eruption pathway.** In the periphery of this zone the follicular fibers, regarded as the **gubernaculum dentis** or **gubernacular cord** (Fig. 6-10), are directed toward the mucosa. Some scientists believe that these fibers guide the teeth in their movements to ensure complete tooth eruption.

Macrophages appear in the eruption pathway tissue. These cells cause the release of hydrolytic enzymes that aid in the destruction of the cells and fibers in this area with the loss of blood vessels and nerves. Osteoclasts are found along the borders of the resorptive bone overlying the teeth. This bone loss adjacent to the teeth keeps pace with the eruptive movements of the teeth (Fig. 6-9). **Osteoclasts** and **osteoblasts** constantly remodel the alveolar bone as the teeth enlarge and move forward in the direction of the growing face.

Although the process of eruption for permanent teeth is similar to that of the primary, the presence of primary teeth roots presents a problem. The resorption of their roots is similar to the process of bone resorption for the emergence of primary teeth. Permanent teeth establish an eruptive path lingual to the primary anterior teeth and the premolars under the primary molars. Permanent molars erupt into the alveolar free space behind primary teeth (Fig. 6-9). Small foramina just posterior to the primary tooth row are evidence of the eruption sites of the anterior permanent teeth (Fig. 6-11). As the roots resorb, the primary crowns are lost or shed (Fig. 6-12). Dentin resorption is similar to bone resorption (Fig. 6-10).

The resorptive process of primary and permanent teeth results from action of osteoclasts that arise from monocytes of the circulating bloodstream. These monocytes appear and fuse with others to form the multinucleated osteoclasts. Their function is to resorb the hard tissue. They do so by first separating the mineral from the collagen matrix through the action of the hydrolytic enzymes secreted by the osteoclasts. This enzymatic action is believed to occur within lacunae, which are de-

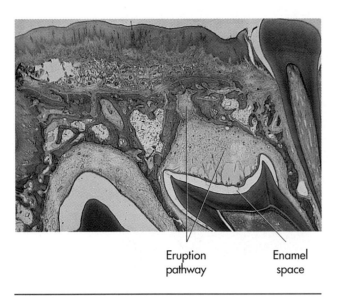

FIG. 6-8 Histology of prefunctional erupting tooth. Observe the appearance of the eruption pathway overlying crown.

Eruption pathway

Enamel space

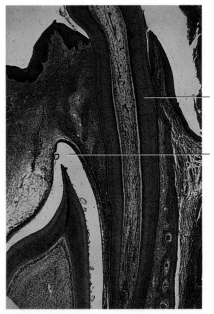

Primary tooth

Erupting permanent tooth crown

FIG. 6-9 Histology of the relation of functional primary tooth root on right to permanent crown nearing eruption on left.

veloped by the osteoclasts. The osteoclast's cell membrane is in contact with the bone and becomes modified by an enfolding process termed the **ruffled border** (Figs. 6-13 and 6-14). This border greatly increases the surface area of the osteoclast and allows the cell to function maximally in bone resorption (Fig. 6-15).

Hard tissue resorption is believed to occur in two phases: the **extracellular phase,** in which the mineral is separated from the collagen and is broken into small fragments (Fig. 6-15), and the **intracellular phase,** in which the osteoclast ingests these mineral fragments and continues the dissolution of this mineral. Crystals appear in cytoplasmic vacuoles of the osteoclast and are gradually digested within them. Resorption of mineral occurs at the ruffled border interface outside the cell, and the mineral is then taken within the cell (Fig. 6-16). Spe-

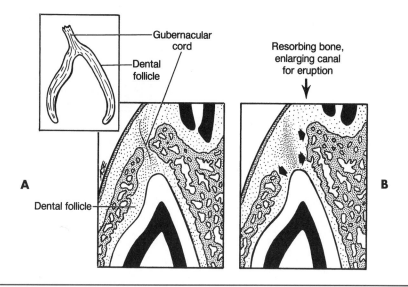

FIG. 6-10 Developing eruption pathway. **A,** Gubernaculum dentis. **B,** Bone resorption in eruption pathway.

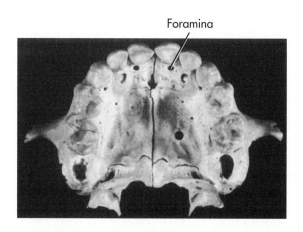

FIG. 6-11 Foramina lingual to maxillary primary incisors. These are sites of eruption for permanent incisors.

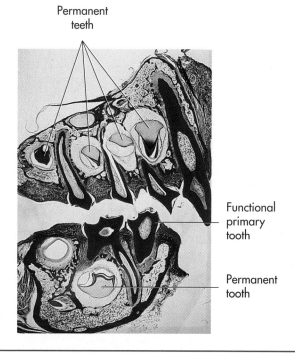

FIG. 6-12 Histology of mixed dentition period. Roots of erupted primary teeth are resorbing. Crowns of developing permanent teeth are below primary teeth.

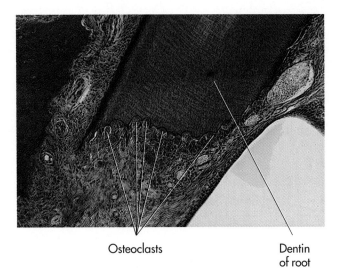

Osteoclasts

Dentin of root

FIG. 6-13 Histology of active resorption sites on primary tooth roots. Osteoclasts in lacunae are shown.

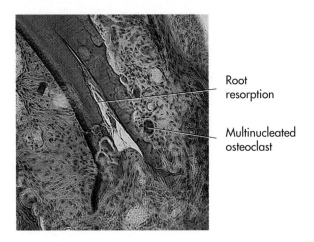

Root resorption

Multinucleated osteoclast

FIG. 6-14 Histology of osteoclasts in resorption lacunae. Observe the large multinucleated cells shown within the lacunae.

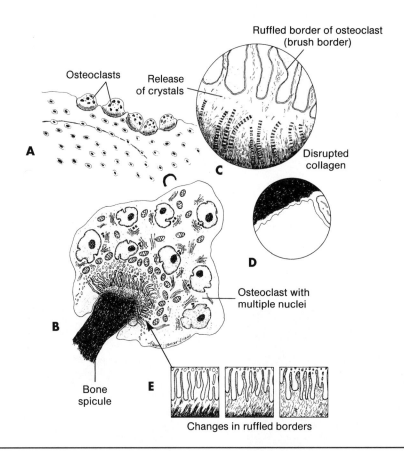

Ruffled border of osteoclast (brush border)

Osteoclasts

Release of crystals

Disrupted collagen

A

C

D

Osteoclast with multiple nuclei

B

Bone spicule

E

Changes in ruffled borders

FIG. 6-15 Osteoclast activity. **A,** Osteoclasts in lacunae on bone surface. **B,** Large multinucleated osteoclast with brush border in contact with bone spicule. **C,** High magnification of ruffled border of osteoclast showing mineral crystals passing into spaces between cell extensions. Unmasked collagen fibers are nearby. **D,** Clear zone on osteoclast surface. **E,** Ruffled border of osteoclast in constant motion or change.

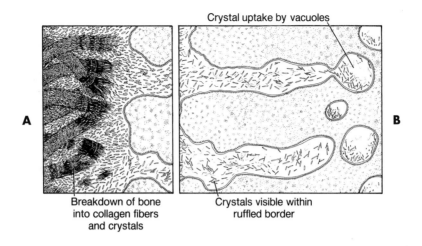

FIG. 6-16 **A,** High magnification of unmasked collagen fibers. Mineral crystals are near osteoclast surface. **B,** Diagram of uptake of crystals into osteoclast vacuoles.

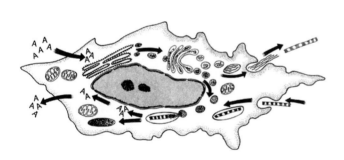

FIG. 6-17 A fibroblast (fibroblast-fibroclast) capable of synthesis of collagen as well as its breakdown. Collagen fibers are phagocytosed into cells and broken down to release amino acids. These amino acids are then used to form new collagen units.

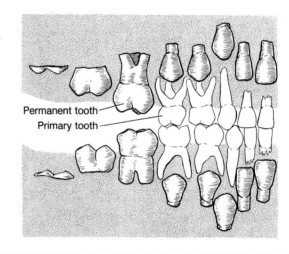

FIG. 6-18 Relationship between primary and permanent teeth during mixed dentition period.

cial fibroblast **(fibroblast-fibroclast)** cells are believed to secondarily destroy the remaining collagen fibers by ingesting them in an intracellular phagolysosome system (Fig. 6-17). Amino acids resulting from this breakdown are used in the formation of collagen within this same cell and can be used in this same area for bone formation. Only the posterior permanent molars, which have no primary predeciduous teeth, erupt through alveolar bone (Fig. 6-18). Fig. 6-19 summarizes what happens in the tissues overlying the teeth during their prefunctional eruptive phase. Bone loss has occurred as the tooth approaches the oral epithelium (Fig. 6-19, A). The tooth organ epithelium makes contact with the oral mucosa (Fig. 6-19, *B* and *C*). This contact causes stretching and

thinning of the oral membrane and finally its rupture and penetration by the tooth (Fig. 6-19, *D* and *E*). Only a thin developmental cuticle then covers the tooth (Fig. 6-19, *E* and *F*). As the tooth emerges farther into the mouth, more crown is exposed, and as clinical contact with the opposing tooth is made, the epithelial attachment shifts to the cervical area (Fig. 6-19, *G*). Clinically, tooth eruption is seen as a blanching of the mucosa, and this condition may persist for several days because the eruptive process is neither rapid nor continuous. Each eruptive movement, however, results in greater exposure of the crown. With successive eruptive movements the area of attached epithelium becomes lower on the clinical crown.

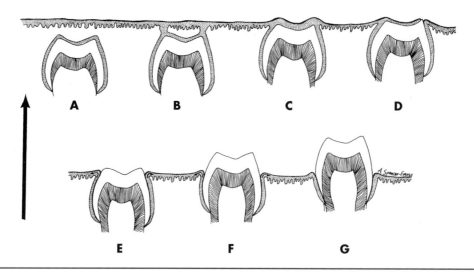

FIG. 6-19 Tooth eruption **A,** Crown penetrating bone and connective tissue. **B,** Contact of crown with oral epithelium. **C,** Fusion of epithelia. **D,** Thinning of epithelia. **E,** Rupture of epithelium. **F,** Crown emergence. **G,** Occlusal contact.

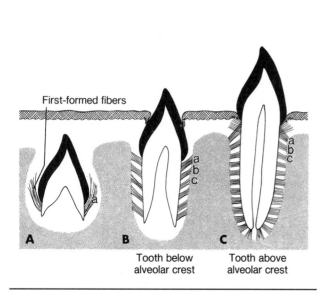

FIG. 6-20 Principal fiber development during tooth eruption. **A,** Origin of fibers at the cervical area. **B,** Fiber development with root growth. **C,** Change in orientation of the fibers with occlusal function. *a,* Initial fiber formation. *b,* Development of secondary fibers. *c,* Further fiber development. Initial fiber groups change direction. Observe the changes in direction of these initial fiber groups.

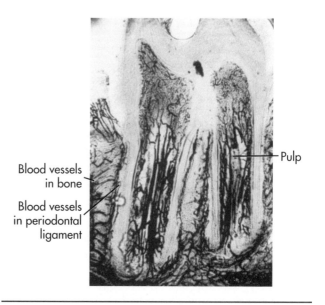

FIG. 6-21 Histology of erupting tooth with vascular injection of India ink to outline the presence of blood vessels in periodontium and tooth pulp.

Surrounding the Teeth

The tissues around the teeth change from delicately fine fibers lying parallel to the surface of the tooth to bundles of fibers attached to the tooth surface and extending toward the periodontium. The first fibers to appear are those in the cervical area as root formation begins (Fig. 6-20, *A*). As the root elongates, bundles of fibers appear on the root surface (Fig. 6-20, *B* and *C*). Fibroblasts are the active cells in both the formation and the degradation of the collagen fibers. With tooth eruption, the alveolar bone crypt increases in height to accommodate the forming root. After the teeth attain functional occlusion, the fibers gain their natural orientation (Fig. 6-20, *C*). Special fibroblasts have been found in the periodontium around the erupting teeth. These fibroblasts have contractile properties. During eruption, collagen fiber for-

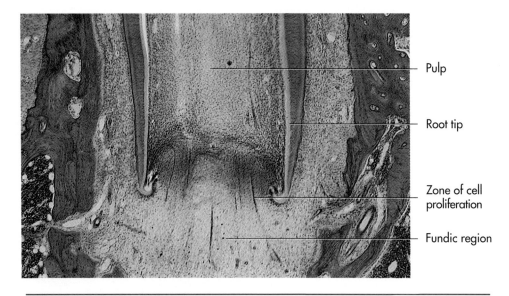

Pulp

Root tip

Zone of cell proliferation

Fundic region

FIG. 6-22   Histology of erupting tooth with immature roots and wide-open apices. As the tooth erupts, a bony ladder fills in fundic region of tooth socket.

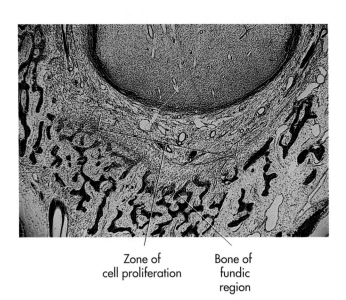

Zone of cell proliferation

Bone of fundic region

FIG. 6-23   Histology of changes in fundic region during tooth eruption. Fine trabeculae of new bone appear near tooth apices.

mation and fiber turnover are rapid, occurring within 24 hours. This mechanism enables fibers to attach and release and attach in rapid succession. Some fibers may detach and reattach later while the tooth moves occlusally as new bone forms around it. Gradually the fibers organize and increase in number and density as the tooth erupts into the oral cavity. Blood vessels then become more dominant in the developing ligament

CLINICAL COMMENT

Teeth are considered submerged when eruption is prevented because of crowding or tipping of the adjacent teeth into the space created by the missing primary tooth. Retained primary teeth may be caused by the lack of development of the permanent successor.

and exert additional pressure on the erupting tooth (Fig. 6-21).

Underlying the Teeth

As the crown of a tooth begins to erupt, it gradually moves occlusally, providing space underlying the tooth for the root to lengthen (Fig. 6-22). In the fundic region these changes in the soft tissue and the bone surrounding the root apex are believed to be largely compensatory for the lengthening of the root. During root formation the dentin of the root apex tapers to a fine edge that terminates in the epithelial diaphragm (Fig. 6-23). Fibroblasts form collagen around the root apex, and these fiber bundles become attached to the cementum as it begins to form on the apical dentin. Fibroblasts appear in great numbers in the fundic area, and some of these fibers form strands that mature into calcified trabeculae. These trabeculae form a network, or bony ladder, at the tooth apex. This is believed to fill the space left behind as the tooth begins eruptive movement (Fig. 6-23). Gradually this delicate bone ladder becomes denser as addi-

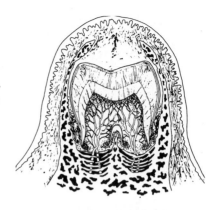

FIG. 6-24 Diagram of a later stage of tooth eruption in fundic region illustrating bone ladder development.

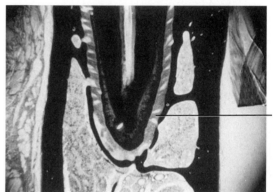

FIG. 6-25 Histology of tooth in functional occlusion to show density of functioning periodontal fibers. Spaces between fiber bundles are for blood vessels and nerves.

Periodontal fiber bundles

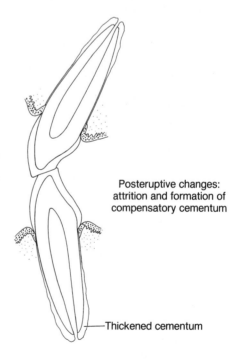

FIG. 6-26 Functional eruptive changes illustrating attrition of incisal surface of enamel and compensatory deposition of cementum in the apical region.

Posteruptive changes: attrition and formation of compensatory cementum

Thickened cementum

tional bony plates appear (Fig. 6-24). The bony plates remain until the teeth are in functional occlusion at the end of this phase. Dense bone then forms around the tooth's apex, and bundles of fibers attach to the apical cementum and extend to the adjacent alveolar bone to provide more support (Fig. 6-25).

FUNCTIONAL ERUPTIVE PHASE

The final eruptive phase takes place after the teeth are functioning and continues as long as the teeth are present in the mouth. During this period of root completion, the height of the alveolar process undergoes a compensating increase. The fundic alveolar plates resorb to adjust for formation of the root tip apex. The root canal narrows as a result of root tip maturation, during which the apical fibers develop to help cushion the forces of occlusal impact. Root completion continues for a considerable length of time, even after the teeth begin to function. This process takes about 1 to 1.5 years for deciduous teeth and 2 to 3 years for permanent teeth.

The most marked changes occur as occlusion is established. At that time the mineral density of the alveolar bone increases and the principal fibers of the periodontal ligament increase in dimension and change orientation in their mature state. These fibers separate into groups oriented about the gingiva, the alveolar crest, and the alveolar surface around the root. Such fibers stabilize the tooth to a greater degree, and the blood vessels become more highly organized in the spaces between the bundles of fibers (Fig. 6-25). Later in life, attrition and abrasion may wear down the occlusal or incisal surface of the teeth, causing the teeth to erupt slightly to compensate for this loss of tooth structure. Any such change results in deposition of cementum on

the root's apex (Fig. 6-26). Cementum is also deposited in the furcation area of a two- or three-rooted tooth.

POSSIBLE CAUSES OF TOOTH ERUPTION

Of the numerous causes of tooth eruption, the most frequently cited are root growth and pulpal pressure. Other important causes are cell proliferation, increased vascularity, and increased bone formation around the teeth. Additional possible causes that have been noted are endocrine influence, vascular changes, and enzymatic degradation. Probably all of these factors have an influencing role, not necessarily independent of one another.

Although not all factors associated with tooth eruption are known, elongation of the root and modification of the alveolar bone and periodontal ligament are thought to be the most important ones. These events are coupled with changes overlying the tooth that produce the eruption pathway. Blood vessels in this area are compressed by the influence of the advancing crown and become nonfunctional. Connective tissue in the eruption pathway gradually disappears as the tooth epithelium and the oral epithelium fuse. In summary, the erupting tooth moves from an area of increased pressure to an area of decreased pressure.

SEQUENCE AND CHRONOLOGY OF TOOTH ERUPTION

The formula for the eruptive sequence of the primary and permanent dentition appears in Table 6-1. Table 6-2 shows the chronologic development and eruption of the primary dentition, and Table 6-3 shows the development and eruption of the permanent dentition.

Table 6-1
Sequence of Tooth Eruption

PRIMARY

	CI	LI	1M	Cu	2M
	L	U	U	U	L
	U	L	L	L	U

PERMANENT

U1M	LCI	UL	LCU	U1Pre	U2Pre	UCu	L2M	L3M
L1M	UCI	LL		L1Pre	L2Pre		U2M	U3M

Table 6-2				
Chronology of Development of the Primary Dentition*				
Primary Teeth Listed in Order of Eruption (Sequence)	Beginning Calcification (Mo in Utero)	Crown Completed Postnatally (Mo)	Appearance in the Oral Cavity (Eruption Time) (Mo)	Root Completed (Yr)
Lower central incisor	3-4	2-3	6-8	1-2
Upper central incisor	3-4	2	7-10	1-2
Upper lateral incisor	4	2-3	8-11	2
Lower lateral incisor	4	3	8-13	1-2
Upper first molar	4	6	12-15	2-3
Lower first molar	4	6	12-16	2-3
Upper canine	4-5	9	16-19	3
Lower canine	4-5	9	17-20	3
Lower second molar	5	10	20-26	3
Upper second molar	5	11	25-28	3

*The normal range of eruption times indicates a wide variation in eruption times. It is important to know that a difference of 1 or 2 months either side of the normal range does not necessarily indicate that a child's eruption time schedule is abnormal. Only deviations considerably out of this range should be considered abnormal.

Table 6-3

Chronology of Development of the Permanent Dentition

Permanent Teeth Listed in Order of Eruption (Sequence)	Beginning Calcification	Crown Completed (Yr)	Appearance in the Oral Cavity (Eruption Time) (Yr)	Root Completed (Yr)
Lower first molar	Birth	3-4	6-7	9-10
Upper first molar	Birth	4-5	6-7	9-10
Lower central incisor	3-4 mo	4	6-7	9
Upper central incisor	3-4 mo	4-5	7-8	10
Lower lateral incisor	3-4 mo	4-5	7-8	9-10
Upper lateral incisor	10-12 mo	4-5	8-9	10-11
Lower canine	4-5 mo	5-6	9-10	12-13
Upper first premolar	1-2 yr	6-7	10-11	12-14
Lower first premolar	1-2 yr	6-7	10-11	12-14
Upper second premolar	2-3 yr	7-8	10-12	13-14
Lower second premolar	2-3 yr	7	11-12	14-15
Upper canine	4-5 mo	6-7	11-12	14-15
Lower second molar	2-3 yr	7-8	11-12	14-15
Upper second molar	2-3 yr	7-8	12-13	15-16
Lower third molar	8-10 yr	12-16	17-20	18-25
Upper third molar	7-9 yr	12-16	18-20	18-25

CLINICAL COMMENT

A lack of eruption may be related to fusion of tooth roots to the bony socket or to the crown of a permanent tooth. The condition is known as ankylosis because the tooth root fuses with underlying hard tissue.

CONSIDER THE PATIENT . . .

A patient complains about a retained primary tooth. She notes the absence of the permanent successor. How could you determine what has occurred?

SHEDDING OF PRIMARY TEETH

Humans are considered **diphyodont** because they possess two dentitions, primary and permanent. Teeth in the primary dentition are smaller and fewer in number than the permanent dentition to conform to the smaller jaws of the young person. Teeth in the permanent dentition are larger, longer, and more numerous, which the larger jaws of the adult can accommodate.

The primary dentition functions from about 2 to 8 years of age. Teeth from both dentitions are present in the **mixed dentition period,** which extends from about 8 to 12 years of age. This is an interesting period because only part of the primary teeth roots are present while they undergo resorption, and only part of the permanent roots are present while they are in the formative stage. In this way, nearly 50 teeth can be accommodated in the jaws during this 4-year span (Fig. 6-12).

The period of tooth shedding follows the mixed dentition period. **Shedding** is the loss of the primary dentition caused by the physiologic resorption of the roots, the loss of the bony supporting structure, and therefore the inability of these teeth to withstand the masticatory forces.

The degeneration of primary pulp tissue is similar to that of the tissues in the eruption pathway with a loss of cells, nerves, and blood vessels. When a primary tooth is extracted, blood is still likely to be in the crown, although only the oral epithelium holds the tooth in the socket. Fig. 6-27 shows the correlation between root growth and eruption. It illustrates changes that occur in the preeruptive *(A, B)*, prefunctional *(C, D)*, and functional eruptive *(E)* stages of the tissues overlying and around the root surface as the tooth develops functionally.

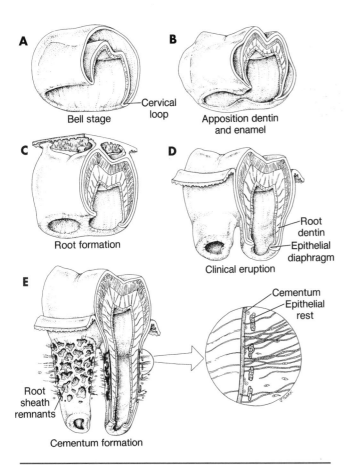

A, Bell stage — Cervical loop

B, Apposition dentin and enamel

C, Root formation

D, Clinical eruption — Root dentin, Epithelial diaphragm

E, Cementum formation — Cementum, Epithelial rest, Root sheath remnants

FIG. 6-27 Summary of tooth eruption. **A,** Early preeruptive changes in enamel organ at bell stage. **B,** Late preeruptive changes as enamel and dentin form. **C,** Early prefunctional changes as tooth moves to oral epithelium. **D,** Late prefunctional changes as tooth emerges into oral cavity. **E,** Functional eruptive phase with clinical contact. Root growth is shown with root sheath detaching from root surface. Epithelial rests and cementum formation by cementoblasts is now occurring.

SELF-EVALUATION QUESTIONS

1. Define tooth eruption and each of its phases.
2. Describe the changes overlying the tooth during eruption.
3. Describe the changes occurring around the tooth during eruption.
4. Describe the significant changes in the area underlying the teeth that relate to eruption.
5. What are the three fundamental causes of tooth shedding?
6. Give the sequence of eruption of the primary and permanent teeth.
7. What is the origin of osteoclasts?
8. Give the sequence of events that occur in hard tissue resorption.
9. Give the chronology of eruption for the primary teeth.
10. Give the chronology of eruption for the permanent teeth.

 CONSIDER THE PATIENT . . .

Discussion: To answer this question, the dentist takes an x-ray film of the area to determine whether the permanent tooth is missing or displaced. In either case the primary tooth is retained in position while the dentist determines the status of the permanent tooth and, if the tooth is present, aids its eruption into the proper place.

ACKNOWLEDGMENT

Dr. N.M. ElNesr contributed to the production of chapters in Avery JK: *Oral Development and Histology,* ed 2, New York, 1994, Thieme Medical. Some of those comments and figures have been used in this chapter.

SUGGESTED READING

Gorski JP, Marks SC Jr: Current concepts of the biology of tooth eruption, *Crit Rev Oral Biol Med* 3:185-206, 1992.

Marks S et al: Tooth eruption a synthesis of experimental observations. In Davidovich Z, editor: *The biological mechanisms of tooth eruption and root resorption,* Birmingham, Ala, 1988, EBSCO Media, pp 161-169.

Moxham BJ: The role of the periodontal ligament in tooth eruption. In Davidovich Z, editor: *The biological mechanism of tooth eruption and root resorption,* Birmingham, Ala, 1988, EBSCO Media, pp 207-233.

Proffit WR: The effect of intermittent forces on eruption. In Davidovich Z, editor: *The biological mechanism of tooth eruption and root resorption,* Birmingham, Ala, 1988, EBSCO Media, pp 187-191.

Wise GE, Marks SC, Cahill DR: Ultrastructural features of the dental follicle associated with the eruption pathway in the dog, *J Oral Pathol* 15:15-26, 1985.

Zajick G: Fibroblast kinetics in the periodontal ligament in the mouse, *Cell Tissue Kinet* 7:479-492, 1974.

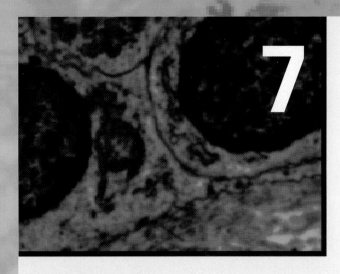

7

Enamel

OVERVIEW

Enamel, the hard protective substance that covers the crown of the tooth, is the hardest biologic tissue in the body. It consequently is able to resist fractures during the stress of mastication. Enamel provides shape and contour to the crowns of teeth and covers the part of the tooth that is exposed to the oral environment.

Enamel is composed of interlocking rods that resist masticatory forces. Enamel rods are deposited in a keyhole shape by the formative ameloblastic cells. Groups of ameloblasts migrate peripherally from the dentinoenamel junction as they form these rods. Ameloblasts take variable paths, which produces a bending of the rods. These cells maintain a relationship as they travel in different directions and produce adjacent rods. The enamel rod configuration viewed in incidental light appears as light and dark bands of rod groups termed **Hunter-Schreger bands.** Because these rods bend in an exaggeratedly twisted manner at the cusp tips, they are called **gnarled enamel.**

All enamel rods are deposited at a daily appositional rate or increment of 4 μm. Such increments are noticeable, like rings in a cross section of a tree, and appear as dark lines known as **striae of Retzius.** The growth lines become apparent on the surface of enamel as ridges, known as **perikymata.** Two structures are noticeable at the dentinoenamel junction: **spindles,** the termination of the dentinal tubules in enamel, and **tufts,** hypocalcified zones caused by the bending of adjacent groups of rods.

Because enamel is composed of bending rods, which in turn are composed of crystals, minute spaces or gaps exist where crystals did not form between rods. This feature causes enamel to be variable in its density and hardness. Therefore some areas of enamel may be more prone to penetration by small particles. This characteristic leads to tooth destruction by dental caries. After enamel is completely formed, no more enamel can be deposited.

PHYSICAL PROPERTIES

Because enamel is very hard, it is also brittle and subject to fracture. Fracture is especially likely to occur if the underlying dentin is carious and has weakened the enamel's foundation.

Enamel is about 96% inorganic mineral in the form of **hydroxyapatite** and 4% water and organic matter. Hydroxyapatite is a crystalline calcium phosphate that is also found in bone, dentin, and cementum. The organic component of enamel is the protein **enamelin,** which is similar to the protein keratin that is found in the skin. The distribution of enamelin between and on the crystals aids enamel permeability. Enamel is grayish white but appears slightly yellow because it is translucent and the underlying dentin is yellowish. Enamel ranges in thickness from a knifelike edge at its cervical margin to about 2.5-mm maximum thickness over the occlusal incisal surface.

CLINICAL COMMENT

Although enamel is the hardest tissue in the human body, it is permeable to some fluids, bacteria, and bacterial products of the oral cavity. Enamel exhibits cracks, checks, and microscopic spaces within and between rods and crystals, allowing penetration.

ROD STRUCTURE

Enamel is composed of rods that extend from their site of origin, at the dentinoenamel junction, to the enamel outer surface (Fig. 7-1). Each rod is formed by four ameloblasts. One ameloblast forms the rod head; a part of two ameloblasts forms the neck; and the tail is formed by a fourth ameloblast. Fig. 7-2 shows the six-sided design that is the shape of the ameloblast in contact with the forming keyhole- or racquet-shaped rod, which is columnar in its long axis. The head of the enamel rod is the broadest part at 5 μm wide, and the elongated thinner portion, or tail, is about 1 μm wide. The rod, including both head and tail, is 9 μm long. The enamel rod is about the same size as a red blood cell (Fig. 7-3).

Each rod is filled with crystals. Those in the head follow the long axis of the rod, and those in the tail lie in the cross axis to the head (Figs. 7-4 and 7-5). The upper right rod head of Fig. 7-4 indicates how the mineral is oriented during the rod's development, which forms the rod head and tail as seen on the left side of the figure. The architecture of the mineral orientation is complex, especially when viewed in any direction other than cross section (Fig. 7-5).

Rods form nearly perpendicular to the dentinoenamel junction and curve slightly toward the cusp tip. This unique rod arrangement also undulates throughout the enamel to the surface. Each rod interdigitates with its neighbor, the head of one rod nestling against the necks of the rods to its left and right (Fig. 7-3). The rods run almost perpendicular to the enamel surface at

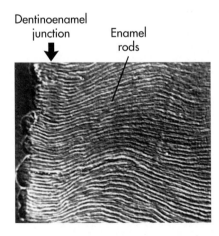

FIG. 7-1 Enamel rods appear wavy in section of enamel as they extend from dentinoenamel junction on left to enamel surface. This picture is possible because section is etched and viewed with scanning electron microscope.

(Courtesy Dr. JW Simmelink, Professor of Oral Biology, School of Dentistry, Case Western Reserve University. From Avery JK: *Oral development and histology,* New York, 1994, Thieme Medical.)

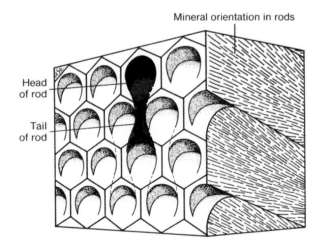

FIG. 7-2 Diagram showing outline of six-sided ameloblasts overlying keyhole-shaped enamel rods. Parts of four cells form each enamel rod. Crystal orientation of three rods can be seen on the side of model.

(Courtesy Dr. JW Simmelink, Professor of Oral Biology, School of Dentistry, Case Western Reserve University. From Avery JK: *Oral development and histology,* New York, 1994, Thieme Medical.)

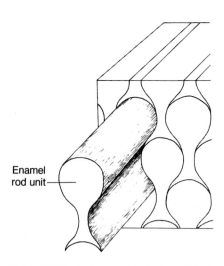

FIG. 7-3 One rod is pulled out to illustrate how individual enamel rods interdigitate with neighboring rods.

(Courtesy Dr. JW Simmelink, Professor of Oral Biology, School of Dentistry, Case Western Reserve University. From Avery JK: *Oral development and histology*, New York, 1994, Thieme Medical.)

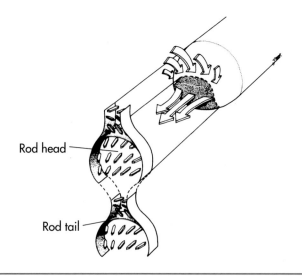

FIG. 7-4 Left side of diagram shows orientation of crystals in the forming rod head and tail. Right part shows, with arrows, how forming crystals pack in the rod from the cell complex.

the cervical region but are gnarled and intertwined near the cusp tips (Fig. 7-6). The surface of each rod is known as the rod sheath, and the center is the core. The rod sheath contains slightly more organic matter than the rod core (Fig. 7-7).

CONSIDER THE PATIENT . . .

A patient has attrition of cusp tips in the enamel of the crowns. What do you expect when you look at the root length? Why would you see this?

Groups of rods bend to the right or left at a slightly different angle than do adjacent groups (Fig. 7-6). It is believed that this feature provides the enamel with strength for mastication and biting. When light is projected at the surface of a thin slab of enamel, light and dark bands appear. These bands are seen because the light transmits along the long axis of one group of rods but not along the adjacent rods, which lie at right angles. This is known as the **Hunter-Schreger bands** phenomenon (Fig. 7-8). These bands are named after the dental scientist who first noted the Schreger band effect microscopically. The repeating pattern from the cervical area to the incisal or occlusal areas can be seen along the long axis of the tooth. Hunter-Schreger bands extend through half to two thirds of the thickness of enamel as shown in a diagram (Fig. 7-6) and a tooth section (Fig. 7-8).

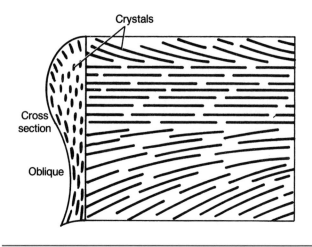

FIG. 7-5 Orientation of crystals in mature enamel rod as indicated by cross section and side of cut rod.

(Courtesy Dr. JW Simmelink, Professor of Oral Biology, School of Dentistry, Case Western Reserve University. From Avery JK: *Oral development and histology*, New York, 1994, Thieme Medical.)

CLINICAL COMMENT

The rods that form enamel are woven during formation into a mass that resists average masticatory impact of 20 to 30 pounds per tooth. Enamel is thin in the cervical areas where masticatory impact is the least and thickest over the areas of crown cusps where impact is greatest.

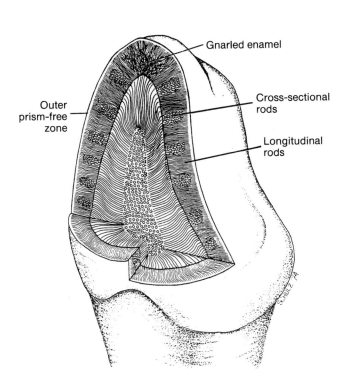

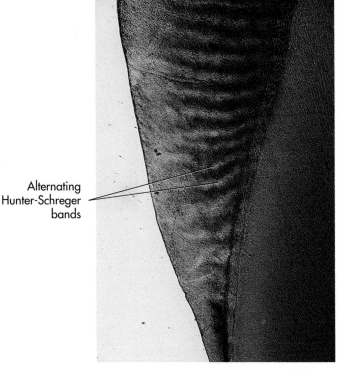

FIG. 7-6 Diagram of enamel rod orientation as shown in both longitudinal and cross section of the crown. Enamel rods are intertwined at cusp tip; this is called gnarled enamel. Groups of outer enamel rods all run nearly perpendicular to the surface of the enamel whereas inner groups of enamel rods alternate. Some appear in cross section while adjacent groups appear longitudinal.

(Courtesy Dr. JW Simmelink, Professor of Oral Biology, School of Dentistry, Case Western Reserve University. From Avery JK: *Oral development and histology,* New York, 1994, Thieme Medical.)

FIG. 7-8 Photomicrograph of enamel taken by reflected light and illustrating phenomena of light and dark (Hunter-Schreger) bands.

INCREMENTAL LINES

The incremental lines **(lines of Retzius)** in enamel are the result of the rhythmic recurrent deposition of the enamel. As the enamel matrix mineralizes, it follows the pattern of matrix deposition and provides the growth lines in enamel (Fig. 7-9). These incremental lines may be accentuated because of a variation in the mineral deposited at the point of enamel hesitation in deposition. In some cases the incremental lines are not visible. With enamel development a row of ameloblasts covering the crown hesitates during deposition. These hesitation lines mark the path of amelogenesis. The spaces between the crystals entrap air molecules, accentuating these lines. Dr. Retzius, who first noted these "growth lines," termed them the **striae of Retzius.**

Part of the enamel of most deciduous teeth is formed before birth and part after birth. Because environment and nutrition change abruptly at the time of birth, a notable line of Retzius occurs at that time. This is known as the **neonatal line** (Fig. 7-10). Although the neonatal line is an accentuated incremental line, it can be seen microscopically that this line is prominent for another reason. The enamel internal to this line is of a different consistency from that external to it. The enamel internal to the line was formed before birth, and the external was formed after

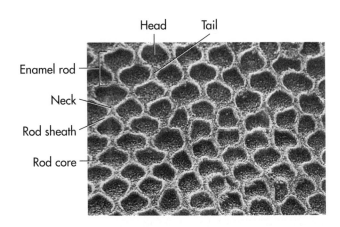

FIG. 7-7 Enamel rods in cross section. Each rod has a sheath and core. The rod sheath surrounds rod head and tail. This enamel sample has been etched to reveal organic matrix.

(Courtesy Dr. JW Simmelink, Professor of Oral Biology, School of Dentistry, Case Western Reserve University. From Avery JK: *Oral development and histology,* New York, 1994, Thieme Medical.)

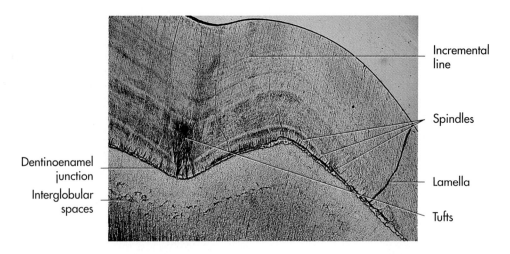

FIG. 7-9   Photomicrograph of dentinoenamel junction showing dentin below and enamel above this junction. Enamel exhibits incremental lines, tufts, spindles, and lamella. Within dentin, band of primary dentin is just below dentinoenamel junction. At lower border of this band of primary dentin is a row of interglobular spaces.

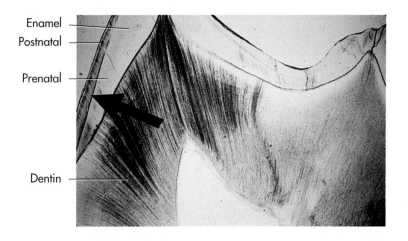

FIG. 7-10   Photomicrograph of section of enamel and dentin of primary tooth by transmitted light. Neonatal line is at point of large arrow. Enamel to the left of this line is a darker stain than enamel to the right of it. The enamel formed before birth is less pigmented and has fewer defects than postnatal enamel. Dentin exhibits numerous dead tracts as dark lines. Dead tracts are tubules filled with air; hence they appear black in transmitted light.

birth. The prenatal enamel has fewer defects than the postnatal. The staining of the postnatal enamel has numerous minute spaces that are stained with pigment (Fig. 7-10).

CLINICAL COMMENT

Enamel is composed of mineral crystals that are the same as those found in dentin, cementum, and bone. Unlike bone and cementum, the mineral crystals in enamel are not replaced once deposited in enamel.

ENAMEL LAMELLAE

Enamel lamellae are cracks in the surface of enamel that are visible to the naked eye (Figs. 7-9 and 7-11). Lamellae extend from the surface of enamel toward the dentinoenamel junction. Some lamellae form during enamel development, creating an organic pathway or tract. Spaces between groups of rods are another example of lamellae and may be caused by stress cracks that occur because of impact or temperature changes. Breathing cold air or drinking hot or cold beverages may cause small checks to occur in enamel, especially enamel weakened by underlying caries. Lamellae are not tubular defects but appear leaflike, extending around the

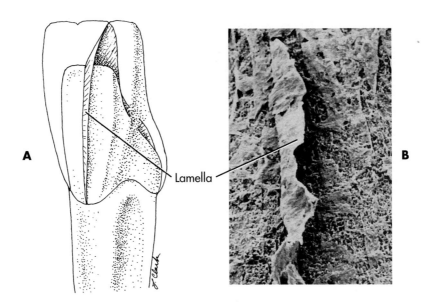

Lamella

FIG. 7-11 **A,** Diagram of possible location of leaflike enamel lamellae extending from the cervical to incisal enamel. **B,** Scanning electron micrograph of lamellae in enamel. (Enamel was decalcified away, and lamellar space was impregnated with resin for its maintenance.)

(Courtesy Dr. JW Simmelink, Professor of Oral Biology, School of Dentistry, Case Western Reserve University. From Avery JK: *Oral development and histology*, New York, 1994, Thieme Medical.)

crown (Fig. 7-11). Lamellae are a possible avenue for dental caries.

CLINICAL COMMENT

Temperature changes from breathing cold air or drinking hot or cold beverages may cause small checks or cracks to develop in enamel. This is especially evident in enamel weakened by underlying caries but can also appear in otherwise normal enamel.

ENAMEL TUFTS

Enamel tufts are another defect in enamel filled with organic material. They are located at the dentinoenamel junction and appear at right angles to it. They can extend one fifth to one tenth of the distance from the dentinoenamel junction to the outer surface of the tooth (Figs. 7-12 and 7-13). Tufts form between groups of enamel rods, which are oriented in slightly different directions at the dentinoenamel junction. These spaces are thus developed between adjacent groups of rods, which are filled with organic material termed **enamelin.** The interface of the junction of dentin and enamel is scalloped, and often tufts arise from these scalloped peaks (Fig. 7-12).

ENAMEL SPINDLES

Spindles arise at the dentinoenamel junction and extend into enamel. These spindles are extensions of dentinal tubules that pass through the junction into enamel (Fig. 7-13). Because dentin forms before enamel, the odontoblastic process occasionally penetrates the junction and enamel forms around this process, forming a tubule. These small tubules may contain a living process of the odontoblast, possibly contributing to the vitality of the dentinoenamel junction. Tubules are found singularly or in groups and are shorter than tufts, only a few millimeters in length. The fingerlike spindles appear quite different than the broader and longer tufts.

SURFACE CHARACTERISTICS

The enamel surface may be smooth or have fine ridges. Such ridges result from the terminiation of the striae of Retzius on the surface of enamel (Fig. 7-14). These surface manifestations are ridges called **perikymata or imbrication lines.** Perikymata are produced by the ends of rod groups accentuated by hesitation of ameloblasts before the next group of rods contact the enamel surface (Fig. 7-15). This manifestation is more prominent on the facial surface of the tooth, near the cervical region (Fig. 7-14). Another feature of outer enamel near its surface is the zone of **prismless enamel,** which is 20 to 40 μm

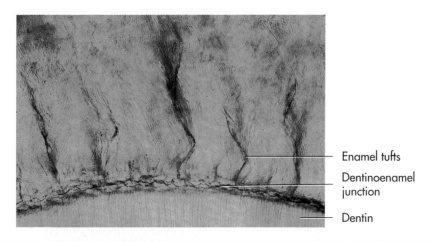

FIG. 7-12 Transmitted light micrograph of dentinoenamel junction area showing enamel tufts. In addition to tufts, scalloped dentinoenamel junction and fine enamel rod structure can be seen between tufts. Below junction are dentinal tubules.

(Courtesy Dr. JW Simmelink, Professor of Oral Biology, School of Dentistry, Case Western Reserve University. From Avery JK: *Oral development and histology,* New York, 1994, Thieme Medical.)

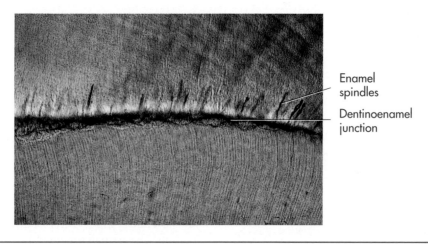

FIG. 7-13 Enamel spindles at dentinoenamel junction are extensions of dentinal tubules that may contain odontoblastic processes in enamel.

(Courtesy Dr. JW Simmelink, Professor of Oral Biology, School of Dentistry, Case Western Reserve University. From Avery JK: *Oral development and histology,* New York, 1994, Thieme Medical.)

 CLINICAL COMMENT

When caries has spread from the tooth's surface to near the dentinoenamel junction, the hypocalcified tufts allow a lateral spread along this junction.

thick. Throughout this zone, no Schreger band effect is noted. This zone is not accentuated except near the cervical region and in deciduous teeth. The prismless zone of enamel is important because it appears as a structure-

less microcrystalline environment of enamel rods oriented nearly perpendicular to the enamel surface. This enhances the integrity of the enamel surface and should be recognized when a bevel for restorations is prepared.

PERMEABILITY

Enamel permeability is a feature of clinical importance. The passage of fluid, bacteria, and bacterial products through enamel is an important consideration in clinical therapy. Permeability of enamel is caused by several fac-

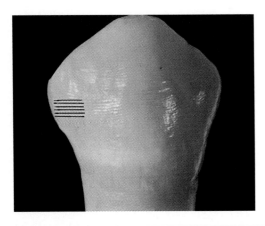

FIG. 7-14　Fine ridges on enamel surface of crown are perikymata or imbrication lines.

(Courtesy Dr. JW Simmelink, Professor of Oral Biology, School of Dentistry, Case Western Reserve University. From Avery JK: *Oral development and histology*, New York, 1994, Thieme Medical.)

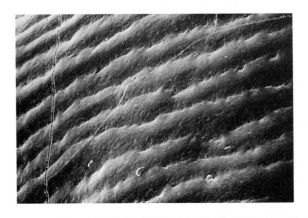

FIG. 7- 15　Scanning electron micrograph of perikymata in Fig. 7-14 at a much higher magnification, which shows alternating ridges and valleys.

(Courtesy Dr. JW Simmelink, Professor of Oral Biology, School of Dentistry, Case Western Reserve University. From Avery JK: *Oral development and histology*, New York, 1994, Thieme Medical.)

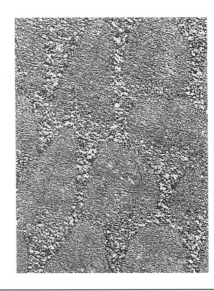

FIG. 7-16　Transmission electron micrograph of a cross section of enamel rods that shows difference in rod sheath and rod core crystal orientation.

(Courtesy Dr. JW Simmelink, Professor of Oral Biology, School of Dentistry, Case Western Reserve University. From Avery JK: *Oral development and histology*, New York, 1994, Thieme Medical.)

tors, some of which are evident as they relate to leakage around faulty restorations and decomposition of the tooth by dental caries. These latter examples need no further explanation, but fluid and fine particles can also pass through unbroken enamel by way of pathways described previously in this chapter, such as lamellae, cracks, tufts, and spindles. These all contribute to the microporosity of enamel. The minute spaces between or around enamel rods and through crystal spaces within rods are also important and are called **microlamellae.** Differences in crystal orientation can cause enamel to have minute spaces, which can be seen at high magnification (Fig. 7-16). Also, surface irregularities, such as those found in central fissures and near the cervical region, are important in influencing permeability.

Enamel and dentin are both composed of hydroxyapatite crystals, although the crystals in enamel are about 30 times larger than those in dentin (Fig. 7-17). Crystal size is a factor in the extreme hardness of enamel in contrast to dentin.

ETCHING

Etching with dilute acids, such as citric acid, may alter the surface of enamel. This dilute acid selectively etches the ends of the enamel rods and provides adherence of a plastic sealant to the surface of enamel rods (Fig. 7-18). The rod sheath resists demineralization to a greater extent than the rod core. The purpose of this procedure is to produce an intact surface and prevent caries.

 CLINICAL COMMENT

Some etched areas of enamel can be remineralized by solutions of sodium fluoride or stannous fluoride. Tests show that the fluoride ion penetrates the porous etched surface enamel. Low levels of fluoride stimulate remineralization.

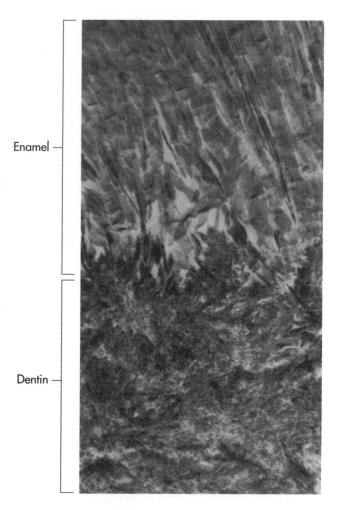

FIG. 7-17 Dentinoenamel junction. Enamel is above and dentin below. Crystallites of enamel and dentin are different in size and orientation. Whereas crystals of human enamel may be 90 nm (900 Å) in width and 0.5 μm in length, those of dentin are only 3 nm (30 Å) in width and 100 nm (1,000 Å) in length. Crystals of dentin are similar in size to bone. (Electron micrograph ×35,000.)

(Courtesy of RM Frank, Professor and Dean, Dr A Brendel, Faculty de Chirurgie Dentaire, Strasbourg, France. From Bhaskar SN: *Orban's oral histology and embryology,* ed 11, St Louis, 1991, Mosby.)

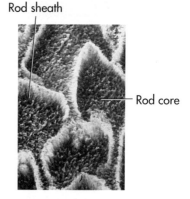

FIG. 7-18 Acid-etched enamel rod core dissolved to greater extent than rod sheath, which provides for attachment of sealant.

SELF-EVALUATION QUESTIONS

1. Describe the shape and size of the enamel rods.
2. Define Hunter-Schreger bands.
3. Define striae of Retzius. What is a synonym?
4. Describe gnarled enamel. Where is it located?
5. What are perikymata and imbrication lines?
6. What are the location and importance of tufts?
7. Define and give the cause of neonatal lines.
8. What is prismless enamel?
9. What is the inorganic component of enamel, dentin, and bone?
10. What is the organic component of enamel?

CONSIDER THE PATIENT. . .

Discussion: A radiograph would reveal a lengthened root with excessive cemental deposition that is due to hypereruption of the tooth. Because of the hypereruption, space is provided for compensating cemental deposition.

SUGGESTED READING

Bhaskar SN, editor: *Orban's oral histology and embryology,* ed 11, St Louis, 1991, Mosby.

Boyd A, Lester KS, Martin LB: Basis of the structure and development of mammalian enamel as seen by electron microscopy, *Scanning Microsc* 2:1479-1490, 1988.

Fernhead RW: *Tooth enamel V,* Yokohama, Japan, 1989, Florence.

Kodaka T, Natajima F, Higashi S: Structure of the so-called "prismless" enamel in human deciduous teeth, *Caries Res* 23:290-296, 1989.

Nylen MU, Termine JD, editors: Tooth enamel III; its development, structure and composition, *J Dent Res* 58(B):675, 1979.

Simmelink JW, Nygaard VK: Ultrastructure of striations in carious human enamel, *Caries Res* 16:279, 1982.

Stack MV, Fernhead RW, editors: Tooth enamel: its composition, properties and fundamental structure, Bristol, UK, 1971, John Wright & Sons.

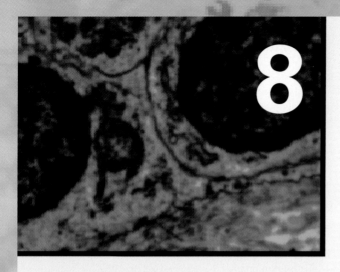

8 Dentin

OVERVIEW

This chapter focuses on dentin, the hard tissue that constitutes the body of the tooth. Dentin is a living tissue not normally exposed to the oral environment. Root dentin is covered by cementum, and crown dentin is covered by enamel. Dentin, like bone, is composed primarily of an organic matrix of collagen fibers and the mineral hydroxyapatite. It is classified as **primary, secondary,** or **tertiary** on the basis of the time of its development and the histologic characteristics of the tissue. Primary dentin is the major component of the crown and root and consists of both **mantle** dentin and **circumpulpal** dentin. Mantle dentin is deposited first, along the dentinoenamel junction, in a band about 150 μm wide. The collagen fibers of this dentin are larger than those of the circumpulpal dentin, which forms later. Mantle dentin is separated from the circumpulpal dentin by a zone of disturbed dentin formation called **globular dentin,** which is noted because of the spaces between the globules, termed **interglobular spaces.** Globular dentin is believed to be a result of deficient mineralization. Dentin continues to form, although the collagen fibers are smaller, until the teeth erupt and reach occlusion. As the teeth begin to function, the dentin is termed **secondary dentin.** Dentin is responsive to the environment. When caries or mechanical trauma affects the pulp, dentin is deposited underlying that area and is termed **response, reparative,** or **tertiary dentin.** This dentin is deposited to protect the pulp. Bordering the pulp is **predentin,** which is newly formed dentin before calcification and maturation. Predentin is composed of collagen fibers, which calcify within 24 hours as the odontoblasts deposit a new band of collagen fibers.

In addition to classifying dentin, this chapter describes properties and characteristics of dentin. Like osteoblasts that form bone, the odontoblasts that form dentin lie on the surface of the forming hard tissue. Unlike bone, the odontoblastic processes exist in tubules and penetrate the dentin from the pulp to the dentinoenamel junction. Dentin, like bone, is deposited by appositional growth and produces **incremental lines.** In addition, a **granular dentin** anomaly appears along the root surface. This anomaly may also be caused by the cementum that forms adjacent to the root dentin during development. The odontoblasts may die because of trauma or old age, and **dead tracts** then develop in dentin. The tubules may later calcify as they fill with mineral. When this occurs, the dentin is termed **sclerotic** or **transparent dentin.**

PHYSICAL PROPERTIES

Dentin, which forms the bulk of the tooth, is yellowish in contrast to the whiter enamel. It appears darker if a root canal has been performed. Dentin is composed of 70% inorganic hydroxyapatite crystals, 20% organic collagen fibers with small amounts of other proteins, and 10% water by weight. With 20% less mineral than enamel, dentin is softer, although it is slightly harder than bone or cementum. Therefore it is more radiolucent than enamel but much more dense or radiopaque than pulp. Dentin is resilient or slightly elastic, which allows the impact of mastication to occur without fracturing the brittle overlying enamel. This resilience is due in part to the presence throughout the matrix of tubules, which extend from the dentinoenamel junction to the pulp.

CLINICAL COMMENT

Metallic restorations, such as gold inlay, crown, or silver amalgam, are excellent thermal conductors. Therefore it is appropriate to place a cement base under these restorations to protect the pulp by minimizing pain conduction.

DENTIN CLASSIFICATION

Dentin includes **primary, secondary,** and **tertiary dentin.** Based on structure, primary dentin is composed of **mantle** and **circumpulpal** dentin. Examples of these classifications are in Fig. 8-1, *A.* Fig. 8-1, *B,* shows the "**S curve**" of the dentinal tubules through primary and secondary dentin. Primary dentin forms the body of the tooth; secondary dentin forms only after tooth eruption and is a narrow band that borders the pulp. Tertiary or reparative dentin is formed only in response to trauma to the pulp.

Primary Dentin

Mantle dentin is the first primary dentin formed. It is deposited first at the dentinoenamel junction (Fig. 8-2) and extends approximately 150 μm from the junction pulpward to the zone of **interglobular** or **globular dentin.** Mantle dentin is so named because it serves as a covering or mantle over the rest of the dentin. **Circumpulpal dentin** directly underlies mantle dentin and comprises the bulk of the tooth's primary dentin. Circumpulpal dentin may be 6 to 8 mm thick in the crown and a little thinner in the roots.

Zones of dentin have structural differences. Mantle dentin is composed of large collagen fibers, some of which are 0.1 to 0.2 μm in diameter, in contrast to the circumpulpal dentinal matrix, which is 50 to 200

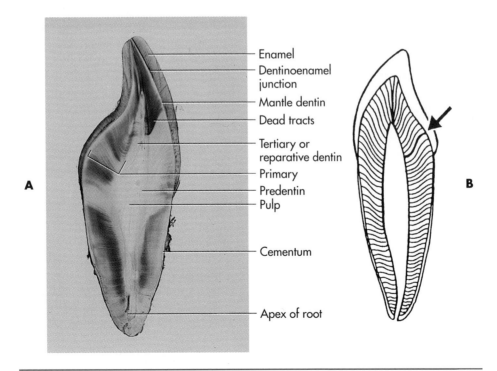

FIG. 8-1   A, Incisor tooth section illustrating structures in enamel, dentin, and cementum. **B,** Diagram of dentin showing S curvature of the dentinal tubules, especially at the arrow.

(From Avery JK, editor: *Oral development and histology,* ed 2, New York, 1994, Thieme Medical.)

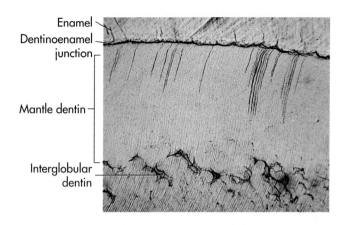

FIG. 8-2   Histology of mantle dentin bounded by dentino-enamel junction above and interglobular dentin below.

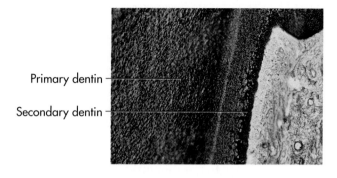

FIG. 8-3   Primary dentin *(left)* and secondary dentin *(right)*. (From Bhaskar SN, editor: *Orban's oral histology and embryology,* ed 11, St Louis, 1991, Mosby.)

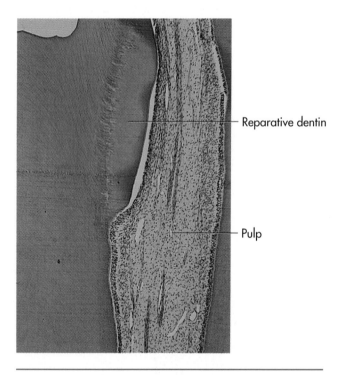

FIG. 8-4   Reparative dentin formed in localized area underlying cavity. Tubules from cavity floor lead to zone of reparative dentin.

nanometers (nm). Thus the fibers in circumpulpal dentin are 10 times smaller than those in mantle dentin. Mantle dentin is also slightly less mineralized and contains fewer defects than circumpulpal dentin. Mantle dentin is nearly free of developmental defects. It interdigitates with enamel at the scalloped dentinoenamel junction peripherally and in the zone of globular dentin centrally. The area of globular dentin usually exists only in the crown but may extend into the root. Such a zone

of dentinal matrix is not completely mineralized, and the area of globular calcospherites has not fused correctly (Figs. 8-2 and 8-6C).

Globular dentin contains hypomineralized areas between the globules, termed **interglobular spaces**. Fig. 8-6 shows examples of various structures in dentin. Interglobular spaces are not true spaces but are less mineralized areas between the calcified globules. The dentinal tubules run without interruption through this zone, indicating a defect in mineralization, not a defect in matrix formation (Fig. 8-2). Interglobular dentin is especially noticeable with vitamin D deficiency, which affects mineralization of teeth and bones. Primary dentin constitutes the bulk of dentin in crowns and roots of teeth. It is characterized by the continuity of tubules from pulp to dentinoenamel junction and by incremental lines that indicate a daily rhythmic deposition pattern of approximately 4 μm of dentin per day.

   CLINICAL COMMENT

The sensitivity of dentin is an important clinical consideration after placement of a restoration that conducts heat or cold. Dentin responds to such stimuli by deposition of reparative dentin and by changes in the dentin tubules underlying the restoration. The sensitivity of the tooth will diminish after a few weeks because of these changes.

Secondary Dentin

Secondary dentin forms internally to primary dentin of the crown and root. It develops after the crown has come into clinical occlusal function and the roots are nearly

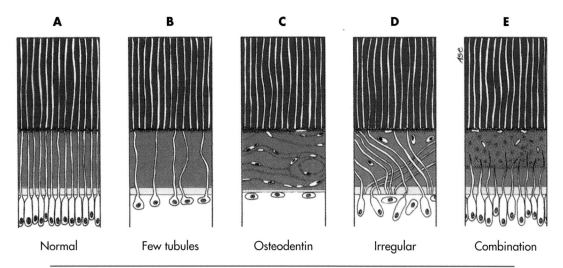

FIG. 8-5 **A,** Normal dentin; **B** to **E,** reparative dentin; **B,** decrease in number of tubules; **C,** cell inclusions; **D,** irregular and twisted tubules; **E,** combination of types.

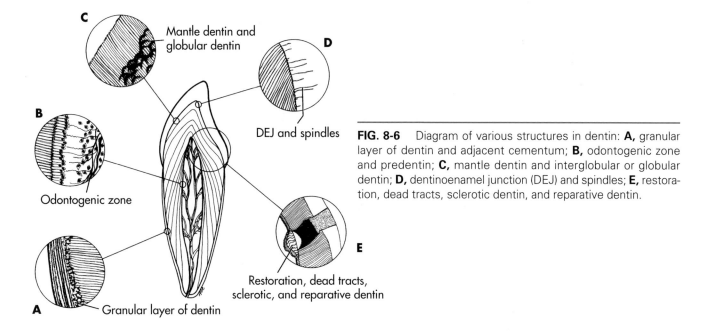

FIG. 8-6 Diagram of various structures in dentin: **A,** granular layer of dentin and adjacent cementum; **B,** odontogenic zone and predentin; **C,** mantle dentin and interglobular or globular dentin; **D,** dentinoenamel junction (DEJ) and spindles; **E,** restoration, dead tracts, sclerotic dentin, and reparative dentin.

completed (Fig. 8-3). This dentin is deposited more slowly than primary dentin, and its incremental lines are only about 1.0 to 1.5 μm apart. Dental scientists theorize that after the crown begins clinical function, the brain signals the dentin to slow the rate of production. This keeps the pulp from being obliterated by the previous rapid rate of dentin formation. The tubules of primary and secondary dentin are generally continuous unless the deposition of secondary dentin is uneven. In molar teeth, for example, more secondary dentin is deposited on the roof and floor of the coronal pulp chamber than on the lateral walls. This leads to protection of the pulpal horns as occlusal function occurs.

Reparative or Tertiary Dentin

Reparative or tertiary dentin results from pulpal stimulation and forms only at the site of odontoblastic activation. Whether the formation is due to attrition, abrasion, caries, or restorative procedures, this dentin is deposited underlying only those stimulated areas. (See Figs. 8-4 and 8-5 on pp 96-97.) It may be deposited rapidly, in which case the resulting dentin appears irregular with sparse and twisted tubules and possible cell inclusions (Fig. 8-5, *B* to *E*). Odontoblasts, fibroblasts, and blood cells have been found in this type of dentin. In contrast,

if it is formed slowly because of fewer stimuli, the dentin appears more regular, much like primary or secondary dentin (Figs. 8-4 and 8-5, *A*). Reparative dentin at times resembles bone more than dentin and is then termed **osteodentin** (Fig. 8-5, *C*). It can also appear as a combination of several types (Fig. 8-5, *E*). Recent terminology suggests that the term **reparative dentin** be used when the original odontoblasts function in deposition and **response dentin** be used when newly recruited odontoblasts begin depositing dentin. The latter case occurs with a more severe injury to the tooth.

CONSIDER THE PATIENT . . .

Case 1: A patient complains of pain in a tooth after placement of a large gold crown. The tooth is very sensitive to hot or cold fluids or foods. Why?

PREDENTIN

Predentin is a band of newly formed, unmineralized matrix of dentin at the pulpal border of the dentin (Fig. 8-7).

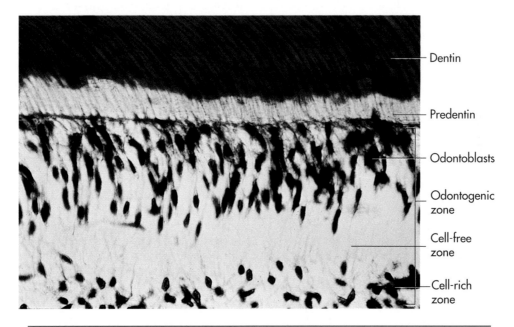

Dentin

Predentin

Odontoblasts

Odontogenic zone

Cell-free zone

Cell-rich zone

FIG. 8-7   Photomicrograph of predentin zone that borders pulp with mature dentin above. Odontogenic zone is below predentin and comprises odontoblasts and cell-free and cell-rich zones.

Predentin is evidence that dentin forms in two stages: first, the organic matrix is deposited, and second, an inorganic mineral substance is added. Mineralization occurs at the predentin-dentin junction, and predentin becomes a new layer of dentin. During primary dentin formation, 4 μm of predentin is deposited and calcified each day. After occlusion and function, this activity decreases to 1.0 to 1.5 μm per day.

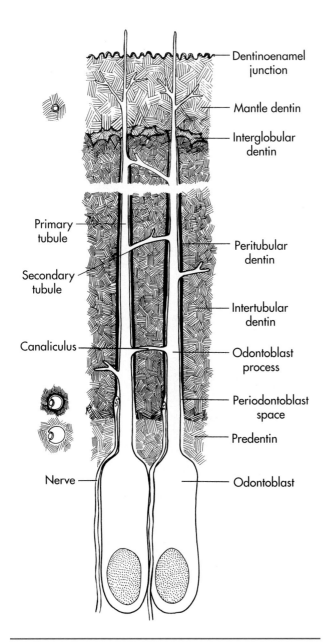

FIG. 8-8 Odontoblast process in the dentinal tubule and extending from the dentinoenamel junction to the pulp. Side branches of processes in tubules are termed canaliculi.

(From Bhaskar SN, editor: *Orban's oral histology and embryology,* ed 11, St Louis, 1991, Mosby.)

TUBULAR AND INTERTUBULAR RELATIONS

Primary and Secondary Tubules

As dentin is formed by odontoblasts, space is provided for the lengthening process of the odontoblast that moves pulpward from the amelodentinal junction. The tubules normally begin at this junction but may extend into the forming enamel matrix. The process begins forming before either enamel or dentin matrix begins forming. Thus the spindles that are extensions of the odontoblastic process extend a short distance into enamel. The odontoblastic process then forms an **S curve**, which extends to the pulp. As the process elongates, it branches and its secondary processes appear at nearly right angles to the main process (Fig. 8-8). These cells and their processes give the dentin vitality. The surface area ratio of the dentinoenamel junction to the pulpal surface is about 1:5. Therefore the tubules are farther apart at the dentinoenamel junction than at the pulpal surface (Figs. 8-1 and 8-8). In addition, the tubules are smaller in diameter in the outer dentin (1 μm) than at the pulpal border (3 to 4 μm). The ratio of the number of tubules at the dentinoenamel junction to the number at the pulpal border is about 4:1. This relates to the odontoblast's gradual increase in size as its process grows in length. Also, more tubules are in the crown than in the root. Approximately 30,000 to 50,000 tubules per square millimeter exist in the dentin near the pulp. The lateral branches of the odontoblastic processes are seen throughout dentin, crown, and root. These lateral branches are termed canaliculi, secondary branches, or microtubules (Fig. 8-8) and are less than 1 μm in diameter. Some of these lateral branches lead to an adjacent dentinal tubule, and some appear to terminate in the intertubular matrix. Each of these secondary tubules contains branches of the odontoblastic process.

Intratubular or Peritubular Dentin

The dentinal matrix that immediately surrounds the dentinal tubule is termed **intratubular** or **peritubular** dentin (Fig. 8-9). Peritubular dentin is present in tubules throughout dentin except near the pulp. It is called peritubular because it is a hypermineralized collar surrounding the tubules. However, because it is formed within and at the expense of the tubules, **intratubular dentin** is a more accurate term. Intratubular dentin is missing from the dentinal tubules in interglobular dentin. This is an area of deficient mineralization like the area of predentin, which is also not calcified. In some areas the hypermineralized intratubular dentin completely fills the tubules, as in the area near the dentinoenamel junction overlying the pulp horns. This condition is also found in the peripheral tubules of the root near the cementum. These are areas of very small tubules and areas where external stimulation may play a role. **Sclerotic dentin** or **transparent dentin** (Fig. 8-10) is the term for dentin with tubules that are completely obliterated. The name is derived from the transparent nature of dentin, which manifests itself when the tubules are no longer present. Sclerotic dentin increases in amount with age and is believed to be another mechanism to protect the pulp, like reparative dentin. Permeability to the pulp

is eliminated in these areas, and sclerotic dentin is found in areas of attrition, abrasion, fracture, and caries of the enamel.

CLINICAL COMMENT

Dentinal tubules increase in size by the loss of intratubular or peritubular dentin. This dentin is subject to decalcification by caries or acid cleansing of the cavity, which removes the smear layer. This dentin is about 40% more highly calcified than the remainder of the dentin.

Intertubular Dentin

The main body of dentin is located between or around the dentinal tubules. Intertubular dentin is the body of dentin, which comprises the crown and root. This dentin consists of the same type of organic matrix fibers (type I collagen fibers and inorganic crystals of hydroxyapatite) as that of intratubular dentin. Intertubular dentin, however, is less highly calcified and changes little throughout life. The collagen fibers of the matrix form a meshwork oriented nearly perpendicular to the intratubular dentin. They exhibit a typical 640-Angstrom (Å) cross banding similar to those of bone or cementum.

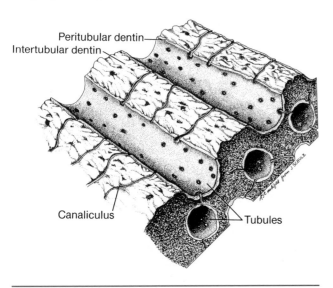

FIG. 8-9 View of dentinal tubules shows peritubular and intertubular dentin. Note that side branches of dentinal tubules are in the intertubular dentin.

(From Bhaskar SN, editor: *Orban's oral histology and embryology,* ed 11, St. Louis, 1991, Mosby.)

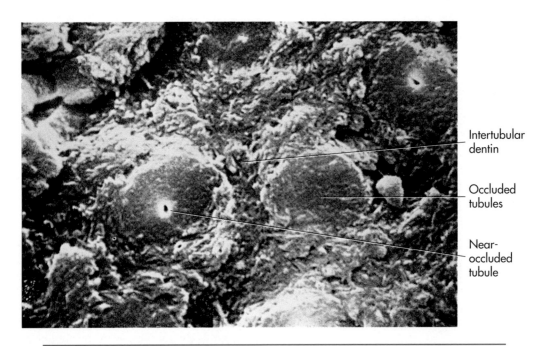

FIG. 8-10 Scanning electron micrograph of sclerotic dentinal tubules. Micrograph shows minute size of nearly occluded dentinal tubules and some completely occluded tubules. Tubule occlusion is a mechanism to protect pulp.

(Courtesy Martin Branstrom, DDS. From Avery JK, editor: *Oral development and histology,* ed 2, New York, 1994, Thieme Medical.)

INCREMENTAL LINES

All dentin is deposited incrementally, which means that as a certain amount of matrix is deposited daily, a hesitation in activity follows. This hesitation in formation results in an alteration of the matrix known as **incremental lines, imbrication lines,** or **lines of von Ebner.** Although daily lines are difficult to distinguish, lines formed by increments over several days (possibly every 5 days), resulting in 20-µm lines, are believed to be the ones von Ebner described (Fig. 8-11). Analysis of soft x-ray films has shown these lines to represent hypocalcified bands, at least in the primary teeth and the permanent first molars, indicating that dentin is formed before birth. Prenatal and postnatal dentin are separated by an accentuated contour line known as the **neonatal line** (Fig. 8-12). This line reflects the abrupt change in environment that occurs at or near birth.

GRANULAR LAYER

When a thin, calcified section of root is studied under transmitted light, a granular-appearing layer of dentin is seen underlying the cementum that covers the root. This layer is known as the **granular layer** or **granular layer of Tomes** (Fig. 8-13). This zone increases slightly in width, proceeding from the cementoenamel junction to the root apex. The zone is believed to be the result of a coalescing and looping of the terminal portions of the dentinal tubules. It is possible that the odontoblast is initially disoriented as it begins dentin formation. The odontoblast turns at right angles to the root surface and proceeds pulpward, causing the dentinal matrix in this area to be defective (Fig. 8-14).

ODONTOBLASTIC CELL PROCESSES

Odontoblastic cell processes are cytoplasmic extensions of the cell body that are positioned at the pulp-dentin border. Opinions vary about whether these processes extend through the entire thickness of dentin. This difference in opinion is caused in part by the difficulty in preserving and visualizing these processes. Recently, improved techniques of immunofluorescence labeling, freeze fracture, and polymer replacement have revealed that these processes extend to the dentinoenamel junction (Fig. 8-15). In some instances they also extend into the enamel for a short distance as enamel spindles (Fig.

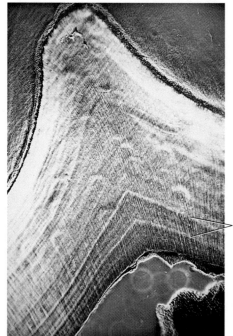

Incremental lines

FIG. 8-11 Microradiograph of 20-µm incremental lines (lines of von Ebner) in dentin. Fine daily incremental lines can be seen microscopically between the 20-µm lines.

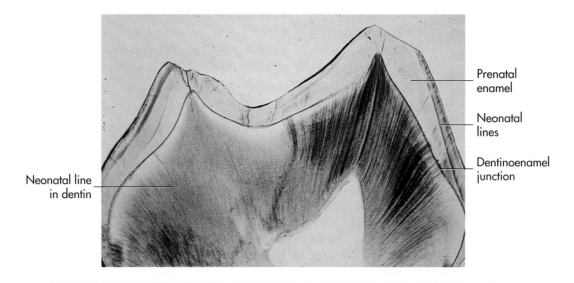

FIG. 8-12   Neonatal line is seen at birth in both enamel and dentin because each is forming at that time. Neonatal line is more easily seen in enamel because of color change between prenatal and postnatal enamel. Dentin has a neonatal line that is difficult to see at this magnification but is located midway through dentin.

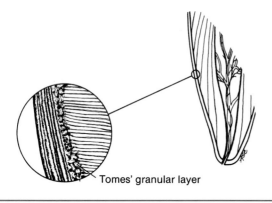

FIG. 8-13   Appearance and location of granular layer of dentin along cementodentinal junction of root.

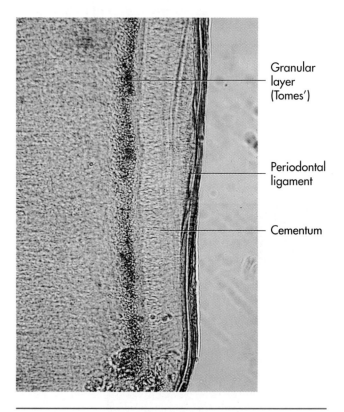

FIG. 8-14   Histologic appearance of granular layer of dentin *(center)* and cementum *(right)*, with periodontal ligament remnants *(far right)*.

8-16). The odontoblastic processes are largest in diameter near the pulp (3 to 4 μm) and taper to 1 μm near the dentinoenamel junction. These processes divide near the dentinoenamel junction to end in several branched processes (Fig. 8-17).

Periodically along the odontoblastic process, lateral branches arise at nearly right angles to the main odontoblastic process, extend into the intertubular dentin, and sometimes extend into adjacent dentinal tubules (Fig. 8-15). Within the odontoblastic process are microtubules, small filaments, occasional mitochondria, and microvesicles. All of these structures are indicative of the protein-synthesizing character of the odontoblast. Collagen is deposited along the predentinal border and to a lesser extent along the tubule wall. Nerve terminals can be seen close to the odontoblastic cell body and within the dentinal tubule in the region of the predentin. These are described in Chapter 9. Loss of the odontoblastic

process usually results in the appearance of **dead tracts** in dentin. In the dentin underlying an area of attrition or a carious lesion, odontoblasts may die and processes disintegrate, producing a group of open tubules that contain debris and spaces. If these tubules are open to over-

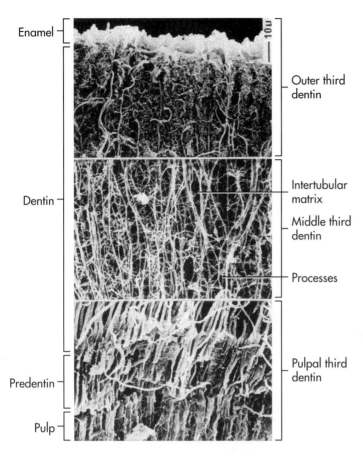

Enamel

Dentin

Predentin

Pulp

Outer third dentin

Intertubular matrix

Middle third dentin

Processes

Pulpal third dentin

FIG. 8-15 Photomicrograph of odontoblasts *(bottom)* with their processes intact and extending upward to dentinoenamel junction *(top)*. Peritubular and intertubular dentinal matrix has been removed, exposing odontoblastic processes.

(Courtesy Takahyde Gunji, DDS.)

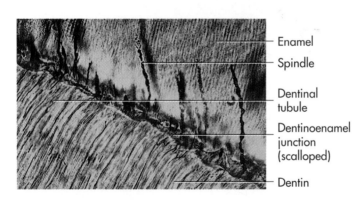

Enamel

Spindle

Dentinal tubule

Dentinoenamel junction (scalloped)

Dentin

FIG. 8-16 Spindles, which are extensions of dentinal tubules, pass across dentinoenamel junction into inner enamel.

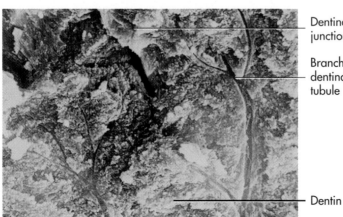

Dentinoenamel junction

Branching dentinal tubule

Dentin

FIG. 8-17 Scanning electron micrograph of dentinal tubules branching near dentinoenamel junction.

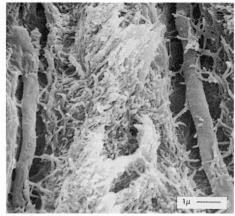

FIG. 8-18 Scanning electron micrograph of dentin near the dentinoenamel junction, illustrating odontoblastic processes. Side branches of odontoblastic process extend into intertubular dentin.

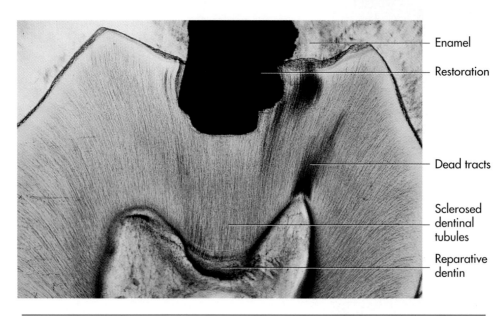

Enamel

Restoration

Dead tracts

Sclerosed dentinal tubules

Reparative dentin

FIG. 8-19 Black dead tracts (open tubules) underlie a black (dense) restoration that appears associated with sclerosed dentinal tubules. Tubules lie adjacent to the reparative dentin, which is seen on the roof of the pulp chamber. Each of these tubules probably resulted from stimulation from the overlying restoration.

lying caries, bacteria may enter them and migrate to the pulp, causing inflammation. The areas of dead tracts may appear black when the teeth are sectioned and viewed by transmitted light because air may penetrate these tubules and create this appearance (Fig. 8-18).

 CONSIDER THE PATIENT . . .

Case 2: A patient asks why carious dentin does not elicit pain during its removal.

DENTINOENAMEL JUNCTION

The junction between dentin and enamel, termed **dentinoenamel junction,** is scalloped, which enhances con-

tact and adherence of the two structurally different tissues. This can be seen microscopically in Figs. 8-13 and 8-16. Scalloping has been found to be accentuated in the cusps where the incisal or occlusal contact is greatest. Features in addition to scalloping that characterize the dentinoenamel junction are enamel spindles and fine branching of the terminal dentinal tubules in the dentin (Figs. 8-16 and 8-17). The odontoblastic processes extend to the dentinoenamel junction unless stimulation has caused a change in the tubule and its contents. Fig. 8-18 shows the processes with their side branches, and Fig. 8-19 gives an example of changes in dentin underlying a restoration. Loss of tubular contents results in dead tracts (black streaks), which indicate air in the tubules. Below the dead tract area in Fig. 8-19 is sclerosed dentin, which protects the pulp from bacteria or bacterial products in the tubules underlying the restoration.

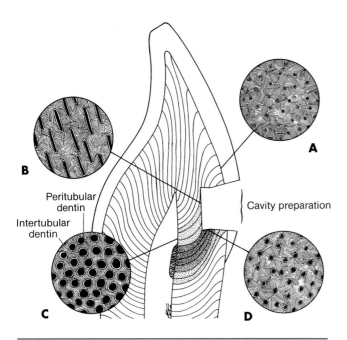

FIG. 8-20 Location and differences in size of dentinal tubules at dentinoenamel junction *(A)* and at pulp *(C)* and relationship between tubules in cavity floor *(B* and *D)* and the pathway of caries through dentin. Size of tubules at pulp border *(C)* can be compared with those in the floor of the cavity *(B* and *D)* and at the dentinoenamel junction *(A)*. Deposition of reparative dentin underlies invading caries.

(From Avery JK, editor: *Oral development and histology,* ed 2, New York, 1994, Thieme Medical.)

CLINICAL COMMENT

Dentin is a vital tissue that contains living cell processes. Because these branching processes permeate the dentin so completely, it is not possible to touch a cavity preparation in dentin with an explorer without inflicting pain.

PERMEABILITY

The outer surface of dentin is approximately five times larger in surface area than the inner surface. Because the tubule diameter is only 1 μm near the dentinoenamel junction, the tubules are farthest apart at this junction. They are, however, much closer together at the pulpal surface because the tubules are larger (3 to 4 μm) and the dentinal surface is five times smaller (Fig. 8-20). The tubules are consequently cone shaped and permit increased permeability from the cavity wall or floor to the pulp. The system of branching tubules increases the permeability. Also, because the peritubular dentin is more highly calcified than is the intertubular, the etching of a cavity causes an increase in the diameter of the tubule. The only feature that protects the pulp is that it has higher osmotic pressure than the area of the dentinoenamel junction. Fluid is constantly being forced outward by this increased pressure of the pulp. Therefore, when some dentinal tubules are cut, a small vesicle of fluid appears on the cut surface of the cavity preparation. Against the direction of this flow, minute particles such as bacteria or bacterial products percolate down the dentinal tubules to the pulp. Again, loss of the odontoblastic process, which produces a dead tract, results in increased permeability. For these reasons, the permeability factor is a major consideration in cleansing of the cavity preparation and the placement of a cavity liner to prevent microleakage. In Fig. 8-20 the shaded area indicating caries signifies that bacteria find the shortest distance to the pulp along the dentinal tubules. The figure also shows the deposition of reparative or response dentin to the cavity preparation.

The tubules of dentin are effectively blocked by the production of a **"smear layer"** on the floor or walls of the cavity during preparation. The smear layer is composed of the fine particles of cut dentinal debris that are produced by cavity preparation. These particles enter the tubules as smear plugs at the cut surface of the cavity preparation. The effectiveness of the plug is dependent on the size of the tubules and the size of the cut particles of dentin.

REPAIR PROCESS

Dentin is laid down throughout life. Pathologic effects of dental caries, attrition, abrasion, and cavity preparation cause changes in dentin. The changes are described as odontoblastic degeneration, formation of dead tracts, calcification of tubules leading to sclerosis, and tertiary or reparative dentin formation. Stimulation of the odontoblasts leads to increased dentinogenesis underlying an area of pathologic change. If the stimulation is mild enough for the odontoblast to survive, new or reparative dentin will be formed. This is believed to be a protective mechanism of the pulp to maintain its vitality. A second situation arises after death and degeneration of the odontoblast. When dead tracts appear, sclerosis of the dentin may occur and further reparative dentin in the pulp forms. In this instance the pulp is again protected by this walling off action, which blocks the tubules underlying the area of trauma (Figs. 8-19 and 8-20). With appropriate coverage, pulps can maintain their vitality. Dead tracts and sclerosis of dentin do not occur if leakage is prevented. An example of this is shown in Fig. 8-21, in which the pulp is viable in the first molar under a full crown. The pulp in the second molar is not visible because the crown was not cut through its center. This unusual section shows teeth and the surrounding supporting bone.

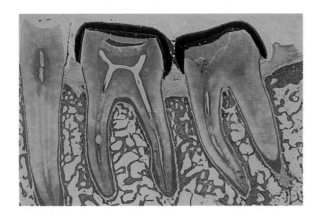

FIG. 8-21 Thin section of two human mandibular molar teeth in situ. Observe the two crowns. Pulp of first molar appears normal with no sign of sclerotic dentin or dead tracts.

(Courtesy Dr Michael Rohrer, University of Oklahoma, School of Dentistry, Department of Oral Pathology.)

CLINICAL COMMENT

The pulp is covered by smear layer dentinal particles, which block the tubules and aid in walling off the pulp, and by the formation of reparative dentin.

SELF-EVALUATION QUESTIONS

1. Name the type of dentin that comprises the greater part of the crown and root.
2. Name the newly formed area of collagen matrix that borders the pulp.
3. Describe the location and composition of the granular layer of dentin.
4. Name several factors that affect the permeability of the dentin.
5. What are the location and composition of mantle dentin?
6. What is the smear layer and what is its importance to permeability of dentin?
7. Why is dentin considered a vital tissue?
8. What is sclerotic dentin and where is it most likely to be seen?
9. What is secondary dentin and when does it form?
10. What is interglobular dentin and how does it form?

CONSIDER THE PATIENT . . .

Discussion 1: Metals are good conductors of heat and cold. (Similar complaints may result after placement of an amalgam or an inlay.) But the dentist can offer the patient assurance that the tooth will respond to the pain with internal healing. The dentist knows that reparative dentin forms slowly and eventually will insulate the pulp nerves from the metal restoration. Within 6 months or a year following such a restoration, the patient may note that the pain no longer exists. This indicates that the reparative dentin has formed.

Discussion 2: The odontoblastic process is believed to function in pain conduction in dentin and is nonliving in carious dentin. During cavity preparation, pain arises only from the adjacent living dentin.

SUGGESTED READING

Bergenholtz G et al: Leakage around dental restorations and its effect on the dental pulp, *Pathology* 11:439, 1982.

Boskey A: The role of extracellular matrix in dentin mineralization, *Crit Rev Oral Biol Med* 2:369-388, 1991.

Holland GR: The odontoblast process: form and function, *J Dent Res* 64:499-514, 1984.

Linde A: Structure and calcification of dentin. In Bonucci E, editor: *Calcification in biological systems*, Boca Raton, Fla, CRC Press, 1992, pp 269-311.

Pashley DH: Dentin permeability and dentin sensitivity, *Proc Finn Dent Soc* 88(S1):31-38, 1992.

Pashley DH: Smear layer: overview of structure and function, *Proc Finn Dent Soc* 88(S1):225-242, 1992.

Szabo J, Trombitas K, Szabo I: The odontoblast processes branches, *Arch Oral Biol* 26:331, 1984.

Trowbridge HO et al: Response to thermal stimulation in human teeth, *J Endocrinol* 66:40, 1980.

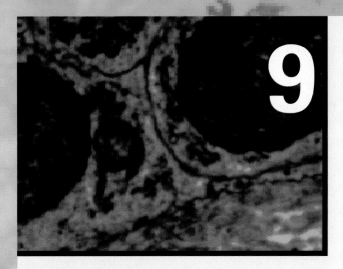

9 Dental Pulp

OVERVIEW

Dental pulp is the soft connective tissue located in the central portion of each tooth. It has a crown (coronal part) and a root (radicular part). Pulp is a delicate, specialized connective tissue containing thin-walled blood vessels, nerves, and nerve endings enclosed within dentin. Each pulp opens into the tissue surrounding the tooth, the periodontium, through the apex of the root canal. Accessory canals may be present at the apex of the tooth.

Pulp has a central zone and a peripheral zone, which are observed in both the coronal and radicular pulp. The central zone contains large arteries, veins, and nerve trunks that enter the pulp from the apical canal and proceed to the coronal pulp chamber. Fibroblasts are the preponderant cell, existing in an intercellular substance of glycosaminoglycans and collagen fibers. Odontoblasts are the second most prevalent cell. The odontogenic zone in the periphery consists of odontoblasts and cell-free and cell-rich zones. Adjacent to the cell-rich zone is a parietal layer of nerves.

Odontoblasts form dentin throughout life, which causes the pulp to grow smaller with time. The terminal blood cells in the periphery are in thin-walled capillaries situated among the odontoblasts. Larger vessels with muscle cell support in their walls exist centrally and are under sympathetic control. Several theories exist concerning pain conduction through dentin. The **hydrodynamic theory** is the most popular. It defines the movement of the odontoblast into contact with pulpal and intratubular nerve endings. Recent findings indicate, however, that odontoblasts are capable of receiving, conducting, and transmitting impulses to nerve endings in close proximity.

Pulp has several functions, such as initiative, formative, protective, nutritive, and reparative activities. All these clinical features are important to the production and maintenance of teeth.

Pulp may regress after trauma or with age and contain diffuse areas of collagen fiber bundles and pulp stones. These pulp stones may be attached, embedded, or free in the pulp tissue. Pulp may also contain diffuse calcifications.

ANATOMY OF THE PULP

Human beings have 52 pulps in their teeth, 20 in the primary dentition and 32 in the permanent (Fig. 9-1). All pulps have similar morphologic characteristics, such as a soft, gelatinous consistency in a chamber surrounded by dentin, which contains the peripheral extensions of the pulpal odontoblasts. The total volume of the pulps of the permanent dentition is approximately 0.38 ml, and the mean volume of a single human tooth is 0.2 ml. The pulps of molar teeth are approximately four times larger than those of the incisors (Fig. 9-1).

Coronal Pulp

The two forms of pulpal tissue are coronal and radicular (Figs. 9-2 and 9-3). **Coronal pulp** occupies the crown of the tooth. It is much larger than root pulp and has a structure different from the root tissue. In general the coronal pulp follows the contour of the outer surface of the crown. Coronal pulp has six surfaces: mesial, distal, buccal, lingual, occlusal, and the floor. Coronal pulp has pulp horns, which are protrusions of pulp that extend into the cusps of the teeth. The number of pulp horns depends on the number of cusps (Fig. 9-1). At the cervi-cal region the coronal pulp joins the root pulp. With age the coronal pulp decreases in size because of continued dentin formation (Fig. 9-2).

Radicular Pulp

Pulpal root canals extend from the cervical region to the apex of the root. **Radicular pulp** of the anterior teeth is singular, whereas the posterior teeth have multiple root pulps. Radicular pulp is tapered or conical and, like coronal pulp, becomes smaller with age because of continued dentinogenesis (Figs. 9-2 and 9-3). The apical canal may become narrowed by cementum deposition.

CLINICAL COMMENT

Radiographic knowledge of the pulp chamber's shape and the extension of pulp horns into the overlying cusps is important in providing safe restorative dentistry. Pulp horns present a potential problem for pulp exposure.

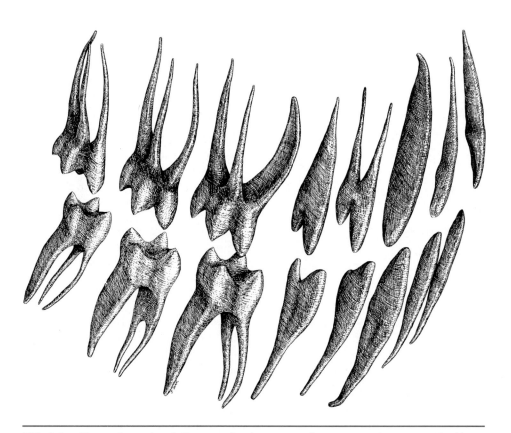

FIG. 9-1 Three-dimensional diagram of pulp organs of permanent human teeth. *Upper row,* Maxillary arch; left central incisor through third molar; *lower row,* mandibular arch; left central incisor through third molar.

(From Bhaskar SN, editor: *Orban's oral histology and embryology,* ed 11, St Louis, 1991, Mosby.)

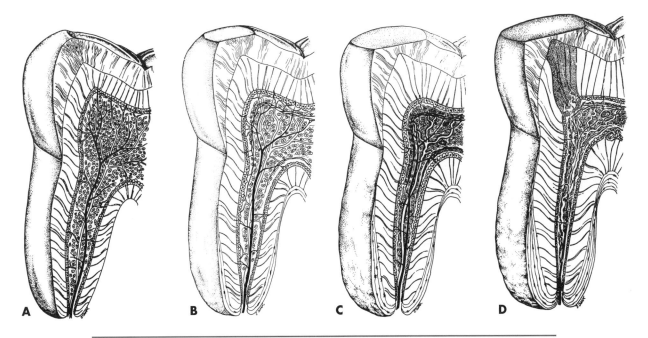

FIG. 9-2 Diagram of series of pulps. **A,** Young stage. **B,** After some attrition. **C,** At middle age. **D,** In old age. Pulp size and number of cells decrease, and fibrous tissue increases. Attrition also affects pulp horn with appearance of dead tracts and sclerotic dentin.

(From Bhaskar SN, editor: *Orban's oral histology and embryology,* ed 11, St Louis, 1991, Mosby.)

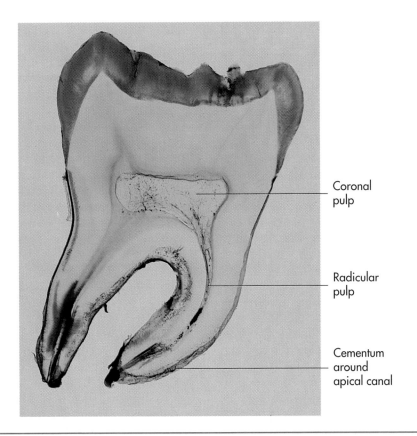

Coronal pulp

Radicular pulp

Cementum around apical canal

FIG. 9-3 Calcified section of older tooth showing decreased size of coronal and root pulp. Pulp horn underlies cusp.

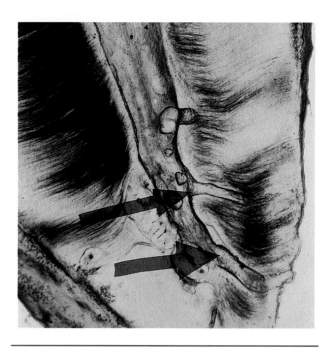

FIG. 9-4 Section of tooth apex illustrating an accessory canal at the upper arrow and main apical canal at the lower arrow.

 CONSIDER THE PATIENT . . .

A patient calls a pink incisor to the dentist's attention. He wants to know what causes this symptom.

Apical Foramina and Accessory Canals

The **apical foramen** is the opening of root pulp into the periodontium. This opening varies from 0.3 to 0.6 mm, being slightly larger in the maxillary teeth than in the mandibular teeth. The apical foramen generally is centrally located in the newly formed root apex but becomes more eccentrically located with age (Figs. 9-3 and 9-4). If several apical canals exist, the larger is designated the apical foramen and the more lateral ones are called the accessory canals (Fig. 9-4). Accessory canals may result from the presence of blood vessels obstructing dentin formation or from a break in the epithelial root sheath to induce initial root formation. The incidence of accessory canals is about 33% in permanent teeth. Accessory canals are located on the lateral sides of the apical region and may be found in the bifurcation area of multirooted teeth. Clinically, accessory canals are important because they represent contact of the pulp with the periodontal tissues. If inflammation of the pulp is present, it can spread to the periodontium or vice versa.

 CLINICAL COMMENT

The presence of accessory pulp canals in an area where periodontal pathologic conditions exist may allow bacteria to spread into the pulp. If a pathologic condition exists in the pulp, on the other hand, it could be disseminated to the periodontium through such an accessory canal.

HISTOLOGY OF PULP

The pulp consists of coronal and root pulp. Coronal pulp is larger and contains many more elements than root pulp. Root pulp acts as a conducting tube to carry blood to and from the coronal area to the apical canal. Both pulp areas contain the same elements, although the cells, fibers, blood vessels, and nerves are more numerous in coronal pulp. Centrally the pulp is composed of large veins, arteries, and nerve trunks surrounded by fibroblasts and collagen fibers embedded in an intercellular matrix (Fig. 9-5, *A*). Peripherally along the dentin in both coronal and radicular pulp are the formative cells of dentin, odontoblasts. The **odontogenic zone** includes these odontoblasts, the **cell-free zone,** and the **cell-rich zone** (Fig. 9-5, *B*). The cell-free zone is known as the **zone of Weil** or **Weil's basal layer.** Adjacent to this zone is a zone of high cell density called the **cell-rich** zone, and pulpal to this zone is the **parietal layer of nerves** (Fig. 9-5, *B*). Thus the peripheral area of pulp is highly organized. The odontogenic zone appears most notably in coronal pulp and relates to the process of dentin formation, although the function of the cell-rich and cell-free zones in this process is still uncertain. In addition to the regions of the central and peripheral pulp is the area of the pulp horns. Here the odontoblasts are crowded and appear palisaded in contrast to their appearance in the remainder of the coronal area (Fig. 9-6). In the middle area, root pulp odontoblasts are short and cuboidal.

Odontoblasts

Odontoblasts line the perimeter of the pulp from the time they begin organizing to form dentin to the time they are in quiescence and no longer producing dentin. Odontoblasts are small and oval when they first differentiate but soon become columnar (Fig. 9-7). These cells then develop processes or extensions around which dentin forms. As the process lengthens, the amount of dentin thickens. Then the odontoblastic process develops many side branches. When these branches develop, space is provided in the dentin for them (Fig. 9-8). Odontoblasts are larger in coronal pulp than in the root

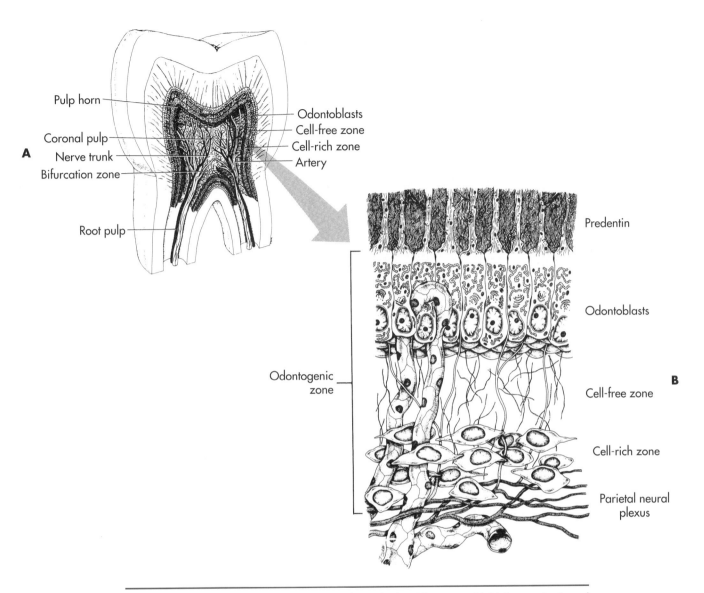

Pulp horn
Coronal pulp
Nerve trunk
Bifurcation zone
Root pulp
Odontoblasts
Cell-free zone
Cell-rich zone
Artery

A

Predentin

Odontoblasts

Odontogenic zone

Cell-free zone

Cell-rich zone

Parietal neural plexus

B

FIG. 9-5 **A,** Diagram of pulp organ illustrating pulpal architecture with high organization of the peripheral pulp and the appearance of centrally located nerve trunks *(dark)* and blood vessels *(light)*. **B,** Odontogenic zone of pulp. *Top to bottom:* Predentin, odontoblasts, cell-free and cell-rich zones, and parietal layer of nerves.

(From Bhaskar SN, editor: *Orban's oral histology and embryology,* ed 11, St Louis, 1991, Mosby.)

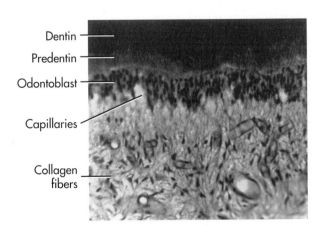

Dentin
Predentin
Odontoblast
Capillaries
Collagen fibers

FIG. 9-6 Photomicrograph of odontoblasts in coronal area of pulp organ. Pulpal capillaries are shown among these cells.

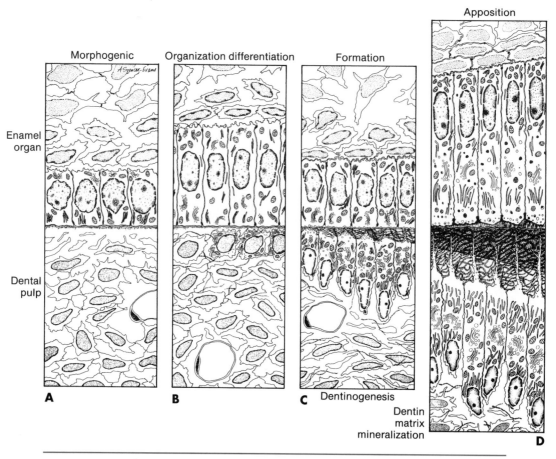

FIG. 9-7 Changes in odontoblast during its differentiation from preodontoblast *(A)* to beginning function *(D)*. In the enamel organ, ameloblast differentiates first and odontoblast second, but odontoblast then forms dentin before ameloblast forms enamel.

and appear columnar in pulp horns (Fig. 9-6). These tall, columnar cells are about 35 μm long in the pulp horns, whereas in radicular pulp they are more cuboidal, and cells of the apical region appear flat. The process of the odontoblast is the largest part of the cell, extending from the pulp to the dentinoenamel junction. In the crown the process could be several millimeters long, but it is shorter in the root.

The active cell has a large nucleus in its basal part and a Golgi's apparatus in its apical part. Abundant rough-surface endoplasmic reticulum and numerous mitochondria are scattered through the cell body (Fig. 9-9). The process arises from the odontoblast at the predentinal border, where the cell constricts as the process enters the dentinal tubule (Fig. 9-8). The process passes through the predentin, where a few mitochondria are located. As it continues into the mineralized dentin, the process is devoid of major organelles but contains filaments and microtubules throughout its length to the dentinoenamel junction. How far the process extends into the dentin has been the subject of much discussion.

Recent evidence indicates that it extends all the way to, and in some instances through, the dentinoenamel junction and into the enamel as spindles (Fig. 9-8).

Three types of junctional complexes are found between adjacent odontoblasts: **tight (zonula occludens), gap,** and **intermediate junctions** (Fig. 9-10). Each junction has a different function. Adhering junctions or desmosomes are beltlike areas around these cells that possibly function in maintaining positional relationship between cells. This also prevents substances in the pulp from passing into the dentin. Gap junctions are openings between odontoblasts for communication of cell electrical impulses and passage of small molecules (Figs. 9-10 and 9-11). In this manner the odontoblasts can have synchronous activity. If stimuli reach the odontoblasts, this information spreads throughout the cell layer by gap junctions. Although odontoblasts are generally believed to live as long as the tooth is viable, inactivity and aging of the odontoblasts result in loss of organelles and a reduction of cell size.

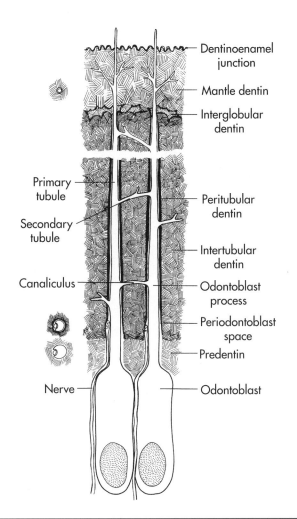

Dentinoenamel junction

Mantle dentin

Interglobular dentin

Primary tubule

Secondary tubule

Canaliculus

Nerve

Peritubular dentin

Intertubular dentin

Odontoblast process

Periodontoblast space

Predentin

Odontoblast

FIG. 9-8 Odontoblast and process extend through entire thickness of dentin into inner enamel, as noted at top of picture. Side branches of odontoblastic process are shown, and cross section of tubules is at left.

 CLINICAL COMMENT

The pulp horns recede with age. This is a protective measure performed by the pulp cells. Also, reparative dentin forms under cavity preparations or other areas of trauma. Cells in the pulp can be called on to become new odontoblasts and form dentin at required sites.

Fibroblasts

Fibroblasts are the most numerous cells in pulp because they are located throughout pulp. These cells are characterized by their functional state. In young pulp, fibroblasts produce collagen fibers and ground substance. At

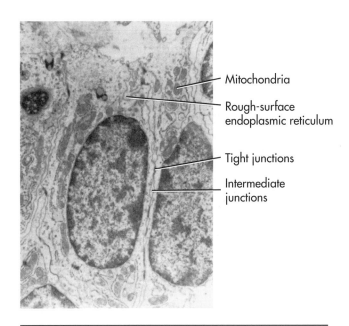

Mitochondria

Rough-surface endoplasmic reticulum

Tight junctions

Intermediate junctions

FIG. 9-9 Electron micrograph of tight, intermediate, and gap junctions, which are located between odontoblasts. Cell organelles may also be seen above the region of nuclei.

(Courtesy Dr Daniel J Chiego. From Avery JK: *Oral development and histology,* ed 2, New York, 1994, Thieme Medical.)

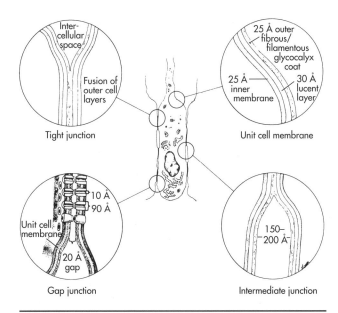

FIG. 9-10 The three types of junctional complexes found between adjacent odontoblasts. Their locations can be noted in central diagram, and an illustration of unit membrane is at upper right.

(From Bhaskar SN, editor: *Orban's oral histology and embryology,* ed 11, St Louis, 1991, Mosby.)

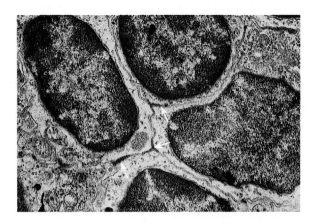

FIG. 9-11 Electron micrograph of junctions between four odontoblasts in the region of cell nuclei. Cell membranes meet at thickened dense-staining zones where junctions are formed, as indicated by arrows. These dark zones are gap junctions that allow passage of small molecules between cells.

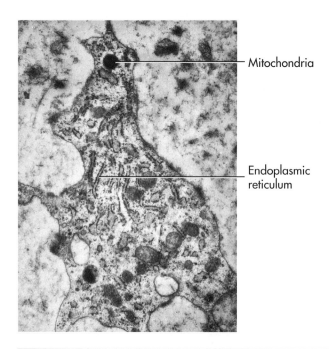

FIG. 9-13 Electron micrograph of pulp fibroblasts showing rough-surface endoplasmic reticulum and mitochondria.

(From Bhaskar SN, editor: *Orban's oral histology and embryology,* ed 11, St Louis, 1991, Mosby.)

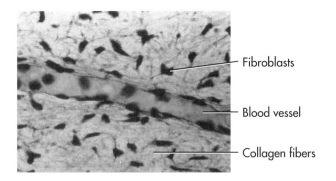

FIG. 9-12 Pulp fibroblasts, collagen fibers, and blood vessels in young pulp.

(Courtesy Dr Daniel J Chiego. From Avery JK: *Oral development and histology,* ed 2, New York, 1994, Thieme Medical.)

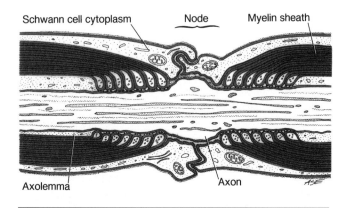

FIG. 9-14 Pulpal nerve axon surrounded by Schwann cell cytoplasm.

that time they have a large oval nucleus that is centrally located and has multiple processes (Fig. 9-12). Higher magnification of a fibroblast (Fig. 9-13) illustrates a Golgi's apparatus, adjacent abundant rough-surface endoplasmic reticulum, and mitochondria. This fibroblast is a protein-producing cell. In aging these cells appear smaller and shaped like a spindle, with few organelles.

Other Pulpal Cells

Nerve cells in the pulp include **Schwann's cells** (Fig. 9-14). These cells form the myelin sheath of nerves and are associated with all pulp nerves. In addition, **endothelial cells** lining the capillaries, veins, and arteries of the pulp can be visualized (Fig. 9-15). Accompanying most blood vessels are **pericytes** and numerous **undifferentiated cells** found in normal pulp. They function as a cell pool and are called into action when new odontoblasts or fibroblasts are needed. For example, this may happen when repara-

tive dentin is needed for a pulp exposure. **Macrophages,** normal constituents of the pulp, function in pulp maintenance because of the turnover of cells in pulp (Fig. 9-16). **Lymphocytes** are also found in pulp-free spaces and probably function in an immune system of pulp. **Erythrocytes, lymphocytes, leukocytes, eosinophils,** and **basophils** are found in pulp blood vessels.

Fibers and Ground Substance

Collagen fibers exist in the extracellular matrix, which surrounds the cells. Collagen originates from the pulpal fibroblasts throughout pulp. Both types I and II collagen have been found in pulp. Type I is probably produced

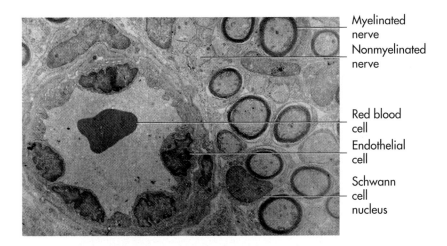

Myelinated
nerve

Nonmyelinated
nerve

Red blood
cell

Endothelial
cell

Schwann
cell
nucleus

FIG. 9-15 Electron micrograph of arteriole in central pulp. Lumen is surrounded by endothelial cells and layer of muscle cells. Endothelial cells constitute the intima, and muscle cells the media. At right are myelinated nerves; large nuclei belong to accompanying Schwann cells.

(Courtesy Dr Daniel J Chiego. From Avery JK: *Oral development and histology,* ed 2, New York, 1994, Thieme Medical.)

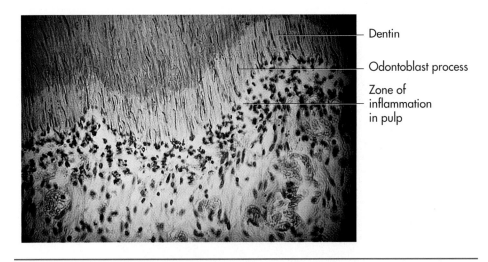

Dentin

Odontoblast process

Zone of
inflammation
in pulp

FIG. 9-16 Area underlying dentin with leukocytes, lymphocytes, and macrophages apparently responding to an irritant that resulted in inflammation. Odontoblastic processes in dentinal tubules are degenerating.

by odontoblasts because this is the type of collagen found in dentin, the tissue that the odontoblasts produce. Type II is probably produced by pulp fibroblasts. In young pulp, fibers are relatively sparse and the tissue appears delicate (Fig. 9-12). Around the fibers is the ground substance of pulp. This substance is the environment that provides life for cells in pulp and throughout the body. If pulp is irritated, fibers may accumulate rapidly. However, older pulp contains more collagen of both bundle and diffuse types (Fig. 9-17).

Vascularity

The pulp organ is highly vascularized with vessels arising from the external carotid arteries to the superior and inferior alveolar arteries. It drains by the same veins. Although the periodontal and pulpal vessels both originate from these vessels, their walls are different. The walls of the periodontal and pulpal vessels become quite thin as they enter the pulp because the pulp is protected within a hard, unyielding container of dentin. These thin-walled arteries and arterioles enter the apical canal and pursue a direct route up the root pulp to the coronal area (Fig. 9-18). Along the way, vessels produce branches that pass peripherally to a plexus that lies in and adjacent to the odontogenic zone of the root (Fig. 9-19). Blood flow is more rapid in the pulp than in most areas of the body, and the blood pressure is quite high. The diameter of the arteries varies from 50 to 100 μm, which equals the size of arterioles in other areas of the body.

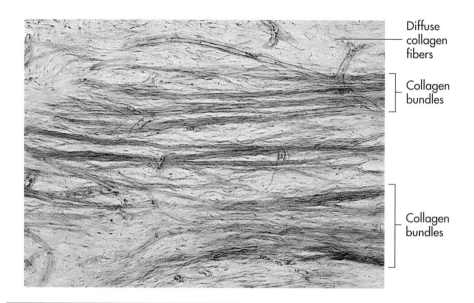

Diffuse
collagen
fibers

Collagen
bundles

Collagen
bundles

FIG. 9-17   Collagen bundles in older pulp organ. Trauma may also have contributed to collagen in this pulp.

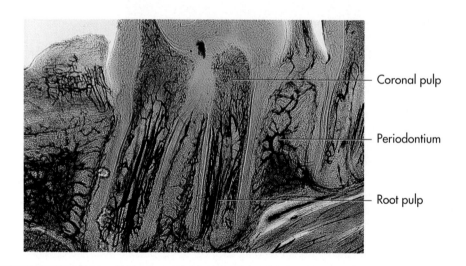

Coronal pulp

Periodontium

Root pulp

FIG. 9-18   India ink injected to illustrate blood vascular organization in pulp and periodontium. Larger vessels conduct blood in the root pulp, and smaller capillaries are in the coronal pulp.

These vessels have three layers: the inner lining, or **intima,** which consists of oval or squamous-shaped endothelial cells surrounded by a closely associated fibrillar basal lamina; a middle layer or **media,** which consists of muscle cells from one to three cell layers thick (Fig. 9-20); and an outer layer, or **adventitia,** which consists of a sparse layer of collagen fibers forming a loose network around the larger arteries.

Smaller arterioles with a single layer of muscle cells range from 20 to 30 μm, and **terminal arterioles** of 10 to 15 μm are also present. **Precapillaries** measuring 8 to 12 μm and **capillaries** measuring 8 to 10 μm in diame-

 CLINICAL COMMENT

The vitality of pulp is due in part to the apical canal's ability to remain open. This opening can become blocked, however, as the tooth ages and cementum becomes deposited around the apical canal. Thin walls of veins are the first structure affected by cemental constriction of the apices; vascular congestion can occur, leading to pulpal necrosis.

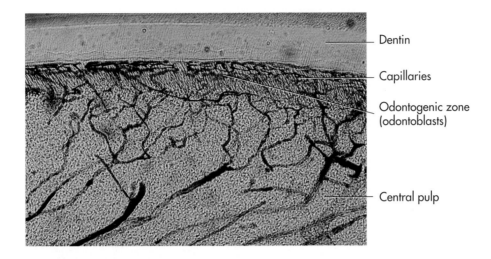

Dentin

Capillaries

Odontogenic zone
(odontoblasts)

Central pulp

FIG. 9-19 India ink injected in blood vessels to illustrate network of capillaries among odontoblasts in odontogenic zone. Dentin, which protects pulp, is seen at top of picture. The central pulp is in lower part of micrograph.

(Courtesy Dr Daniel J Chiego. From Avery JK: *Oral development and histology,* ed 2, New York, 1994, Thieme Medical.)

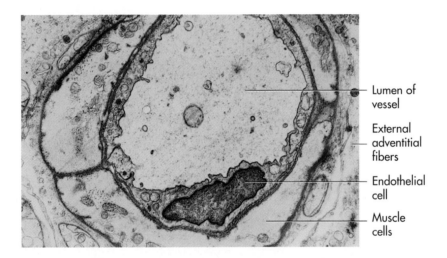

Lumen of
vessel

External
adventitial
fibers

Endothelial
cell

Muscle
cells

FIG. 9-20 Ultrastructure of a pulp arteriole. Central lumen is surrounded by endothelial cells; a nucleus is seen below. These cells compose the intima layer. Surrounding the intima is a layer of muscle cells that form the media. External adventitial fibers are also present.

(Courtesy Dr Daniel J Chiego. From Avery JK: *Oral development and histology,* ed 2, New York, 1994, Thieme Medical.)

ter are present in the peripheral pulp. Capillaries are endothelial-lined tubes that form a network among the odontoblasts (Fig. 9-19). Numerous investigators have shown that lymphatic vessels are present in pulp. These vessels are thin walled, irregularly shaped, and larger than capillaries and have an incomplete lamina supporting the intima and media.

Nerves

Several large nerves enter the apical canal of each molar and premolar, and single nerves enter the anterior teeth. These nerve trunks traverse the radicular pulp, proceed to the coronal area, and branch as they extend peripherally (Fig. 9-21). Nonmyelinated axons also enter with the myelinated axons, but they are smaller. A young molar may have as many as 350 to 700 myelinated axons and 1000 to 2000 nonmyelinated axons entering the apex.

The large nerve trunks are invested with Schwann's cells (Figs. 9-14 and 9-15). Later, as the pulp organ matures, the subodontoblastic plexus is apparent in the roof and lateral walls of the coronal pulp and, to a lesser extent, the root canals. This network, comprising both myelinated and nonmyelinated axons, is known as the **parietal layer** of nerves or nerve **plexus of Raschkow**

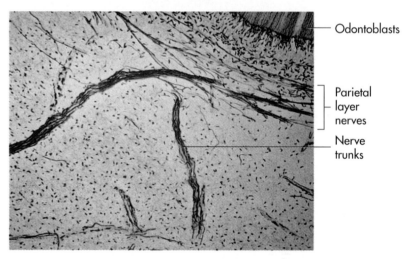

FIG. 9-21 Nerve trunks pass from radicular pulp into coronal area. These nerves extend to periphery, where they form plexus of nerves adjacent to odontogenic zone at top of micrograph.

(From Bhaskar SN, editor: *Orban's oral histology and embryology,* ed 11, St Louis, 1991, Mosby.)

FIG. 9-22 Myelinated nerves extending into parietal nerve plexus in peripheral pulp. From this area they extend between odontoblasts to terminate among them or in dentinal tubules.

(Courtesy Dr Daniel J Chiego. From Avery JK: *Oral development and histology,* ed 2, New York, 1994, Thieme Medical.)

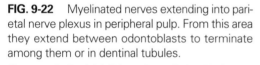

(Figs. 9-21 and 9-22). From the parietal layer the nerves pass into the odontogenic zone and then terminate among the odontoblasts or extend into the dentinal tubules with the odontoblastic process.

Nerve Endings

Most pulpal nerve endings are in the odontogenic region of the pulp horns. Some terminate on or in association with the odontoblasts (Figs. 9-23 and 9-24). Others are found in the predentinal tubules, usually in the region of pulp horns or roof of the coronal area (Fig. 9-24). These nerve endings are presumed to function in pain reception. Few nerve endings are located along the larger muscular blood vessels in the central pulp. All these nerve endings have a similar appearance and are highly vascular. They are believed to function in regulation of blood flow, constriction, or dilation of large blood vessels of the pulp.

PAIN AND THE PULP-DENTIN COMPLEX

Pain is a function of the high concentration of nerve endings within the tooth. Pulp is highly sensitive to temperature changes, electrical and chemical stimuli, and pressure as applied to the inner enamel, dentin, or pulp. Teeth are one of the few body structures that perceive only the modality of pain. The close relationship between nerve endings and the odontoblasts and their

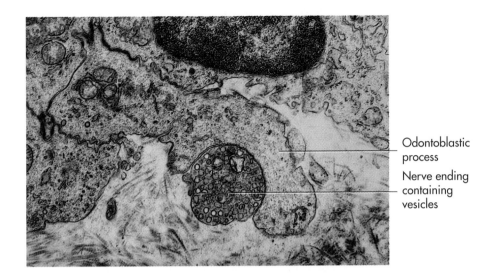

FIG. 9-23 Ultrastructure of nerve ending in close contact with odontoblastic process in predentin. Nerve contains small vesicles believed to contain a neurotransmitter substance. Nerve terminal interdigitates with odontoblastic process.

(From Bhaskar SN, editor: *Orban's oral histology and embryology,* ed 11, St Louis, 1991, Mosby.)

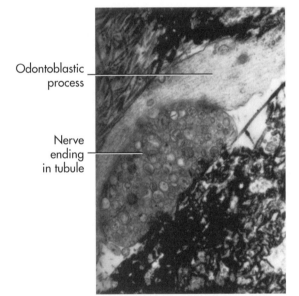

FIG. 9-24 Vesiculated nerve terminal in a dentinal tubule making contact with odontoblastic process. Nerve and process are close to each other. Dark-stained mineral of dentin is shown above and below tubule.

processes is significant. Moreover, the nerve endings in the dentinal tubules and the pulp may be some distance from where the pain is perceived, at the dentinoenamel junction and the inner enamel. Several theories attempt to explain this phenomenon.

The first theory is called the **direct innervation theory,** which is based on the belief that the nerves extend to the dentinoenamel junction. However, studies have not shown nerves present at this junction (Fig. 9-25).

In a second theory, other scientists believe the odontoblastic process is the receptor and that it conducts the pain to nerve endings in the peripheral pulp and in the dentinal tubules. This theory has been termed the **transduction theory** (Fig. 9-25).

A third theory, the **hydrodynamic theory,** was developed to explain the transmission of pain through the thickness of dentin (Fig. 9-25). This theory is based on the premise that when dentin is stimulated, fluid and the odontoblastic process move within the tubules, making contact with the nerve endings in the inner dentin and adjacent pulp. When these nerve endings are contacted, they deform and act as mechanoreceptors to produce an impulse. Several factors support this theory. For example, when a stimulus such as cold is applied to the dentin, the odontoblastic process moves outward, but when heat is applied, the odontoblastic process moves inward. Other evidence is seen in the close relationship of the nerve endings and the odontoblastic process.

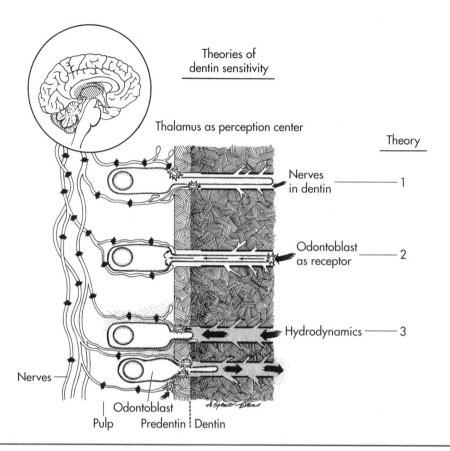

FIG. 9-25 Summary of theories on passage of nerve impulses through dentin. At top, impulses are shown stimulating nerves in dentin; this is termed the direct stimulation theory. In center, odontoblast is depicted as receptor passing impulses to nerves in peripheral pulp and hence on to brain, which is the transduction theory. At bottom, diagram displays concept of fluid and odontoblast movement. This movement causes pressure on the nerve endings, which stimulates them. The odontoblast thus acts as a mechanoreceptor to nerve endings, which in turn conduct impulses to the brain. This is termed the hydrodynamic theory.

(From Bhaskar SN, editor: *Orban's oral histology and embryology,* ed 11, St Louis, 1991, Mosby.)

The odontoblast is a unique cell that forms dentin throughout life. It forms reparative dentin, for example, in response to various stimuli. In addition, it plays a role in conducting stimuli through dentin and in affecting nerve endings in the peripheral pulp.

FUNCTIONS OF THE PULP

Pulp has several functions, none of which is more important than providing vitality to the teeth with its cells, blood vessels, and nerves. The loss of pulp after a root canal does not mean the tooth will be lost; on the contrary, the tooth will function without pain. The tooth, however, has lost the protective mechanism its pulp nerves provided.

Pulp has several other functions. It is **inductive** because in early development the pulp (papilla) interacts

with the oral epithelium and initiates tooth formation. Pulp organs are **formative** because odontoblasts of the pulp form the dentin that surrounds and protects pulp. Pulp is **protective** in its response to stimuli, such as heat, cold, pressure, and operative cutting procedures. The formation of sclerotic dentin, the process of mineral depo-

CLINICAL COMMENT

A cracked tooth may result from masticatory impact on a hard object. It can cause a fracture of a restoration margin. As a result, bacterial organisms or their toxins may penetrate the tooth and cause inflammation of the pulp, pain, and eventually pulpal pathosis.

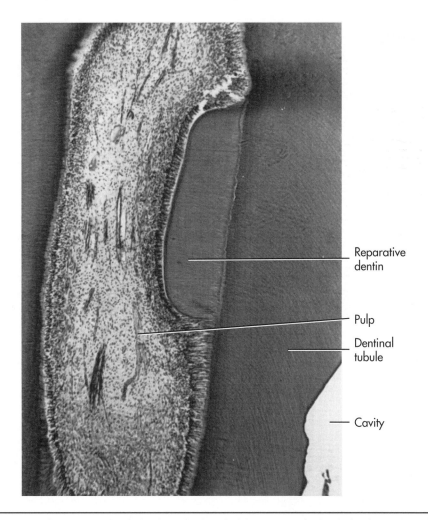

Reparative
dentin

Pulp

Dentinal
tubule

Cavity

FIG. 9-26 Reparative dentin is deposited underlying areas of stimulation by caries, abrasion, cavity preparation, and restorations. It is limited to area underlying dental tubules leading from the cavity floor.

(Courtesy Dr Daniel J Chiego. From Avery JK: *Oral development and histology,* ed 2, New York, 1994, Thieme Medical.)

sition in the tubules, originates in pulp and protects pulp from invasion of bacteria and bacterial products. Pulp is **nutritive** because it carries oxygen and nutrition to the developing and functioning tooth. Finally, pulp has the ability to be **reparative** (Fig. 9-26) through its response to operative cutting or dental caries by the formation of reparative dentin.

REGRESSIVE CHANGES

Numerous regressive changes in the pulp and surrounding dentin are related to environmental stimuli and to aging. It is often difficult to determine which factor has caused the specific change seen. As the tooth ages, pulp decreases in size because of the continued deposition of dentin. This decrease in size usually occurs because of uniform deposition around the entire perimeter of the pulpal border (Fig. 9-27). In addition, changes occur in the dentin with both aging and injury. Areas of dentinal changes, such as dead tracts and mineral deposits, appear in zones of trauma. Reparative dentin usually forms under traumatized areas (Fig. 9-27). In addition, as a result of both aging and trauma, pulpal cells decrease in general, as do cellular perinuclear cytoplasm and organelles in the cytoplasm, such as mitochondria and endoplasmic reticulum. This indicates cell activity has decreased. Therefore aging decreases the ability of the pulp to respond to injury and to repair itself. With injury, however, deposition of dentin appears in a specific location (Fig. 9-27).

Fibrous Changes

Fibrosis, which is seen in some pulps more than others, is believed to be caused more by injury than by aging. In some cases, diffuse fibrosis with collagen fibers appears throughout the pulp. Occasionally, the fibers nearly

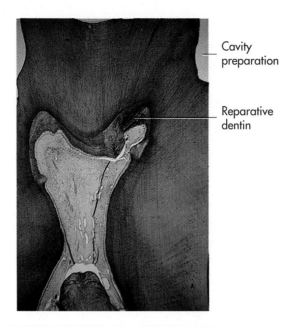

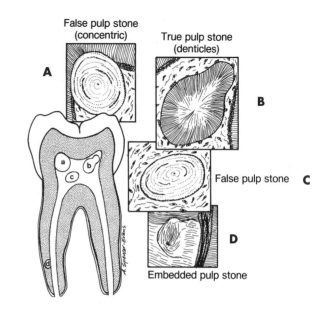

FIG. 9-27   Reparative dentin underlying cavity preparation on mesial-occlusal-distal aspects of crown. Reparative dentin on roof and sides of coronal pulp chamber underlie cut dentinal tubules that lead from cavity preparation.

(Courtesy Dr Daniel J Chiego. From Avery JK: *Oral development and histology,* ed 2, New York, 1994, Thieme Medical.)

FIG. 9-29   Diagram of pulp stones. **A,** False attached denticle. **B,** True denticle with tubules. **C,** False free denticle. **D,** Embedded denticle.

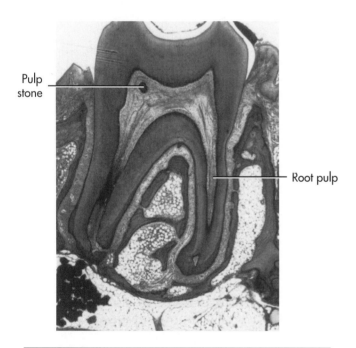

FIG. 9-28   Fibrous changes in pulp. A pulp stone appears in coronal area of molar tooth.

obliterate the pulp. What mechanism causes this condition is not certain, although it is believed caused by pulpal injury, at least in part. Scarring caused by injury is an important factor. One characteristic of aging is an increase in collagen fibers, which become more evident

with the decreasing size of the pulp (Fig. 9-17). Some pulps contain diffuse areas of collagen, and others have bundles of them probably because of injury, as well as unknown systemic factors.

Pulp Stones

Pulp stones or **denticles** are round to oval calcified masses appearing in either the canal or coronal portions of the pulp organ (Fig. 9-28). They appear in teeth that have suffered injury, as well as in otherwise normal pulps. Pulp stones also occur in unerupted, as well as erupted, teeth. These denticles are noted in most pulps of permanent teeth, especially in individuals more than 50 years of age. They are classified according to their structure as true or false. **True denticles** have dental tubules like dentin. Odontoblasts may be on the surface of these denticles, and their processes are evident in their tubules. **False denticles** are concentric layers of calcified tissue (Fig. 9-29). In the center of these false stones may be a group of cells that appear necrotic. These cells are believed to serve as the nidus of denticle formation.

All denticles begin small and grow, sometimes nearly obliterating the pulp. Denticles may appear free in pulp, attached to dentin, or embedded in dentin. Therefore they are classified as **free, attached,** or **embedded denticles.** One pulp may have all three types (Fig. 9-29). Investigators believe that a free denticle may become attached and later embedded as dentin is deposited around the denticle. Most denticles are false stones that are free in the pulp.

Diffuse Calcifications

Diffuse calcifications appear as irregular calcified deposits along collagen fiber bundles or blood vessels in the pulp. This is considered a pathologic condition and usually appears as a sprinkling of or occasionally large masses of mineral. They appear more often in the root canal than in the coronal area of the pulp.

SELF-EVALUATION QUESTIONS

1. Describe the characteristics of the odontogenic zone.
2. Compare the odontoblast in coronal pulp with the odontoblast in root pulp.
3. What are the most prominent cells of pulp and what are their functions?
4. What are five other cell types found in normal pulp?
5. Describe the various blood vessels of pulp and how they differ from blood vessels of the periodontium.
6. Give descriptions and locations of nerve endings in pulp.
7. Name five functions of pulp.
8. Name and describe various types of denticles.
9. What are the types of junctional complexes found between odontoblasts?
10. Name and describe the types of reparative dentin.

CONSIDER THE PATIENT . . .

Discussion: This condition can be caused by internal resorption of the root and crown dentin. The crown appears pink because the transparent enamel reveals the blood vessels in the pulp.

SUGGESTED READING

Avery JK: *Oral development and histology*, ed 2, New York, 1994, Thieme Medical.

Avery, JK: Pulp. In Bhaskar SN, editor: *Orban's oral histology and embryology*, ed 11, St Louis, 1991, Mosby, p 139.

Avery JK, Chiego DJ Jr: Cholinergic system and the dental pulp. In Inoki R, Kudo T, Olgart L, editors: *Dynamic aspects of dental pulp: molecular biology, pharmacology and pathophysiology*, New York, 1990, Chapman & Hall, pp 297-332.

Baume LJ: The biology of pulp and dentine. In Myers H, editor: *Monographs in oral science*, vol 8, New York, 1980, S Karger.

Ten Cate AR: *Oral histology, development, structure and function*, ed 4, St Louis, 1994, Mosby.

Yamada T et al: The extent of the odontoblastic process in normal and carious human dentin, *J Dent Res* 62:798, 1983.

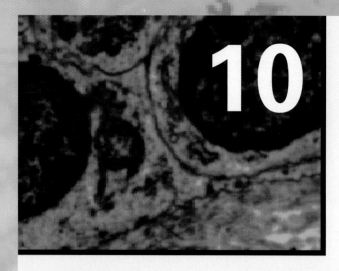

10

Cementum

OVERVIEW

Cementum, which is the focus of this chapter, has two major functions. It seals the tubules of root dentin and serves as an attachment for periodontal fibers to keep the tooth in its socket. Cementum has the ability to reverse root resorption by means of deposition as it forms a smooth patch on the cemental surface.

Two types of hard tissue cover tooth roots. The first, called **intermediate cementum,** is a homogenous layer originating from epithelial root sheath cells. The second, called **cellular-acellular cementum,** is a thicker deposit of a bonelike substance produced by cementoblasts that differentiate from the periodontal ligament fibroblasts. The latter is laid down in increments, usually an acellular layer followed by a cellular layer. Cementum simulates bone by displaying cells within lacunae and cell processes within canaliculi. Cementum also exhibits incremental lines but does not have the vascular and neural filament characteristics of bone. As a result the cementum has unique characteristics, such as lack of neural sensitivity and a greater ability than bone to resist resorption. Both of these are important clinical features. Aging cementum exhibits a rough and irregular surface caused by resorption of the cemental surface. This cementum also is associated with free, attached, or embedded cementicles. These oval to round stones are similar to the denticles in pulp. They are calcified bodies that may be embedded, attached to cementum, or free in the periodontal ligament.

ROLE OF CEMENTUM ON THE ROOT SURFACE

The hard tissue that covers the entire root surface is very thin but manages to carry out two important functions. First, it seals the surface of the root dentin and covers the ends of the open dental tubules. Second, perforating fibers of the periodontal ligament become embedded in the cementum. These fibers function as an attachment for the periodontal ligament fibers to the tooth root and aid in maintaining the tooth in its socket. This chapter discusses sealing of the root surface (Fig. 10-1), and Chapter 12 discusses the attachment fibers.

DEVELOPMENT OF CEMENTUM

The first cementum deposited on the root's surface is called **intermediate cementum** and is formed by the inner epithelial root sheath cells that formed during root dentin formation. This deposition occurs before the root sheath cell layer disintegrates (Fig. 10-2). Intermediate cementum is situated between the granular dentin layer of Tomes and the secondary cementum that is formed by the cementoblasts. These cementoblasts arise from the periodontal ligament fibroblasts. The thin layer of intermediate cementum is approximately 10 nm thick. After being deposited, this layer mineralizes to a greater extent than the adjacent dentin or the cellular-acellular cementum. Under proper magnification a thin line of radiopacity is seen covering the root.

The **cellular-acellular cementum** is a specialized hard tissue covering the root surfaces of teeth (Figs. 10-2 and 10-3). The initial thin layer of this cementum is acellular and is deposited on intermediate cementum. Subsequent layers alternate between cellular and acellular. Thus ce-

mentum is deposited incrementally. Both grossly and histologically this cementum resembles bone because it is a hard tissue with cells contained in lacunae that exhibit canaliculi (Fig. 10-2). However, unlike bone, cementum does not contain blood vessels, nerves, or haversian or Volkmann's canals, which are the nutrient canals containing blood vessels and nerves in bone (Fig. 10-3).

Cementum is limited to the roots of teeth. In 60% of cases, cementum is formed on the cervical enamel for a short distance; in 30% it stops at the cervical line just meeting the enamel; and in 10% a small gap exists between them. This order of frequency is known as **OMG**, or overlap, meet, and gap (Fig. 10-4 and Table 10-1).

INTERMEDIATE CEMENTUM

Intermediate cementum is a thin, noncellular, amorphous layer of hard tissue approximately 10 μm thick. It is deposited by the inner layer of the epithelial cells of the root sheath. Deposition occurs immediately before the epithelial root cells disintegrate as a sheet and migrate away from the root into the periodontal tissue (Fig. 10-2). Recently most authors have used the term **intermediate cementum,** although some prefer **cementoid**

CLINICAL COMMENT

Cementum functions as a covering for the root surface, a seal for the open dentinal tubules, and an attachment for the periodontal fibers that hold the tooth in its socket.

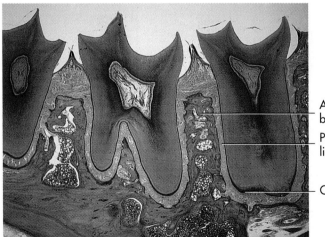

Alveolar bone

Periodontal ligament

Cementum

FIG. 10-1 Relation of root to periodontium. Cementum is shown on the root apex. It covers entire root surface overlying dentin.

(From Avery JK: *Oral development and histology,* New York, 1994, Thieme Medical.)

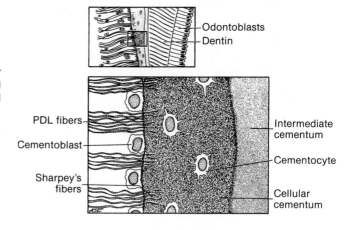

FIG. 10-2 Intermediate cementum is on right, overlying dentin. Cellular cementum is in center of field, and periodontal ligament (PDL) fibers are on left.

(From Avery JK: *Oral development and histology,* New York, 1994, Thieme Medical.)

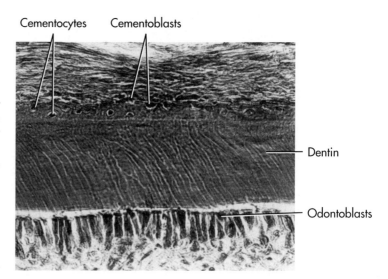

FIG. 10-3 Early cementum deposition on root dentin. Some cementoblasts get enmeshed in cementum matrix and become cementocytes living in lacunae.

(From Avery JK: *Oral development and histology,* New York, 1994, Thieme Medical.)

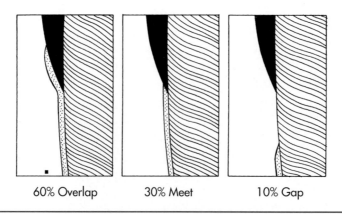

FIG. 10-4 Relation of cementum to enamel at cementoenamel junction. Overlap, meet, and gap (OMG) is the order of frequency of these conditions.

(From Avery JK: *Oral development and histology,* New York, 1994, Thieme Medical.)

Table 10-1

Relationship of Cementum to Enamel at the Cementoenamel Junction	
Relationship	Percentage of Cases
Cementum overlaps enamel	60
Cementum meets enamel	30
Small gap exists between cementum and enamel	10

layer. The latter term is confusing because the initial layer of cementum is called cementoid, like osteoid in Bone.

Intermediate cementum is the first layer of hard tissue deposited, and it seals the tubules of dentin. Because of its epithelial origin, intermediate cementum is composed of enamelin protein rather than collagen, which is the protein typical of cellular or secondary cementum. Intermediate cementum is completely formed before deposition of the secondary cementum begins. As an amorphous, noncellular layer, it is similar to the aprismatic enamel layer on the crown surface of teeth. This cementum calcifies to a greater extent than either the adjacent cellular cementum or the dentin and therefore has a harder consistency (Fig. 10-2).

CELLULAR AND ACELLULAR CEMENTUM

Cementum is deposited directly on the surface of the intermediate cementum at a thickness of about 30 to 60 μm at the cervical region of the crown (Figs. 10-3 and 10-5). It increases gradually to a thickness of 150 to 200 μm at the root apex (Fig. 10-6).

The cementum appears to be more cellular as the thickness increases, probably to maintain its viability (Fig. 10-7). The thin layer near the cervical region requires no cells to maintain viability because fluids bathe its surface.

Cementum forms more slowly than the adjacent dentin (Fig. 10-5). After the inner epithelial root sheath cells stimulate the formation of the root dentin, they deposit the intermediate cementum on the surface of the dentin. These cells then begin to degenerate and migrate from the root surface into the periodontal ligament. Then the cementoblasts, which originate from the periodontal ligament, begin to form increments of cementum along the root surface.

Cementum is always thickest at the apex of the root (Fig. 10-6). Cementum forms through the deposit in increments of a collagenous matrix that then becomes secondarily mineralized (see Chapter 5). The young matrix is called cementoid, and its formation is similar to that of bone from osteoid and dentin from predentin.

Some cementoblasts become incorporated in the forming cementum along the developing front as ce-

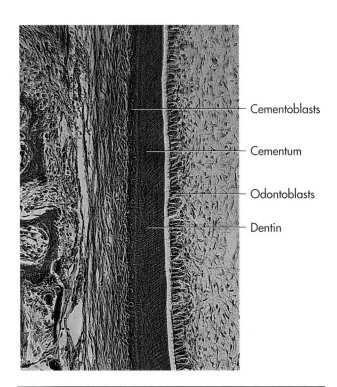

FIG. 10-5 Development of cellular cementum. Epithelial root sheath cells have moved from root surface to position in periodontal ligament. Cementoblasts are forming cementum along left side of band of dentin and cementum.

(From Avery JK: *Oral development and histology,* New York, 1994, Thieme Medical.)

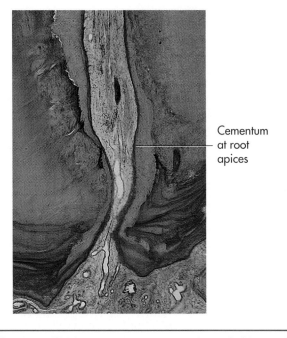

FIG. 10-6 Thick cementum on root apices of older tooth. Cementum deposited around apical foramen in an older person may nearly obliterate foramen. Cementum is lining the pulpal wall near the apex.

(From Avery JK: *Oral development and histology,* New York, 1994, Thieme Medical.)

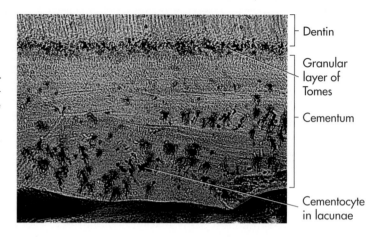

FIG. 10-7   Histology of granular layer of Tomes and lacunae in cementum. Cementum near the apex has the greatest number of lacunae.

(From Avery JK: *Oral development and histology,* New York, 1994, Thieme Medical.)

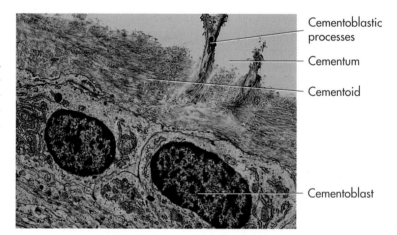

FIG. 10-8   Ultrastructure of early cementum. Cementoblasts become cementocytes as their processes are incorporated in the matrix. Cementocytes are located in cementum and do not appear in this photomicrograph.

(From Avery JK: *Oral development and histology,* New York, 1994, Thieme Medical.)

mentum continues to form around the cementoblasts (Figs. 10-7 to 10-11). These cells are then termed cementocytes because they reside in lacunae and appear most notably in the thick apical cementum (Fig. 10-7). The cementocytes found deep in the cementum are polygonal and have fewer organelles (Fig. 10-9).

Although many blood vessels are near the surface, none actually enters the cementum. In laboratory tests, cementum is slightly more permeable to dyes than bone or dentin. However, the permeability of viable cementum is unknown. Cementum is deposited in increments, resulting in incremental lines similar to those of bone, dentin, and enamel (Fig. 10-12). Cementum has many characteristics of hard tissue, although some elements are absent. Therefore cementum is not exactly like any other tissue in the human body. A thin layer of acellular cementum covers the cervical half of the root surface to a distance of approximately 20 μm. A deposit of cellular cementum then covers the acellular layer on the cervical root to a total thickness of 50 μm. Cellular cementum is then deposited on the apical root dentin to a thickness of 150 to 200 μm.

Without the presence of nerves, cellular cementum is insensitive to pain, which is an important clinical feature. Cementum is also more resistant to resorption than bone, and the lack of cementum vascularity may be part of the reason.

Deep within cementum, many lacunae appear empty, implying that these cells gradually die. Some of these cells have long processes that lie in canaliculi and are in contact with adjacent cementocytes (Figs. 10-7 to 10-10). Near the surface of cementum, the cells appear active with organelles such as Golgi's apparatus, rough surface endoplasmic reticulum, and mitochondria, which are all associated with protein secretion (Fig. 10-10). Layers of cellular cementum may alternate with noncellular layers in their formation, although the reason is unknown. Deeper in the cementum the cells may be less active (Fig. 10-9).

The collagen fibers formed within the cementum are associated with the cementum's function on the root's surface. More superficially, cementum has bundles of noncalcified fibers that are associated with the function of attachment of periodontal fibers. These perforating fibers are called extrinsic fiber bundles of cementum.

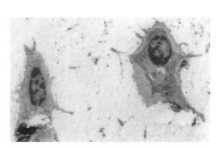

FIG. 10-9 Ultrastructure of two cementocytes deep in cementum. These cells contain few organelles and appear to be inactive.

(From Avery JK: *Oral development and histology,* New York, 1994, Thieme Medical.)

Lacuna   Cell process

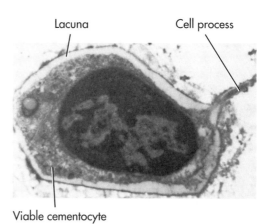

Viable cementocyte

FIG. 10-10 Ultrastructure of cementocyte near surface of cementum. Cementocytes in this region appear viable and relate to adjacent cementocytes by their processes.

(From Avery JK: *Oral development and histology,* New York, 1994, Thieme Medical.)

Alveolar bone

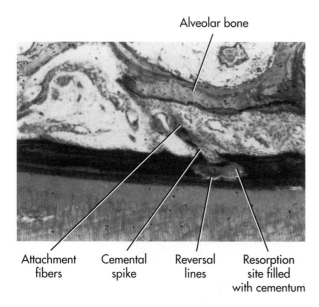

Attachment fibers   Cemental spike   Reversal lines   Resorption site filled with cementum

FIG. 10-11 Aging cementum showing projection of spikes into ligament. Reversal line indicates root resorption and repair. Cementum builds up around bundles of attachment fibers.

(From Avery JK: *Oral development and histology,* New York, 1994, Thieme Medical.)

Alveolar bone ⎤

Periodontal ligament ⎤

Dental cementum ⎤

Dentin ⎤

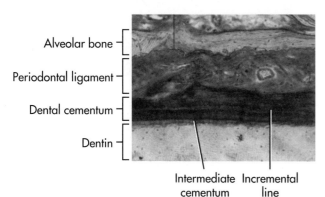

Intermediate cementum   Incremental line

FIG. 10-12 Histology of cementum on root surface. Horizontal incremental lines in cementum appear similar to those of bone, dentin, or enamel.

PHYSICAL PROPERTIES

As one group of hard connective tissues, cementum contains slightly less mineral than dentin or bone (Table 10-2). Cementum is slightly less hard than dentin. It is yellow and can be distinguished from enamel because cementum, unlike enamel, has no luster. Cementum is slightly lighter in color than dentin, which makes it difficult to distinguish between the two. It is softer than dentin, however, which aids in its identification.

AGING OF CEMENTUM

With aging the relatively smooth surface of cementum becomes more irregular (Fig. 10-11). This is caused by the calcification of some ligament fiber bundles where they were attached to the cementum. Such occurrences appear on most surfaces of cementum, but to no greater

degree near the apical zone. In aging a continuing increase of cementum in the apical zone may obstruct the apical canal (Fig. 10-6).

Microscopically, only the lacunae near the surface may have cells that appear viable, whereas deeper lacunae appear empty. Cementum resorption is one characteristic of aging cementum (Fig. 10-11). Resorption be-

CONSIDER THE PATIENT . . .

An older patient notes that root exposure seems common in her contemporaries. She has also noticed this condition in her son who has periodontal disease. She asks why this condition is shared by both groups of people.

CLINICAL COMMENT

Cellular cementum appears similar to bone in structure but does not contain any nerves. Therefore cementum is nonsensitive. Scaling, when necessary, does not produce pain. However, if cementum is removed, exposure of underlying dentin results in sensitivity.

Table 10-2

Organic and Mineral Composition of Cementum, Dentin, and Bone

Substance	Percentage Organic Material (Collagen)	Percentage Mineral (Calcium, Phosphorus)
Cementum	50-55	45-50
Dentin	30	65.5
Bone	30-35	60-65

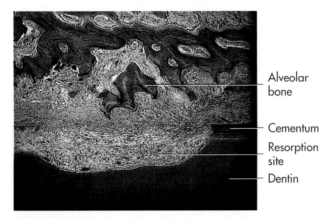

FIG. 10-13 Cemental and dentin resorption with periodontal soft tissue occupying the area. Alveolar bone develops in this space to compensate for root loss. Length of periodontal fibers is thus maintained.

(From Avery JK: *Oral development and histology*, New York, 1994, Thieme Medical.)

Labels: Alveolar bone; Cementum; Resorption site; Dentin

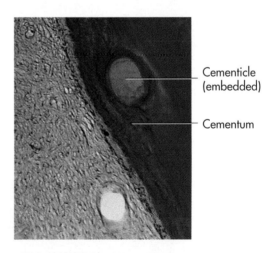

FIG. 10-14 Embedded cementicle. Cementicles may be found as free, attached, or embedded cementicles. They may begin free but gradually become attached and then become deeply embedded in the cementum.

(From Avery JK: *Oral development and histology*, New York, 1994, Thieme Medical.)

Labels: Cementicle (embedded); Cementum

comes active for a period and then may stop. Deposition of cementum occurs in that period, creating reversal lines (Fig. 10-11). Resorption can also occur in root dentin, and cemental repair can cover this defect (Fig. 10-13).

CEMENTICLES

A cementicle is a calcified ovoid or round nodule found in the periodontal ligament. Cementicles may be found singly or in groups near the surface of the cementum (Figs. 10-14 and 10-15). The origin of a cementicle may be a nidus of epithelial cells that are composed of calcium phosphate and collagen in the same amount as cementum (45% to 50% inorganic and 50% to 55% organic). Cementicles may be free in the ligament, attached, or embedded in the cementum (Figs. 10-14 and 10-15). They are more prevalent along the root in an aging person, although they may also be found at a site of trauma.

CEMENTAL REPAIR

Cemental repair is a protective function of the cementoblasts after resorption of root dentin or cementum. These cells are programmed to maintain a smooth surface of the root. Defects arise because of trauma of various kinds, such as traumatic occlusion, tooth movement, and hypereruption caused by the loss of an opposing tooth. Loss of cementum is accompanied by a loss of attachment fibers to the root surface. When this occurs, repair cementum may be deposited by cementoblasts in the defect. After this happens, the attachment fibers readily appear (Fig. 10-11). A cemental deposit means the development of a reversal line. This is seen at the point where resorption stops and deposition begins (Fig. 10-16). Attachment fibers are found embedded in the repair cementum (Fig. 10-11). In an older individual the surface cementum no longer exhibits a smooth surface (Fig. 10-15).

CLINICAL COMMENT

Cementum is resistant to resorption in younger tissues. This is the reason that orthodontic tooth movement results in alveolar bone resorption rather than tooth root loss. Cemental repair is an important root protective mechanism.

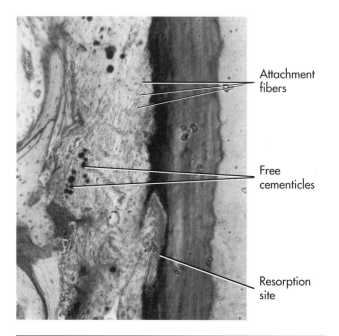

FIG. 10-15 Two groups of free cementicles in periodontal ligament. Resorption area in the cementum is at right.

(From Avery JK: *Oral development and histology,* New York, 1994, Thieme Medical.)

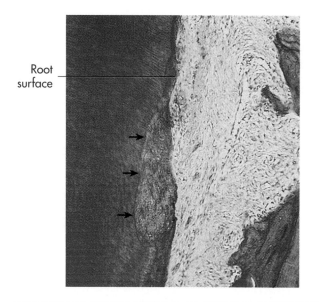

FIG. 10-16 Reversal line in cementum, indicated by arrows. Root surface is again smooth as a result of this deposit.

(From Avery JK: *Oral development and histology,* New York, 1994, Thieme Medical.)

CONSIDER THE PATIENT . . .

Discussion: Root exposure is common in both aging and periodontal disease. In either condition, when there is an apical migration of the epithelial attachment, exposure of cementum and dentin occurs. Pain is associated with exposed dentin and cementum because dentinal tubules open into pulp, where nerves are located. Also, cementum is thin or nonexistent on the cervical root. Patients with root exposure should be careful. Root caries is also common in root exposure. This occurs because the exposed cementum and dentin are less resistant to caries than is enamel. The pain decreases in time because pulpal odontoblasts respond to the stimuli of exposed dentinal tubules with deposition of reparative dentin.

SELF-EVALUATION QUESTIONS

1. What is the origin of intermediate cementum?
2. Where on the root is cementum thinnest and where is it thickest?
3. Name three types of cementicles.
4. Describe the appearance of healed root surfaces.
5. Why is cementum insensitive to pain?
6. What is the function of cementum?
7. What is the origin of cementoblasts and cementocytes?
8. Name two characteristics of aging cementum.
9. What are the percentages that cementum overlaps, meets, or gaps enamel?
10. What are some reasons for cemental resorption?

SUGGESTED READING

Braverman D, Everhardt D, Stoll S: Antigens found in cementum exposed to periodontal disease, *J Periodontol* 59:656, 1979.

Furseth R, Johansen E: The mineral phase of sound and carious human dental cementum studied by electron microscopy, *Acta Odontol Scand* 28:305, 1970.

Jones J, Boyde A: Study of human root cementum as prepared for and examined in the scanning electron microscope, *Z Zellforsch* 130:318, 1972.

Lisodeskog S, Hammerstrom L: Evidence in human teeth of noninvasive factor in cementum or periodontal ligament, *Scand J Dent Res* 88:161, 1980.

Schroeder HE: *Oral structure biology,* New York, 1991, Thieme Medical, pp 187, 290.

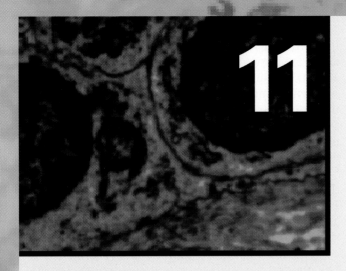

11 Periodontium: Periodontal Ligament

OVERVIEW

The periodontal ligament is a fibrous connective tissue between the alveolar bone proper and the cementum covering the root. This ligament covers the root of the tooth and connects with the tissue of the gingiva. The periodontal ligament occupies the periodontal space and is composed of fibers, cells, and intercellular substance. The latter consists of collagen fibers and ground substance, which in turn contains proteins and polysaccharides. The periodontium develops from dental follicular tissue that surrounds the tooth. The cells forming the ligament fibers, alveolar bone, and cementum develop from the follicle. The periodontium has a thickness of 0.15 to 0.38 mm, is thinnest in the midroot zone, and decreases slightly in thickness with age. The ligament is composed of collagen fiber bundles that attach the cementum to the alveolar bone proper. Interstitial spaces contain the blood vessels and nerve trunks, which communicate freely with vessels and nerves at the apex of the roots and the alveolar bone. This tissue is highly cellular, containing fibro-blasts and vascular, neural, bone, and cemental cells. The primary function of the periodontal ligament is support for the teeth. The ligament also transmits neural input to the masticatory apparatus and has a nutritive function essential to maintaining the liga-ment's health, which has important clinical implications.

ORGANIZATION OF THE PERIODONTAL LIGAMENT

Two groups of principal fibers are named according to their location with respect to the teeth. The **gingival group** is located around the necks of the teeth, and the **dentoalveolar group** surrounds the roots of the teeth (Fig. 11-1). These principal fibers are bundles of collagen fibers strategically positioned at inclinations important to their functions along the root surface from the cervical region to the tooth's apex (Fig. 11-1, *1* to *6*). The collagen bundles are embedded in the cementum of the root and extend into the alveolar bone. Therefore they act as a suspensory ligament for the teeth.

Between each group of fibers is a space termed the **interstitial space** (Fig. 11-2), which is not actually a space. Interstitial spaces contain a network of blood vessels, nerves, and lymphatics that maintain the vitality of the periodontal ligament and a network of finer fibers that interlace in the spaces, as well as support the dense collagen fiber bundles. The interstitial spaces' function relates to the constant stretching and contraction of the fiber bundles during mastication. Most supporting fibers are collagenous, but a few have been described as elastic

like and of a structure different than collagen. These are termed **oxytalan fibers** (Fig. 11-3). Oxytalan fibers are small in diameter and appear to interface with the collagen bundles, supporting the collagen bundles and the blood vessel walls. These are fine, elastic-like fibers that stain with special stains, which reveal their location to be almost longitudinal within the ligament when viewed through a light microscope (Fig. 11-3).

Gingival Fiber Group

The principal fibers of the periodontal ligament in the gingival area are known as the **gingival fibers.** They consist of four groups of fibers, each having a different orientation and all supporting the gingiva (Fig. 11-4). The **free gingival** fibers arise from the surface of the cementum in the cervical region and pass into the free gingiva. The **attached gingival** fibers arise from the alveolar crest and pass into the attached gingiva. The **circular** or **circumferential** fibers are continuous around the neck of the tooth and resist gingival displacement. The **alveolar crest** fibers arise from the cementum at the neck of the tooth and terminate in the alveolar crest. **Transseptal** fibers originate in the cervical region of each crown and extend to similar locations on the

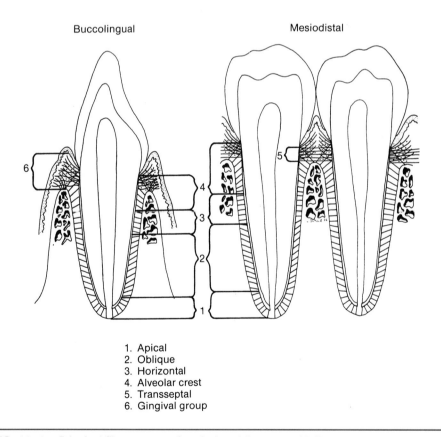

Buccolingual   Mesiodistal

1. Apical
2. Oblique
3. Horizontal
4. Alveolar crest
5. Transseptal
6. Gingival group

FIG. 11- 1 Principal fiber groups of periodontal ligament. All fibers listed in buccolingual plane are also present in mesiodistal plane. Transseptal fiber group number 5, however, is seen only in mesiodistal plane as fibers that are attached tooth to tooth. No other principal fibers are so situated.

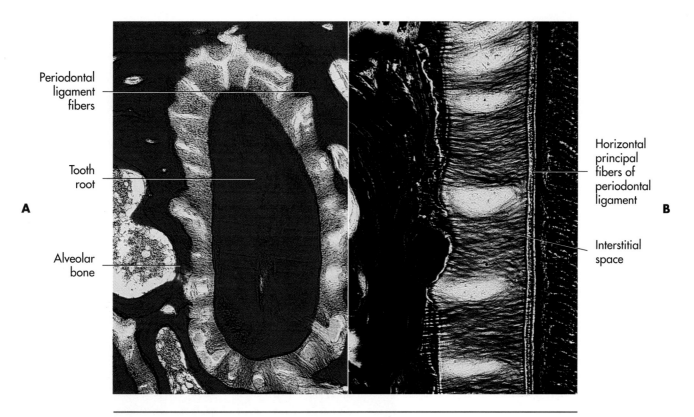

A

B

Periodontal ligament fibers

Tooth root

Alveolar bone

Horizontal principal fibers of periodontal ligament

Interstitial space

FIG. 11-2　**A,** Appearance of principal fiber bundles and interstitial spaces in periodontal ligament as they appear in cross-sectional plane. **B,** Periodontal ligament and interstitial spaces in plane longitudinal to tooth.

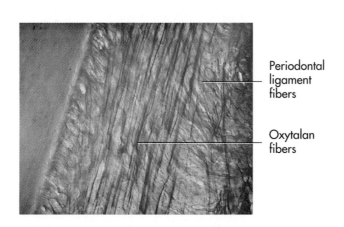

Periodontal ligament fibers

Oxytalan fibers

FIG. 11-3　Histologic appearance of longitudinally oriented oxytalan fibers in periodontal ligament.

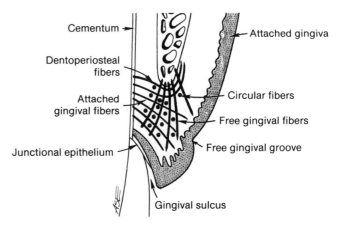

Cementum

Dentoperiosteal fibers

Attached gingival fibers

Junctional epithelium

Attached gingiva

Circular fibers

Free gingival fibers

Free gingival groove

Gingival sulcus

FIG. 11-4　The four groups of gingival fibers. Dentogingival fibers extend from cervical cementum into free and attached gingiva. Alveologingival fibers extend from alveolar crest into gingiva. Circular fibers surround teeth, and dentoperiosteal group extends from cervical cementum into alveolar crest.

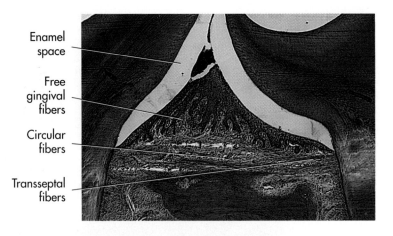

FIG. 11-5 Histology of gingival fibers in interproximal area. Transseptal fiber group extends from mesial of one tooth to distal of adjacent tooth. Relationship of free gingival and circular fibers to transseptal fibers is shown.

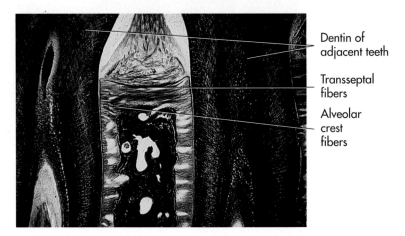

FIG. 11-6 Histology of alveolar crest fibers extending from cementum of cervical region to alveolar bone. Periodontal fibers penetrate alveolar bone, and transseptal fibers extend from tooth on the left to the right.

Table 11-1		
Principal Fibers		
Fiber Group	Location of Attachment	Function
GINGIVAL FIBER GROUP		
Transseptal	Cervical tooth to tooth mesial or distal to it	Resist tooth separation mesial distal
Attached gingival	Cervical tooth to attached gingiva	Resist gingival displacement
Free gingival	Cervical tooth to free gingiva	Resist gingival displacement
Circumferential	Continuous around neck of tooth	Resist gingival displacement
DENTOALVEOLAR FIBER GROUP		
Apical	Apex of root of fundic alveolar bone proper	Resist vertical forces
Oblique	Apical one third of root to adjacent alveolar bone proper	Resist vertical and intrusive forces
Horizontal	Midroot to adjacent alveolar bone proper	Resist horizontal and tipping forces
Alveolar crest	Cervical root to alveolar crest of alveolar bone proper	Resist vertical and intrusive forces
Interradicular	Between roots to alveolar bone proper	Resist vertical and lateral movement

mesial and distal surfaces of each adjacent tooth (Figs. 11-5 and 11-6). This fiber group functions in resistance to the separation of each tooth. Fig. 11-6 shows that transseptal fibers are found in the mesiodistal plane and are not present in the buccolingual plane. All of these fiber groups are illustrated in Fig. 11-1 and listed in Table 11-1.

Dentoalveolar Fiber Group

The dentoalveolar fiber group consists of five differently oriented principal fiber groups named according to their origin and insertion in the dentoalveolar process. The **alveolar crest group** originates at the cervical area, just below the dentinoenamel junction, and extends to the alveolar crest, as well as into the gingival connective tis-

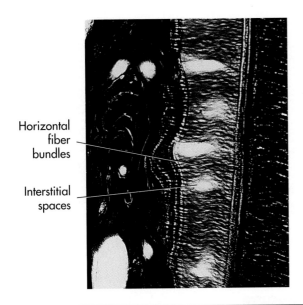

Horizontal fiber bundles

Interstitial spaces

FIG. 11-7 Histologic appearance of horizontal fiber bundles. Observe the bundles perpendicular to root and alveolar bone surface; their perforating fibers are embedded in both the bone and cemental surfaces.

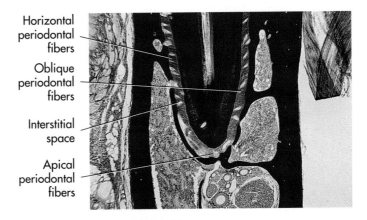

Horizontal periodontal fibers

Oblique periodontal fibers

Interstitial space

Apical periodontal fibers

FIG. 11-8 Histology of horizontal, oblique, and apical fiber groups of periodontal ligament. Angulation is shown for each of these bundle groups, which resist forces of mastication.

sue (Fig. 11-6). These fibers resist intrusive forces. The **horizontal fiber group** extends in a horizontal direction from the midroot cementum to the adjacent alveolar bone proper. These fibers resist tipping of the teeth, as illustrated in Fig. 11-7. The **oblique fiber group** extends in an oblique direction from the area just above the apical zone of the root upward to the alveolar bone (Fig. 11-8), and the fibers resist vertical or intrusive masticatory forces. The **apical fiber group** extends perpendicular from the surface of the root apices to the adjacent **fundic alveolar bone,** which surrounds the apex of the tooth root. Apical fibers resist vertical and extrusive forces applied to the tooth (Fig. 11-8). Another group of fibers that are located between the roots of multirooted teeth is termed **interradicular fibers.** Such fibers extend perpendicular to the tooth's surface and to the adjacent alveolar bone (Fig. 11-9) and resist vertical and lateral forces. For a summary, these fibers are enumerated in Table 11-1.

 CLINICAL COMMENT

Healthy periodontal tissues are of significant importance to the health of dental patients. Chronic periodontal disease and dental caries can lead to infusion of bacteria into the bloodstream.

Interstitial Spaces

The principal fibers make up the structural and functional bulk of the periodontal ligament. They are positioned at regular intervals along the gingival-apical extent of the periodontal ligament. Between each bundle of ligament fibers an interstitial space appears. These spaces appear in both the cross-sectional and longitudinal planes of the ligament (Fig. 11-2). The regularity of these spaces clearly relates to the vascular and neural needs of the functioning ligament. Interstitial spaces appear designed to carry these vascular and neural structures both by encircling the tooth at regular intervals and by connecting with the vessels that run longitudinal to the root (Figs. 11-10 and 11-11). These interstitial spaces are designed to withstand the impact of masticatory forces. The collagenous fiber bundles that surround these spaces are arranged at angles to the surfaces of the spaces, providing support for their maintenance. These spaces are compressed during mastication or tension, as noted in Fig. 11-12. For this reason, their position and support by fiber bundles are important. A network of fine fibers within these spaces can be seen supporting the nerves and nerve endings that occupy these spaces (Figs. 11-13 and 11-14).

Vascular System

The periodontal ligament has a rich blood supply that arises from the inferior and superior alveolar arteries and from branches of the facial artery from the external carotid. These vessels supply the alveolar bone and anastomose freely with the periodontal ligament. The vascular plexus that extends into the ligament traverses from the apical areas to the gingival areas with loops that surround the teeth at regular intervals (Fig. 11-10, *B*). Fig. 11-10, *A,* shows the density and complexity of the liga-

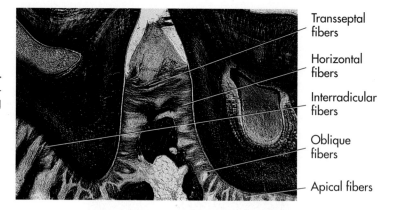

FIG. 11-9 Histology of interradicular fiber groups located between roots and alveolar bone of multirooted teeth.

Transseptal fibers

Horizontal fibers

Interradicular fibers

Oblique fibers

Apical fibers

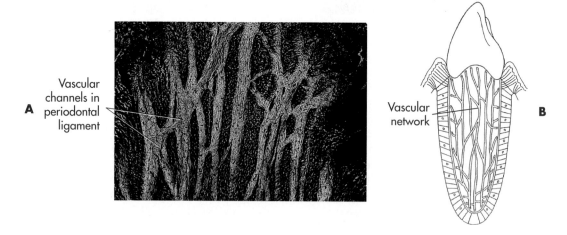

Vascular channels in periodontal ligament

A

Vascular network

B

FIG. 11-10 **A,** Histology of periodontal ligament in longitudinal plane, showing continuity of the interstitial system in center of ligament with lateral connections throughout circumferential interstitial spaces. **B,** Diagram of organized network of blood vessels in ligament. Both arteries (white) and veins (black) vascularize ligament.

FIG. 11-11 Vascular supply of alveolar bone, periodontal ligament, and tooth pulp as seen after injection of vessels with carbon and clearing of the tissues. Bone is on left, periodontal ligament in center, dentin to the right of center, and pulp on right.

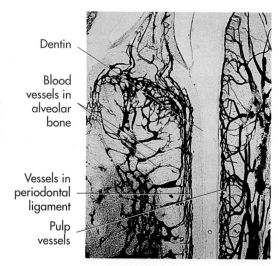

Dentin

Blood vessels in alveolar bone

Vessels in periodontal ligament

Pulp vessels

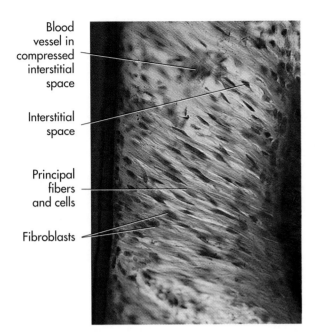

Blood vessel in compressed interstitial space

Interstitial space

Principal fibers and cells

Fibroblasts

FIG. 11-12 Histology of periodontal ligament illustrating tension. Note diminished interstitial spaces and flattening of cells when fibers are stretched.

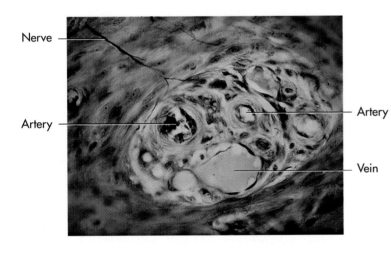

Nerve

Artery

Artery

Vein

FIG. 11-13 Interstitial space viewed at high magnification. At upper left, nerve enters interstitial space from ligament. Within interstitial space are the thick-walled artery and thin-walled veins. Beside the artery and veins are several nerve trunks.

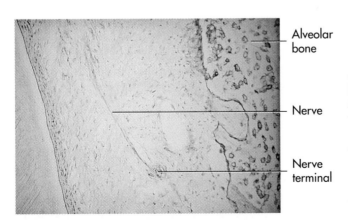

Alveolar bone

Nerve

Nerve terminal

FIG. 11-14 A nerve trunk traversing periodontal ligament along surface of alveolar bone on right. At lower extremity of the trunk is an encapsulated pressure receptor (modified pacinian). These pressure receptor endings sense density of food during mastication.

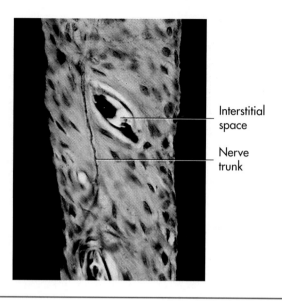

Interstitial space

Nerve trunk

FIG. 11-15 Nerve trunk passing from apical region toward gingival area. Fibers of periodontal ligament wrap around interstitial space.

ment. When the alveolar bone and tooth have been sectioned and the vascular plexus has been injected with carbon particles and then cleared, the orientation and relationship of these vessels can be demonstrated (Fig. 11-11). Both arterioles and venules traverse these tissues, carrying blood to and away from them. Arteriovenous shunts have been demonstrated in the periodontal ligaments that provide direct connections between the arterial and venous blood supply without having to go through a capillary network. Capillaries are evident throughout the principal fiber bundles. The ligament is highly active, undergoing compaction and extension as mastication takes place. Evidence of the ligament activity is seen in cell turnover, in its ability to modify in tooth movement, and in its ability to heal. These conditions relate to the rich vascular supply of the ligament.

CLINICAL COMMENT

The suspensory apparatus of the teeth is organized to protect the blood vessels from undue compression. Pressure receptors in the ligament are thus protective during mastication.

Neural System

The larger nerve trunks of the periodontal ligament are found in the central zone of the tooth's long axis (Fig. 11-15). Branches of these trunks pass into the ligament and alveolar bone at intervals along the path to the gingival tissues. Most nerve trunks and finer nerves are ob-

served in the interstitial spaces, either in the tracts that traverse the ligament longitudinal to the tooth's surface or within any of the spaces between bundles along the root (Fig. 11-13). Nerve terminals are noted throughout the ligament and especially in bundles of principal fibers. Encapsulated pressure receptors and aciniform, fine pain receptors are in greatest numbers (Fig. 11-14). These terminals are known to function during masticatory activity.

CLINICAL COMMENT

Maintaining normal tissue vitality through disease prevention and constant maintenance is important. Oral health is dependent on the combination of professional care and patient participation.

CELLS OF PERIODONTAL LIGAMENT

Fibroblasts, Osteoblasts, and Cementoblasts

Several types of cells located in the ligament have formative, supportive, and resorptive functions. **Fibroblasts** are the most numerous seen in the periodontal ligament because of the high collagen density of this tissue. The abundance of fibroblasts allows rapid replacement of fibers (Fig. 11-12). Recent investigations show that fibroblasts, in addition to forming new collagen fibers, function in the breakdown of worn-out fibers. Fibers are ingested and broken down into amino acids. These amino acids are taken up by other cells and recycled into the formation of new collagen fibers. **Osteoblasts** are located along the surface of the alveolar bone. As bone is continually turning over, the osteoblasts are busy forming new bone in the area of the alveolar bone proper. All osteoblasts differentiate locally from mesenchymal cells as the need for osteoblasts arises. **Cementoblasts** appear along the surface of the cementum. Cementum is constantly being formed as new principal fibers are embedded along the root surface. Cemental resorption may also occur for a number of reasons, such as changes in occlusal relationships or tooth movement, resulting in new cementoblasts becoming active in the repair of resorbed cementum or dentin of the root.

Macrophages and Osteoclasts

Macrophages found in the ligament are important defense cells in this location. Macrophages have mobility, as well as phagocytic function. They take up dead cells, bacteria, and foreign bodies. Some fibroblasts become macrophagic in the periodontal ligament because they have the ability to destroy collagen, as well as form it (Fig. 11-16). This activity relates to the high metabolic function of the periodontal ligament. Two types

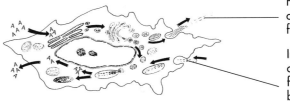

Formation
of new
fibers

Ingestion
of collagen
fibers and
breakdown
into amino
acids

FIG. 11-16 Fibroblasts are present in periodontal ligament in great numbers. It is probable that some of these cells function in forming as well as destroying collagen fibers as need arises.

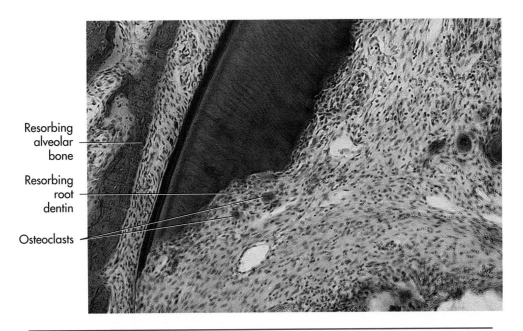

Resorbing
alveolar
bone

Resorbing
root
dentin

Osteoclasts

FIG. 11-17 Osteoclastic action on alveolar bone and on root dentin can be seen in this micrograph. Tooth roots *(at left)* and alveolar bone *(at right)* are undergoing resorption in preparation for eruption of tooth in permanent dentition. In lower right corner is a follicle surrounding erupting permanent tooth crown. Osteoclasts are much larger than any other cell in field.

of fibroblasts may exist—those that only form collagen and those that form and destroy collagen. Macrophages, lymphocytes, leukocytes, and plasma cells may also appear in the periodontium when it is stressed by disease.

Osteoclasts, in instances of both tooth movement and periodontal disease, may function in bone resorption (Fig. 11-17). They appear as a normal consequence of tipping or bodily movement of a tooth (Fig. 11-18). Osteoclasts originate from monocytes within the blood vascular system and become multinucleated cells seen in lacunae of resorption sites in hard tissue (Fig. 11-17).

Epithelial Rests

Epithelial rests are normal constituents of the periodontal ligament and are seen throughout life. Epithelial cells are scattered throughout the ligament, but in the early life of the tooth they are seen along the root surface. Epithelial rests may appear as resting, proliferating, or de-

generating cell masses. They also may be characterized as going through extensive periods of dormancy. These rests are composed of a mass of epithelial cells, some four to six in number, although there may be more in cases where they are proliferating. The cells are believed to originate in the remnants of the root sheath. However, epithelial rests may continue to proliferate from the epithelial cells lining the gingival crevice. They can be observed along the root surface as seen in Fig. 11-19.

Intercellular Tissue

Intercellular tissue surrounds and protects the cells of the periodontal ligament and is the product of these cells. This extracellular matrix (ECM) is composed of water, glycoproteins, and proteoglycans, which surround the collagen fibers. These protein and polysaccharide substances provide the cells with vital substances that arise from the blood capillaries and return catabolites from these cells to the vessels.

FIG. 11-18   Diagram of tooth tipping that may occur in orthodontic tooth movement or naturally as a result of malocclusion. As tooth crown moves to left, root moves to right. As ligament zones marked *A* are compressed, zones marked *B* are stretched. Osteoclasts appear in *A* zones, accompanying bone resorption, and osteoblasts will appear in *B* zones with bone formation.

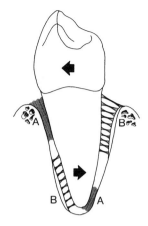

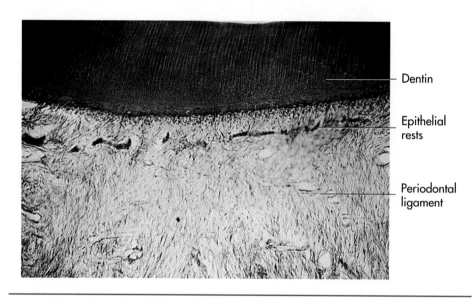

Dentin

Epithelial rests

Periodontal ligament

FIG. 11-19   Epithelial rests appear in periodontal ligament near the cementum covering dentin at the top of the micrograph. This is a young specimen; thus rests are large and distinctive.

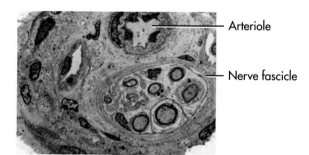

Arteriole

Nerve fascicle

FIG. 11-20   Ultrastructure of an interstitial space with nerve bundle *(lower right)* and arterioles *(above)*.

FUNCTIONS OF PERIODONTAL LIGAMENT

Supportive

The most important function of the periodontal ligament is support of the teeth. Failure of this function results in tooth loss. Every time the teeth are clenched, as in mastication, the periodontal fibers are stretched and then relaxed. This system is highly efficient to compensate for the thousands of times this ligament is called into action.

Sensory

The periodontal ligament is supplied with abundant receptors and nerves that sense any movement in function. When receptors sense pressure, the nerves send signals to the brain, which informs the masticatory apparatus, including the temporomandibular joint and muscles of mastication.

Nutritive

The blood vessels of the ligament provide the essential nutrients for the ligament's vitality and for the hard tissue of cementum and alveolar bone. All cells, such as fibroblasts, osteoblasts, cementoblasts, and even the resorptive osteoclasts and macrophage cells, require the nutrition that is carried by the blood vessels of the ligament (Fig. 11-20).

When an orthodontic appliance or an occlusal problem causes compaction and compression, a constriction of the blood vessels may occur. This results in a lack of vascular continuity, which leads to a diminishing of cells in the area, and the tissue becomes ischemic. The tissue then begins to appear glasslike and is described as a "hyalinized" area. Continued pressure usually leads to the appearance of osteoclasts at this site, with the loss of alveolar bone. This condition then may create space for blood vessels to grow back into this area. The periodontium therefore responds as a coordinated unit.

Maintenance

Periodontal tissues function in maintenance of the masticatory apparatus because these tissues heal readily. The interaction of the mesenchymal cells with their intercellular environment is a continuous process. These tissues function for a lifetime if health is maintained and appropriate care is provided.

CONSIDER THE PATIENT . . .

A patient asks about prevention of periodontal disease. What can the patient do to prevent a future problem?

CLINICAL COMMENT

Renewal capability is an important characteristic of the periodontal ligament fibers. The periodontal fibroblasts provide maintenance of the system when repair is needed.

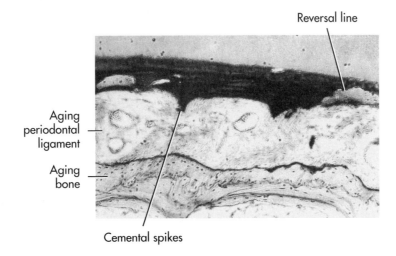

Reversal line

Aging periodontal ligament

Aging bone

Cemental spikes

FIG. 11-21   Aging periodontal ligament, cementum, and alveolar bone. Number of fiber bundles has decreased. Cemental and bone spikes are shown, which are caused by excessive deposition around depleted fiber bundles.

AGING OF LIGAMENT

Aging occurs in ligamentous tissue as in all other tissues of the body. Cell number and cell activity decrease as aging takes place. In aging cementum and alveolar bone, scalloping occurs (Fig. 11-21). Some fibers are attached to the peaks of these scallops rather than over the entire surface. This is one of the more remarkable changes that occur in the aging of supporting structures of the teeth. Activity of these tissues is likely to decrease during the aging process because of restricted diets, and therefore normal functional stimulation of these tissues is diminished. With aging a healthier periodontium can result from general good health of the individual and good oral hygiene. A loss of gingival height related to gingival and periodontal disease promotes destructive changes. Unfortunately, at that time, the presence of a low-grade inflammation may be characteristic of the gingival tissue.

SELF-EVALUATION QUESTIONS

1. Describe the function and location of the principal fiber groups in the gingival group.
2. Describe the function and location of the principal fiber groups in the dentoalveolar group.
3. Describe the function and location of the interstitial system of the periodontal ligament.
4. Describe the vascular system of the periodontal ligament.
5. Describe the types and locations of the nerves and nerve endings in the periodontal tissues.
6. Name the cells and their functions in the periodontal ligament.
7. What are the three types of epithelial cell rests, and where are they found?
8. Discuss the several functions of the periodontal ligament.
9. What are oxytalan fibers, and what are their function and location?
10. Describe the characteristics of aging in the periodontal ligament.

CONSIDER THE PATIENT . . .

Discussion: The patient's role is very important. Patients assist the dental professional in the maintenance of the periodontal structures. These tissues are very susceptible to poor oral hygiene, and therefore deterioration of the periodontium results.

SUGGESTED READING

Bonucci E: New knowledge on the origin, function and fate of osteoclasts, *Clin Orthop* 158:252, 1982.

Jones SJ, Boyde AA: Study of human root cementum surfaces as prepared for and examined in the scanning electron microscope, *Z Zellforsch* 130:318, 1972.

Marchi F: Secretory granules in cells producing fibrillar collagen. In Davidovich Z, editor: *The biological mechanisms of tooth eruption and root resorption*, Birmingham, Ala, 1988, EBESCO Media, pp 53-59.

Marks SC, Jr: The origin of osteoclasts; evidence of clinical applications and investigative challenges of an extraskeletal source, *J Oral Pathol* 12:226, 1983.

Melcher AH: Periodontal ligament. In Bhaskar SN, editor: *Orban's oral histology and embryology*, ed 10, St Louis, 1986, Mosby.

Nakamura TK, Hanal H, Nakamura MT: Ultrastructure of encapsulated nerve terminals in human periodontal ligaments, *J Oral Biol* 24:126, 1982.

Schroeder HE: *Oral structure biology*, New York, 1991, Thieme Medical, pp 187, 290.

Ten Cate AR, Deporter DA: The role of the fibroblast in collagen turnover in the functioning periodontal ligament of the mouse, *Arch Oral Biol* 19:339, 1974.

Ten Cate AR, Mills C: The development of the periodontium: the origin of alveolar bone, *Anat Rec* 173:69, 1972.

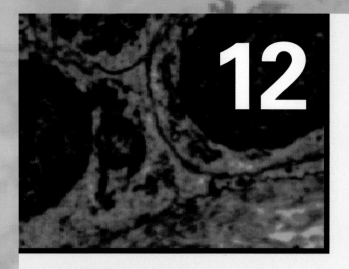

12

Periodontium: Alveolar Process and Cementum

OVERVIEW

This chapter describes the hard tissues of the periodontium, which are cementum and alveolar bone. The alveolar process is the bony part of the maxilla and mandible that has the primary function of supporting the teeth. Alveolar bone is composed of alveolar bone proper, which is attached to the fibers embedded in the roots of the teeth. Supporting bone is the bone covering the mandible, and it serves as cortical plates that give support to the alveolar bone proper. This alveolar bone is in the process of continuous turnover, which enables the tissue to be responsive to manipulation, such as tooth movement resulting from normal physiologic function or orthodontic treatment. Cementum functions as the means of fiber attachment to the tooth roots. These fibers have the ability to form and resorb, which are necessary for support during tooth movement. If teeth are moving in a straight line or rotating, all parts of the suspensory apparatus must change simultaneously. This phenomenon first took place during tooth eruption and continues to function for both the primary and secondary dentition. Tooth function is a prerequisite for the maintenance of the alveolar bone and cementum. Bone loss occurs during aging or periods of inactivity, resulting in possible tooth mobilization. With loss of alveolar bone, loss of periodontal fibers occurs as well. Periodontal disease can cause these conditions with possible tooth loss that could result in an edentulous jaw.

ALVEOLAR PROCESS

The alveolar process is the part of the maxilla and mandible that supports the roots of teeth and is composed of **alveolar bone proper** and **supporting bone** (Fig. 12-1). Alveolar bone proper is the bone lining the tooth socket. In clinical radiographic terms it is defined as the **lamina dura**. Dense bone serves as the attachment bone that surrounds the roots of the teeth. Supporting bone is, as the name implies, the bone that serves as a dense cortical plate to sustain the alveolar bone proper. This cortical plate covers the surface of the maxilla and mandible and supports the alveolar bone proper. The supporting cancellous bone underlies and supports the dense cortical bone (Figs. 12-1 and 12-2). The existence of alveolar bone is entirely dependent upon the presence of teeth. Alveolar bone develops initially as a protection to the soft developing teeth and later, as the roots develop, as a support to the teeth. Finally, as the teeth are lost, the alveolar bone resorbs. Teeth are responsible not only for the development but also for the maintenance of the alveolar process of the mandible (see Fig. 3-21). The coronal border of the alveolar process is known as the **alveolar crest** (Fig. 12-2). This crest is normally located approximately 1.2 to 1.5 mm below the dentinoenamel junction of the teeth. It is rounded on the anterior region and nearly flat in the molar area. When teeth are in buccolingual version, the alveolar crest may be thin or missing. The area of bone loss where an apical root penetrates the cortical bone is known as a **fenestration**, and bone loss in the coronal area of the root is termed a **dehiscence** (Fig. 12-3).

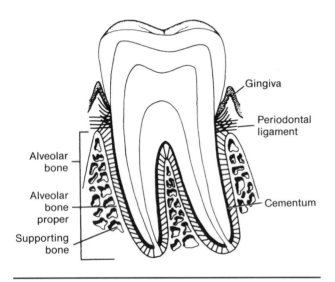

FIG. 12-1 Alveolar bone proper, supporting bone, and cementum of periodontium.

CLINICAL COMMENT

The lamina dura is an important diagnostic landmark in determining the health of the periapical tissues. Loss of density usually means infection, inflammation, and resorption of this bony socket lining.

Alveolar Bone Proper

The compact or dense bone that lines the tooth socket is of two types when viewed microscopically. This bone either contains perforating fibers from the periodontal ligament or is similar to compact bone found elsewhere in the body. Perforating fibers or **Sharpey's fibers** are bundles of collagen fibers embedded in the alveolar bone proper. These fibers are at right angles or oblique to the surface of the alveolar bone proper and along the root of the tooth (Fig. 12-1). The fiber bundles inserting in the bone are regularly spaced and appear similar to

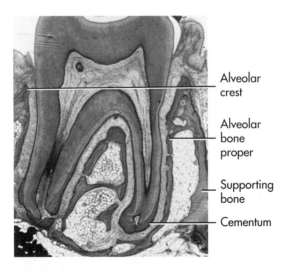

FIG. 12-2 Histology of tooth and its supportive tissues showing relationships among alveolar bone proper, supporting bone, and cementum covering roots.

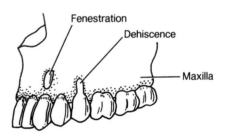

FIG. 12-3 Loss of alveolar bone adjacent to tooth. Loss near root apices is termed fenestration, whereas bone loss in region of cervical root is termed dehiscence.

those that insert into the root surface cementum (Figs. 12-4 and 12-5). These perforating fibers are not limited to periodontal bone. They also appear in the body where ligaments or tendons attach to cartilage or bone.

Because bone of the alveolar process is regularly penetrated by collagen fiber bundles, it can be appropriately termed bundle bone. Bundle bone, being synonymous with alveolar bone proper or lamina dura, appears more dense radiographically than the adjacent supportive bone (Fig. 12-6). This density is probably due to the mineral content or orientation of the bone crystals surrounding the fiber bundles. Blood vessels and nerves penetrate the lamina dura through small foramina. Because the mineral density is sufficient, this bone appears opaque in radiographs (Fig. 12-6). Tension on the perforating fibers during mastication is believed to stimulate this bone and is considered important in its maintenance.

Not all alveolar bone proper appears as bundle bone because the bone lining the socket is constantly being remodeled for adaptation to the stresses of occlusal impact. Newly formed bone does not have perforating fibers (Fig. 12-7). Teeth are constantly moving (drifting) within their sockets, resulting in loss of some fibers. Other fibers continually form and initially attach to the bone's surface and later become embedded.

Supporting Compact Bone

Supporting compact bone of the alveolar process is similar to **haversian bone** found elsewhere in the body (Fig.

12-8). Compact bone of the alveolar process extends over the lingual surface of the mandible and maxilla beside the tongue. Compact bone also covers the buccal surface of the mandible or maxilla adjacent to the lining of the cheek. Compact or cortical bone contains osteons with radiating lamellae accentuated by lacunae, which contain the osteocytes in living bone (Fig. 12-9). Haversian and Volkmann's canals form a continuous system of nutrient canals that radiate throughout the bone. The haversian canals extend through the long axis of the bone, and Volkmann's canals enter haversian canals at

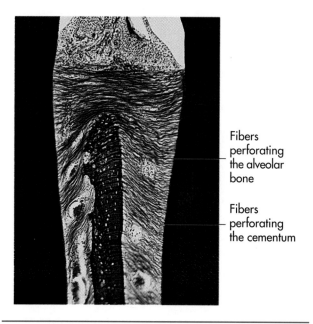

Fibers perforating the alveolar bone

Fibers perforating the cementum

FIG. 12-5 Histology of perforating fiber bundles (Sharpey's). Uniformity of position of numerous fibers in cemental and bony surfaces is shown. Fiber bundles of bone are larger and less numerous than fibers entering cemental surface.

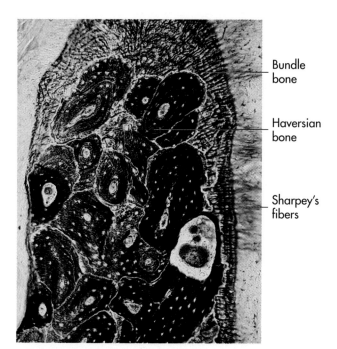

Bundle bone

Haversian bone

Sharpey's fibers

FIG. 12-4   Histology of alveolar crest area illustrating bundle bone with penetrating (Sharpey's) fibers and haversian-type supporting bone.

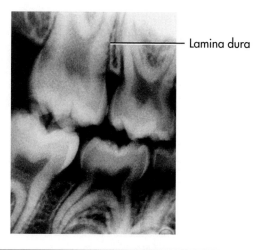

Lamina dura

FIG. 12-6   Radiograph of alveolar bone illustrating lamina dura, the radiodense bone lining tooth sockets.

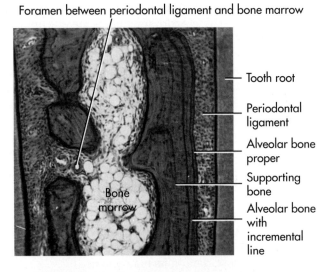

FIG. 12-7 Histology of alveolar bone proper and supporting bone. Foramina communicate between periodontal ligament and marrow spaces in supporting bone on the left.

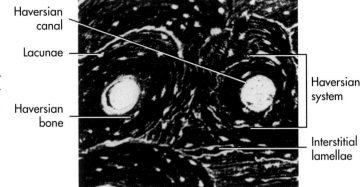

FIG. 12-8 Micrograph of alveolar bone showing concentric haversian system, interstitial lamellae, and lacunae.

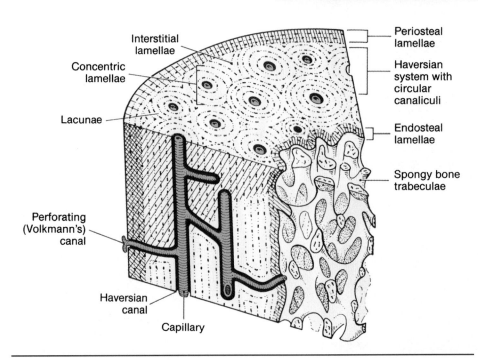

FIG. 12-9 Diagram of haversian systems of compact bone similar to compact bone throughout body. Periosteal lamellae cover the surface of mandible and numerous haversian systems containing blood vessels interconnected by Volkmann's canals. Lacunae containing osteocytes surround the haversian canals.

right angles. These canals form a nutrient network throughout bone. Bone cells or osteocytes are present in many of the lacunae and provide the maintenance and viability of the bone (Fig. 12-9).

Supporting Cancellous Bone

The cancellous or spongy bone supporting the alveolar bone proper of the alveolar process is composed generally of heavy trabeculae or plates of bone with bone marrow spaces between them. Bone marrow contains blood-forming elements, osteogenic cells, and adipose tissues (Fig. 12-7). The supporting bone of the maxilla in particular is filled with marrow tissue, which contains immature red blood cells and leukocytes, especially in the molar region posterior to the maxillary sinus. Bone marrow, found in bones throughout the body, is one of the largest organs in the body and represents approximately 4.5% of body weight.

CEMENTAL SUPPORT

Cementum functions as a support by attaching to perforating fibers of the periodontal ligament at the root surface. The surface of cementum functions like bundle bone because the perforating fibers cover the entire surface of the roots (Fig. 12-5). Some areas of the cementum are inactive, with the absence of fiber bundles, or they undergo surface resorption (Fig. 12-10). The collagen fiber bundles of cementum are smaller in size but more numerous than the bundles of alveolar bone proper (Fig. 12-5). The principal fiber bundle system of the periodontal ligament is balanced in function, although distributed differently on the two surfaces.

One characteristic of the two surfaces, bone and cementum, is their ability to resorb and later to rebuild hard tissue. Cementum is more resistant to resorption than bone, hence the ability to move teeth through bone without the loss of the tooth surface. Some investigators claim that an autoinvasive factor in cementum contributes to this resistance. Other investigators believe the absence of a blood supply in cementum, unlike bone, is important to this resistance. The distribution of penetrating fibers over the surface of the cementum could also relate to resorption. Cementum will resorb, as will dentin, in cases of stress caused by traumatic occlusion or of tooth movement resulting from drift or orthodontic treatment. During exfoliation of primary teeth, root loss is considered a normal process. This process of normal physiologic root and cemental resorption is due to permanent tooth eruption.

TOOTH MOVEMENT

Physiologic movement

The eruptive process involves major remodeling of the alveolar process to compensate for root growth and changes in positional relations of the primary and permanent teeth. Repositioning of teeth occurs, for example, during facial growth. Movement occurs in facial and buccal directions as the arches increase in dimension (Fig. 12-11). The height of the alveolus changes in relation to root growth as part of the facial growth process. Accommodation is made for increased dimension of the permanent teeth. In one situation, **leeway space** (Fig. 12-12) is created in the arches by the replacement of larger primary molars by smaller permanent premolars.

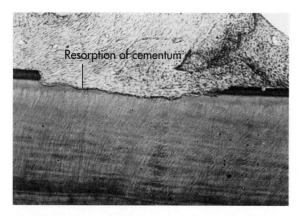

FIG. 12-10 Cemental loss by resorption, which has also destroyed adjacent alveolar bone.

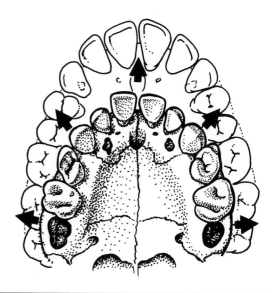

FIG. 12-11 Growth of face results in migration of teeth laterally and anteriorly with an increasing dimension of arch posteriorly as permanent molars develop and erupt.

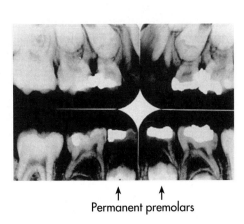

Permanent premolars

FIG. 12-12 Radiograph of permanent premolars replacing primary molars. Smaller premolar produces leeway space in arch.

(Courtesy Dr DC Johnson. From Avery JK: *Oral development and histology*, New York, 1994, Thieme Medical.)

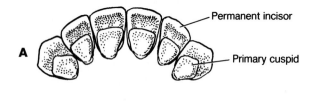

Permanent incisor

Primary cuspid

A

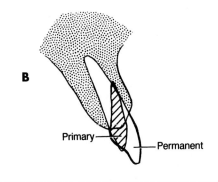

B

Primary — Permanent

FIG. 12-13 **A,** Comparison of interdental spacing of primary and permanent incisor teeth. **B,** Inclination comparison of anterior primary and permanent teeth.

This important situation helps compensate for the **incisor liability factor,** which is the replacement of the smaller primary incisors with larger permanent ones (Fig. 12-13). Part of this increase is compensated by the inclination of the permanent incisors (Fig. 12-13, *B*). Also important is **mesial drift,** a significant occurrence during the mixed dentition period. When the teeth are clenched during normal masticatory function, an ante-

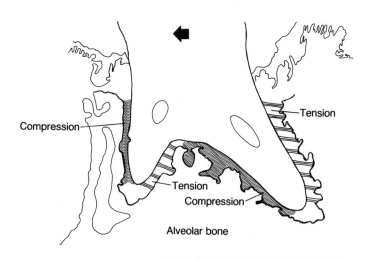

Compression

Tension

Tension

Compression

Alveolar bone

FIG. 12-14 Tooth movement to left with zones of compression along advancing root surface and tension along trailing root surface.

rior force is exerted on the teeth because most cusps are inclined anteriorly and their occlusal inclined planes therefore produce an anterior force. This is due in part to proximal wear. Summation of these forces defines the principle of mesial drift of the teeth. The alveolar process compensates for tooth-related factors, such as increased arch size, as well as effects of occlusal function. The effect of tooth loss or hypereruption is mesial drift, which can result in disruption of normal occlusal function.

  CONSIDER THE PATIENT . . .

A patient asks what would occur if cementum were more easily resorbable than alveolar bone.

Orthodontic movement

Tooth movement by orthodontics is possible only if bone resorption takes place in the direction in which the tooth is being moved. Such movement causes pressure on the surface of the alveolar bone in the direction of tooth movement. Tooth movement also causes tension on the periodontal ligament on the opposite surface of the root. These stresses cause activation of cells and changes in the vascular and neural tissue along the bone and cemental surfaces that are mediated through the periodontal ligament (Fig. 12-14). The alveolar bone and cementum show remarkable ability to be modified. As bone resorption occurs on one surface of the lamina dura, or bone lining the socket, the tooth is allowed to move in that direction and bone consequently forms on

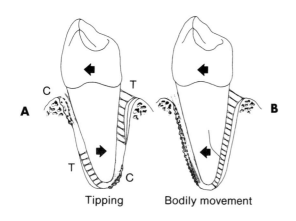

FIG. 12-15 Tipping of tooth crown to left causes root to compress *(C)* the ligament at upper left and lower right. Tension *(T)* occurs at upper right and lower left. Bodily movement *(B)* of crown and root to left causes compression on ligament, bone resorption along entire surface of advancing root, and bone formation of tension surface on right.

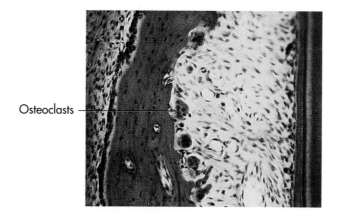

FIG. 12-16 Histology of compression zone of periodontal ligament. Osteoclasts remove bone to relieve compression.

CLINICAL COMMENT

The rate of mesial drift varies from 0.05 to 0.7 mm per year. This may be related to dietary factors and age.

the opposite side of the socket. This stabilizes the tooth in a new position.

For example, if a tooth is tipped, as in Fig. 12-15, *A*, several areas of the periodontium are compressed and several exhibit tension. The **tipping** movement is necessary to accomplish the change in occlusion desired. Pressure applied on a specific point on the tooth causes compression in a limited area between the root and the bone. However, a tooth may need to be moved by **bodily movement,** in which case the root is moved in the same direction, affecting the entire surface of the socket. Compression changes occur in the ligament along the advancing root surface, and tension changes occur in the ligament fibers, bone, and cementum along the opposite surface (Fig. 12-15, *B*). The situation is the same whether a single-rooted tooth or a multiple-rooted tooth is involved. In the multiple-rooted tooth, movement is complicated by the bifurcation bone, which has the additional bony surface related to pressure and tension (see Fig. 12-4).

When compression is too great or too rapid, it causes **hyalinization** of the ligament. The vascularity is excluded, and the ligament appears colorless or "hyalinized." Tooth movement is limited by the rate of resorption, meaning cells that respond to the needs of com-

pression and tension must be mobilized. On the compression surface, bone removal is requisite, so the osteoclasts must become organized. These cells originate from monocytes in the bloodstream. The osteoclasts organize rapidly, appearing within a few hours after tooth movement begins (Fig. 12-16).

Bone loss may occur on the bony surface of the socket, the cementum of the root surface, or both. This action may be reversed by deposition of bone or cementum in the area of resorption. The process of deposition in a resorption zone is known as an **area of reversal.** The area where deposition begins, in this site, is termed a **reversal line.**

On the tension side of the root, collagen fibers appear stretched and the cells become oriented in the direction of the tension (Fig. 12-17). As this occurs, the force of tension is transmitted into a biologic force characterized by the appearance of cells that are responsive to these needs. Fibroblasts, osteoclasts, and cementoblasts arise from mesenchymal cells in this area and begin to function. Many fibroblasts are present that function in collagen renewal. Osteoblasts, in turn, synthesize bone proteins necessary for producing osteoid. These osteoblasts also mineralize the bone matrix. As tension continues, bone develops along the alveolar bone and cemental surfaces around the stretched perforating fibers (Fig. 12-18).

Other types of tooth movement include **rotation** and a combination of tipping and rotation. In addition, **intrusion** or **extrusion** of a tooth may be necessary. Fig. 12-19 illustrates a case of tooth movement over the long term. Fingerlike projections of bone follow the path of tooth movement. This bone growth is a result of tension. The principles of compression and tension are similar in all cases. The plasticity of the alveolar process is remarkable.

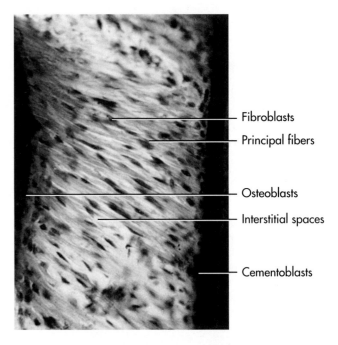

FIG. 12-17 Histology of tension zone of periodontal ligament. Stretched fibers and a number of osteoblasts and cementoblasts are along surface of hard tissue.

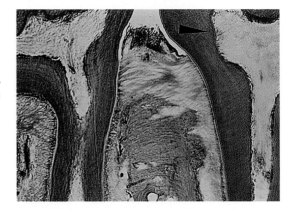

FIG. 12-18 Interproximal zone of two molar teeth. Tooth movement to right *(arrowhead)* causes compression of ligament on left and tension on right. Bone formation appears along alveolar bone on right as a result.

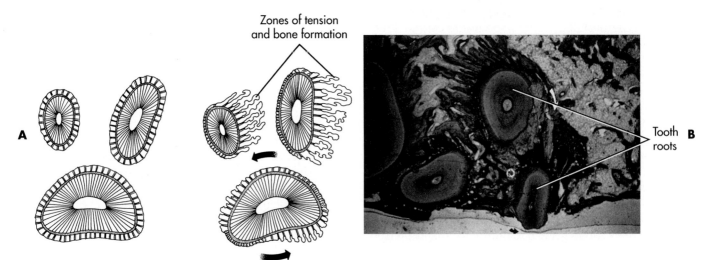

FIG. 12-19 **A,** Rotation of maxillary molar. Large lower root moves less than upper two roots. Bone forms along trailing root surfaces, and resorption occurs on advancing bony surface. **B,** Histology of rotation of maxillary molar illustrating loss of bone along advancing surfaces and bone formation along tension (trailing) surfaces. In addition to rotation, tooth is moving away from zone of tension.

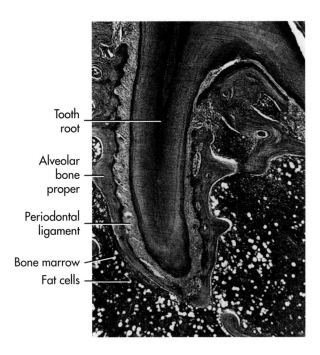

Tooth root

Alveolar bone proper

Periodontal ligament

Bone marrow

Fat cells

FIG. 12-20 Histology of aging alveolar bone illustrating scalloping of alveolar bone proper and infiltration of fat cells in marrow spaces.

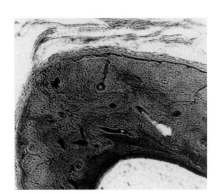

FIG. 12-21 Histology of edentulous ridge after loss of tooth-bearing alveolar bone. Compact bone of mandible is dense. This bone shows little evidence of osteoporosis.

 CLINICAL COMMENT

Patients may be concerned about tooth mobility even when it is within normal limits. The mobility of individual teeth varies. Teeth are slightly more mobile in the morning than later in the day.

AGING OF ALVEOLAR BONE AND CEMENTUM

A comparison of young and old alveolar bone reveals a shift with age from dense bone and smooth-walled sockets to osteoporotic bone and sockets with rough, jagged walls. Aging brings bone loss with fewer fiber bundles being inserted in the bone and cementum. Hard tissue then forms around the fibers in support of these bundles, creating a scalloped surface (Fig. 12-20). During aging fewer viable cells are in the lacunae and the marrow spaces become infiltrated with fat cells. Osteoporosis then becomes more apparent, and the support of the teeth is further diminished.

EDENTULOUS JAWS

Several facts are known about the loss of teeth, although much remains to be learned about changes in the bony alveolar process after tooth loss. First, it is recognized that alveolar bone volume decreases. This is evident from the general loss of the alveolar process with tooth extraction. Next some loss of the internal structure of the bone occurs, resulting in open spaces and fewer trabeculae in the cancellous supporting bone (Fig. 12-21). Osteoporosis may then become more evident. Little change occurs in the location of blood vessels, nerves, glands, and fatty zone in the aging edentulous jaws or in dense compact bone of the mandible beneath the alveolar bone (Fig. 12-21).

CLINICAL COMMENT

Tooth movement can be monitored through radiographic examination, and changes in the interproximal bone density or dimension can also be evaluated. The orthodontist depends on this type of information to follow bone formation and resorption. Radiographs of the hard tissues are also useful in evaluating aging changes. Recognizing changes in the color of the gingival and alveolar mucosa is another valuable index of tissue health.

SELF-EVALUATION QUESTIONS

1. The cortical plates are described as what type of bone?
2. What is the origin of osteoclasts and osteoblasts, and how rapidly can they be mobilized?
3. Define mesial drift and describe some consequences of its occurrence.
4. What is a reversal line and how is it evidenced?
5. Describe an aging periodontium and list the features seen.
6. Describe the difference in tipping and bodily movement.
7. Supporting bone comprises what parts of the mandible?
8. Describe the cells that function in compression and tension.
9. What is the life length of the alveolar bone?
10. In what manner do masticatory stress forces placed on bundle bone differ from those placed on haversian bone?

CONSIDER THE PATIENT . . .

Discussion: Tooth movement, such as mesial drift or orthodontic treatment, could not occur. With tooth movement, cemental and root loss would occur.

SUGGESTED READING

Berkowitz BKB, Moxham BJ, Newman HN, editors: *The periodontal ligament in health and disease,* Oxford, UK, 1982, Pergamon.

Bonucci E: New knowledge on the origin, function, and fate of osteoclasts, *Clin Orthop* 158:252, 1982.

Lisodeskog S, Hammerstrom L: Evidence in human teeth of anti-invasive factor in cementum or periodontal ligament, *Scand J Dent Res* 88:161, 1980.

Marks SC Jr: The microanatomy of the human edentulous maxillae, *Aust Dent J* 23:69, 1978.

Schroeder HE: *Oral structure biology,* New York, 1991, Thieme Medical, pp 197-200.

Severson JS et al: A histologic study of age changes in the adult human periodontal joint (ligament), *J Periodontol* 49:189, 1978.

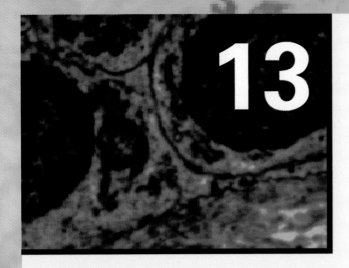

13 Temporo-mandibular Joint

OVERVIEW

This chapter discusses articulation between the condyles of the mandible and temporomandibular fossa of the temporal bone. The temporomandibular joint (TMJ) allows the mandibular condyles to move in both gliding and hinge actions. Therefore instead of being a stationary hinge, the joint slides along the inclined plane while functioning also as a hinge joint. The complex motion of the joint can be observed during mastication. TMJ problems can be associated with pain in the related muscles of the jaws and neck.

The anatomy, histology, and function of the various structures related to jaw function are described in this chapter. The TMJ includes (1) the right and left condylar heads of the mandible, (2) the articulating surfaces of the mandibular condyles and the temporal fossae, (3) a disk that intervenes between the fossa and condyle, and (4) a capsule and supportive ligaments. The capsule enclosing this joint serves as a stabilizer, making complex function possible.

The fibrous articular disk divides the joint in two. The upper half is involved in sliding action, and the lower functions as a hinge action. The joint is supported anteriorly by a tendinous attachment of the capsule and the lateral pterygoid muscle, laterally by the lateral or temporomandibular ligament, medially by the sphenomandibular ligament, and posteriorly by the stylomandibular ligament. The TMJ functions as a ginglymoarthrodial joint, indicating that it moves as a sliding and hinge joint.

Myofacial pain dysfunction (MPD) is a syndrome that has received attention. It has been defined as a complex problem relating to neuromuscular concepts, occlusal concepts, muscle balance, tooth morphology, and guidance and psychophysiologic factors. Much remains to be learned about the normal and abnormal stomatognathic system.

STRUCTURE

Mandibular Condyle

The right and left heads of the mandibular condyles articulate in the temporomandibular or glenoid fossae. At birth the heads of the condyles are round and covered with a thick layer of cartilage. The cartilage front is uneven with spikes of cartilage projecting into the underlying marrow space. Bone forms around these spikes of cartilage so that the head of the condyle is porous (Fig. 13-1, *A*). During development the condyle grows in a lateral direction, changing into an ovoid shape by maturity, which is attained at age 25 (Fig. 13-1, *B*). The oval condyle consists of a smooth, bony surface, which is covered with a layer of fibrous connective tissue in the adult. The cartilage serves as a growth site in the condyle. New cartilage cells arise from near the surface of the perichondrium, which covers the condyle. The cartilage cells grow and divide, and the cells deeper in the cartilage die as the cartilage that surrounds these cells calcifies (Fig. 13-2, *A*). The calcified cartilage is then replaced by bone from the underlying ramus (Fig. 13-2, *B*). This process continues during development with a gradual thinning of the cartilage layer, and at maturity the cartilage has been replaced by bone (Fig. 13-2, *C*).

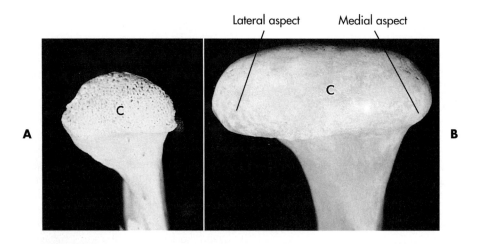

FIG. 13-1   A, Condyle *(C)* of a 6-year-old. Perforations on surface are created by cartilage cap, which is missing because of tissue preparation. **B,** In the adult, smooth bony surface of condyle *(C)* illustrates lateral growth.

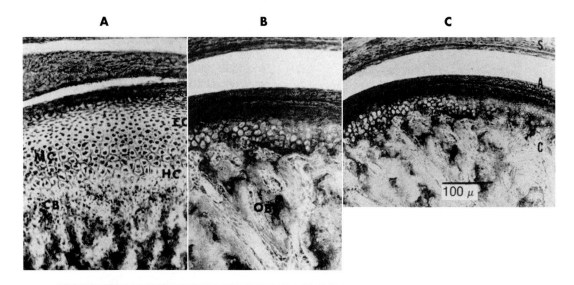

FIG. 13-2   A, Histology of condyle showing wide band of cartilage that appears during postnatal period. *EC,* Reserve cartilage zone; *MC,* multiplication cartilage zone; *HC,* hypertrophy cartilage zone. **B,** Cartilage has thinned considerably. *OB,* Bone formation. **C,** Thin cartilage zone underlying perichondrium in 18-year-old.

The heads of the condyles and the heads of the long bones differ in that long bones form secondary ossification centers (Fig. 13-3). Secondary ossification centers produce cartilage-bone junctions termed epiphyseal lines, where the lengthening of long bone occurs. No epiphyseal line is formed in the condyles. The heads of the condyles, however, accomplish growth much like that of long bones. Differentiation of new cartilage cells first appears, then cartilage matrix around these cells develops, which is then replaced by bone. Another difference in long bones is that the cartilage cells are organized in long rows as they approach the bony junction, whereas in the condyles the chondroblasts are scattered.

The chondroblasts go through similar changes of cell enlargement, cartilage matrix calcification, and bony replacement (Fig. 13-3). This ability to modify the shape of the condyles through cartilage-bone remodeling allows adaptation to functional stress.

Temporomandibular Fossa

The fossa is composed of an anterior part in the form of an eminence and a posterior part, a depression or cavity on the inferior part of the temporal bone. This fossa is located at the posterior medial aspect of the zygomatic arch (Fig. 13-4). The anterior wall of the fossa is smooth and forms a tubercle in which the condyles slide during

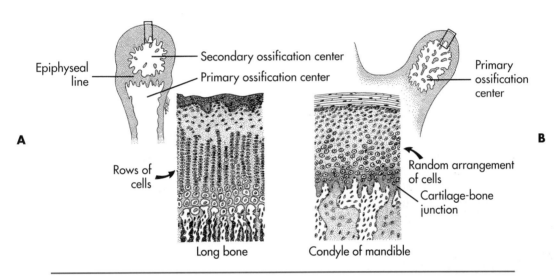

FIG. 13-3   **A,** Cartilage of long bone showing straight vertical rows of cartilage cells, young cells to maturing ones, top to bottom. Bone replaces cartilage at junction of these two tissues. **B,** Random arrangement of cells in condyle, which accomplishes same function as structured rows of cells. As in long bone, at the conclusion of process in condyle, bone replaces cartilage at junction shown.

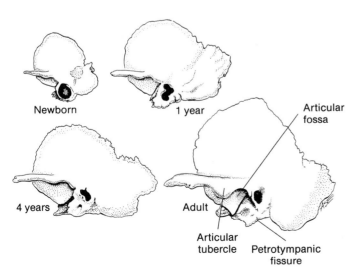

FIG. 13-4   Development of glenoid (temporomandibular) fossa from birth to maturity. Articular fossa deepens during development as condylar head enlarges laterally.

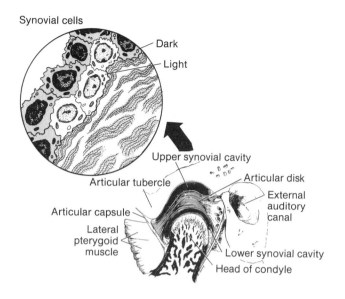

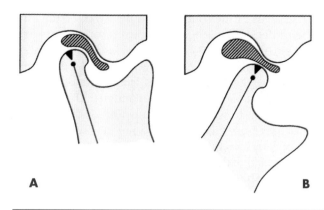

FIG. 13-7   The two actions of temporomandibular joint. **A,** Pathway of movement of condylar head along slope of articular eminence. **B,** Rotary movement of condyle as mouth is opened. Actions occur simultaneously.

FIG. 13-5   Temporomandibular joint with thin anterior and thicker posterior articular disk. Observe position of capsule anteriorly and posteriorly and upper and lower synovial compartments in relation to lateral pterygoid muscle and external auditory canal. Upper and lower compartments are both lined with synovial cells. In the upper diagram are examples of light and dark synovial cells, which function to lubricate movements of condyles.

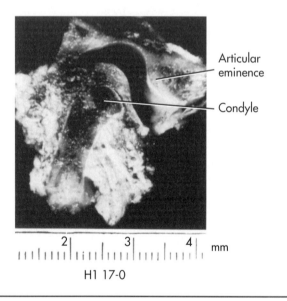

FIG. 13-6   Lateral view of gross appearance of temporomandibular joint at 17 years of age showing size of articular fossa and attachment of muscles to the condyle.

(Courtesy Dr DW Wright. From Avery JK: *Oral development and histology,* New York, 1994, Thieme Medical.)

articulation. On the posterior wall of the fossa is the petrotympanic fissure. This is the junction of the temporal and parietal bones. Some authors report that the origin of elastic fibers, which insert into the posterior part of the disk, is on the posterior wall of this fissure. These

elastic fibers may function in retraction of the disk. The temporomandibular fossa is where the condyles are positioned at rest (Fig. 13-4).

Upper and Lower Compartments

The temporomandibular joint cavity is divided into upper and lower compartments by the articular disk (Fig. 13-5). The upper compartment is bound by the articular fossa above and by the disk below. The lateral, medial, and posterior boundaries are enclosed by the capsule that outlines the TMJ. The lower compartment is bound superiorly by the disk and inferiorly by the head of the disk. The two compartments differ in action. In the upper compartment is a gliding action between the condylar head and the articular eminence, and in the lower compartment is a hinge action between the undersurface of the disk and the rotating surface of the head of the condyle (Figs. 13-5 and 13-6).

Articular Disk

The articular disk is a dense, collagenous, fibrous pad between the condylar heads and the articular surfaces (Figs. 13-5 and 13-6). When the jaw opens, each condylar head moves from the articular fossa and slides along the articular plane to the articular eminence while resting on the intervening articular disk (Fig. 13-7, *A*). The head of the condyle rotates during the sliding action (Fig. 13-7, *B*). This allows the two movements of the TMJ, which are a smooth, **gliding** action and a **hinge** action. The articular disk is a soft pad of fibrous tissue. It is thin and avascular in its center, but thicker and vascular around the margin (Fig. 13-8). The articular disk attaches to the inner wall of the capsule anteriorly and posteriorly, but not medially and laterally, which is where it attaches to the head of the condyle. This structural design requires the disk to be immobile when the head of the condyle moves.

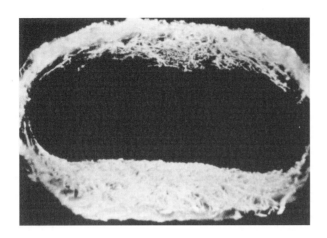

FIG. 13-8 Articular disk with vascular channels injected with latex and surrounding tissue removed. This preparation illustrates that the vascular network is only in periphery of disk, especially in posterior area as shown below, and not to any extent in center of disk.

(Courtesy Dr CC Boyer. From Avery JK: *Oral development and histology*, New York, 1994, Thieme Medical.)

The disk is covered with a thin layer of synovial cells and is known as a **synovial membrane.** This membrane secretes a synovial fluid, which moistens both the upper and lower surfaces of the articular pad and the lining of both compartments (Fig. 13-9). The synovial membrane lining is associated with numerous capillaries and lymphatics along the surface of the disk, especially in the periphery. Synovial fluid is a distillate of the blood, having a high viscosity that provides lubrication and allows freedom of condylar movement. The disk can perforate in its center, or the center can contain a few cartilage cells and islands of cartilage, especially in older age.

CLINICAL COMMENT

The TMJ is a complex and precisely integrated bilateral joint that functions in speech, mastication, and deglutition. You can perceive the downward and forward sliding action of the condylar heads by placing the fingers on them as you open the jaw. This sliding action can also be felt during symmetric protrusion and retrusion or asymmetric lateral shift.

Capsule and Ligaments

A fibrous capsule encloses the TMJ like a cuff. This capsule is composed of an inner lining, or synovial layer, and an outer loose ligamentous layer that is fibrous and tough and supports articulatory movements. The attach-

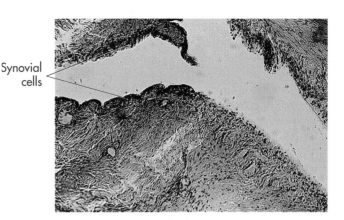

FIG. 13-9 Histology of lateral posterior aspects of disk illustrating dark-stained synovial cells that line joint cavity and disk.

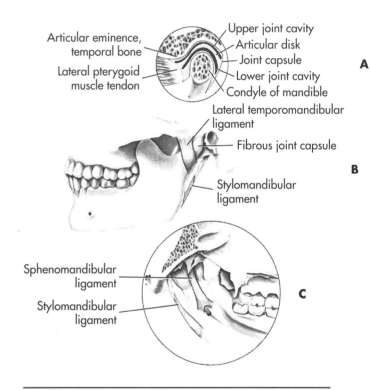

FIG. 13-10 Components of temporomandibular joint (TMJ). **A,** Relationship of TMJ compartments and capsular ligament. **B,** Lateral view of lateral fibrous joint capsule showing relationship of stylomandibular ligament to mandible. **C,** Medial view illustrating location and attachment of sphenomandibular ligament of TMJ.

ment superiorly is to the temporal bone around the limits of the articular eminence and the fossa, and the capsule attaches around the neck of the condyle (Fig. 13-10, *A*). Fibers of the capsule fuse with the fibers of the lateral pterygoid muscle anteriorly, and laterally the capsule is strengthened by the **lateral ligament** or **temporomandibular ligament** (Fig. 13-10, *B*). Medially the **sphenomandibular ligament** supports the joint (Fig. 13-10, *C*). This ligament arises superiorly from the spine of the sphenoid bone and extends downward on the medial side of the ramus to insert on the **lingula,** which is a spine of bone arising from the rim of the mandibular foramen (Fig. 13-10, *C*). Posteriorly the **stylomandibular ligament** arises from the styloid process and inserts on the posterior border of the ramus (Fig. 13-10, *B* and *C*). The lateral ligament and the capsule work in concert to support the joint and limit excursions of the condyles to the normal range. The other two ligaments, the sphenomandibular and stylomandibular,

also serve as support. Mandibular movements involve interplay of the morphology of the teeth and the action of muscles and ligaments surrounding the TMJ.

Vascular Supply

The blood supply to the TMJ is from four arteries, including (1) branches of the **superficial temporal,** (2) **deep auricular,** (3) **anterior tympanic,** and (4) **ascending pharyngeal** (Fig. 13-11). All of these vessels converge on the joint, penetrate the capsule, and send branches into the network of vessels in the periphery of the disk and the posterior area of the joint. Fig. 13-8 shows that the disk is oval and has more blood vessels in the anterior and posterior areas than the lateral or medial surfaces. Interestingly, the blood vessels do not enter the fibrous covering of the head of the condyle (Fig. 13-12) as do blood vessels in some other joints.

Innervation

The nerve supply to the TMJ arises from the branches of the mandibular division of the trigeminal nerve, specifically the **auriculotemporal, masseteric,** and **deep temporal** branches (Fig. 13-12). These are the same nerves supplying the muscles of mastication that function with this joint movement, and so they help ensure coordination of function of the muscles and joint. Both large myelinated and smaller nonmyelinated nerves enter the capsule and disk, and they supply all surfaces of the condylar head, fossa, disk, and capsule (Fig. 13-12). Pain, temperature, touch, and deep pressure nerve terminals are found within the joint. Elaborate encapsulated terminals have been found in the connective tissue associated with the synovial folds and in the disk. Fig. 13-13 shows four types of nerve terminals located in the TMJ.

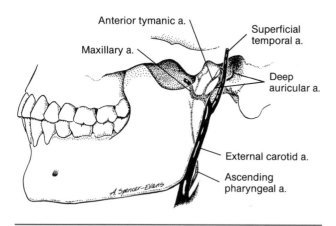

FIG. 13-11 Vascular supply of temporomandibular joint (TMJ). External carotid artery serves TMJ through branches of ascending pharyngeal and superficial temporal arteries. From the maxillary artery come auricular and anterior tympanic arteries, which also supply the joint.

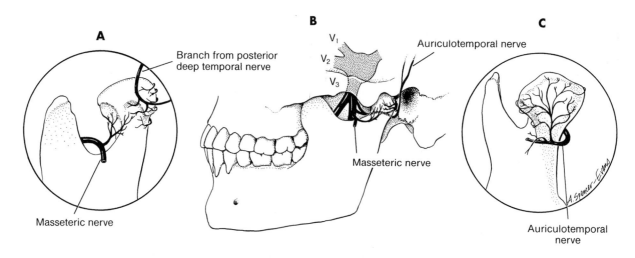

FIG. 13-12 Nerve supply to temporomandibular joint (TMJ). Mandibular division of fifth nerve supplies all surfaces of TMJ through auricular temporal, masseteric, and deep temporal branches. **A,** Anterior view. **B,** Lateral view. **C,** Posterior view.

Muscles of Mastication

The eight powerful muscles of mastication include four on each side of the jaw. Each muscle has a different location, and therefore the direction of fiber contraction results in a different functional relationship. Three of the muscles on each side—the medial pterygoid, the masseter, and the temporalis—exert vertical forces in closing the jaw, whereas the lateral pterygoid muscles protract the mandible and stabilize the joint. These muscles do not function alone but work as a group with the suprahyoid muscles and tongue muscles. Free movements of the mandible relate to the interplay of masticatory muscles and the morphology of the teeth, whereas masticatory movement is the synergistic action of the three groups of muscles—the elevators, depressors, and protractors—that function together and at different times during mastication of food. Following are more details about the muscles of mastication:

1. The **medial pterygoid** arises from the medial surface of the lateral pterygoid plate and inserts on the inferior surface of the ramus and on the angle of the mandible. The blood supply is from the maxillary artery, and the nerve supply is from the mandibular division of the trigeminal nerve. This muscle protracts and elevates the mandible (Figs. 13-14 and 13-15).

2. The **lateral pterygoid** has two heads, the upper arising from the greater wing of the sphenoid and the lower from the pterygoid plate. They insert into the front of the neck of the condyle and the capsule (Fig. 13-15). The blood supply is from the maxillary artery, and the nerve supply is from the ptery-

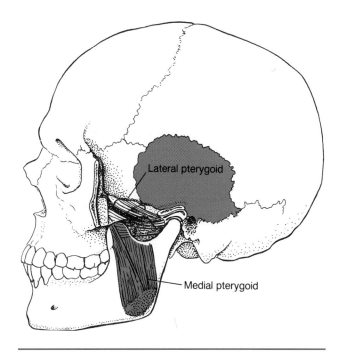

FIG. 13-14 Lateral view of medial pterygoid muscle of mastication. Medial pterygoid functions in elevation and protraction of condyle. This muscle functions in concert with masseteric muscle, forming a sling.

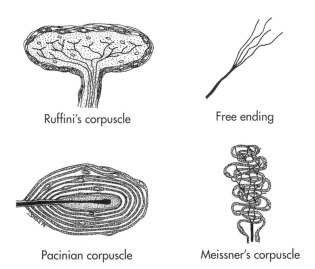

Ruffini's corpuscle   Free ending

Pacinian corpuscle   Meissner's corpuscle

FIG. 13-13 Types of nerve endings in temporomandibular joint. The four types are Ruffini's or temperature endings; the pacinian, which is a pressure receptor; free nerve endings, which are pain endings; and Meissner's corpuscles, which are touch receptors. These are representative of variety of receptors found in capsule, disk, and soft tissues of joint.

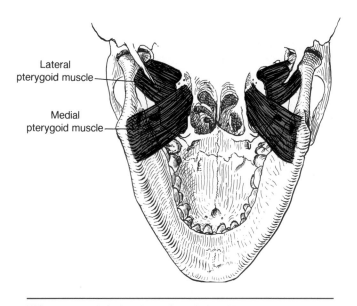

FIG. 13-15 Inferior view of medial and lateral pterygoids to illustrate attachments to mandible and base of skull. Medial pterygoid arises from lateral pterygoid plate and inserts in the inferior angle of mandible. Lateral pterygoid arises from greater wing of sphenoid and the lower head from lateral pterygoid plate. These muscles insert in neck of condyle and capsule.

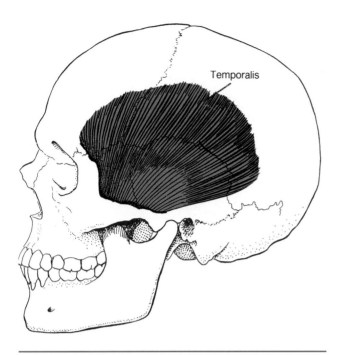

FIG. 13-16 Temporalis muscle of mastication. Temporalis muscle functions in elevation of the jaw, retraction of the mandible, clenching of the teeth, and side-to-side movements of the jaw.

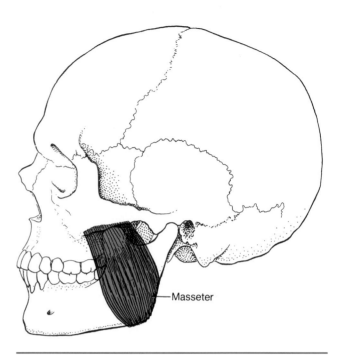

FIG. 13-17 Masseter muscle of mastication. Function of masseter muscle is to elevate jaw, clench teeth, and assist in side-to-side movement of jaw.

goid branch of the mandibular nerve. Both heads of this muscle protrude the mandible and pull the articular disk forward (Figs. 13-14 and 13-15).

3. The **temporalis** muscle fibers originate from the floor of the temporal fossa and temporal fascia. These muscle fibers insert on the anterior border of the coronoid process and anterior border of the ramus of the mandible (Fig. 13-16). The blood supply is from the superficial temporal and maxillary arteries, and the nerve supply is from the deep temporal branches of the mandibular nerve. The temporalis muscle elevates and retracts the mandible and clenches the teeth.

4. The **masseter** muscle has a deep and superficial part. The superficial fibers originate from the anterior two thirds of the lower border of the zygomatic arch, and the deep fibers from the medial surface of the same arch. The superficial fibers are at right angles to the occlusal plane of the posterior teeth, and the deep fibers are directed down and slightly anteriorly. This muscle inserts into the lateral surface of the coronoid process of the mandible, the upper half of the ramus, and the angle of the mandible. The blood supply is from the superficial temporal and the maxillary arteries, and the nerve supply comes from the mandibular division of the trigeminal nerve. The masseter muscle elevates the jaw and clenches the teeth (Fig. 13-17).

CLINICAL COMMENT

A functional relationship of the occlusion of the teeth is expressed through the muscles of mastication. A detailed history and physical examination help the clinician provide an accurate diagnosis. Clinicians must rely on their own judgment in the treatment of patients with TMJ pain.

CONSIDER THE PATIENT . . .

A patient is experiencing severe TMJ discomfort. What treatment is needed? What methods of pain alleviation could be employed during treatment?

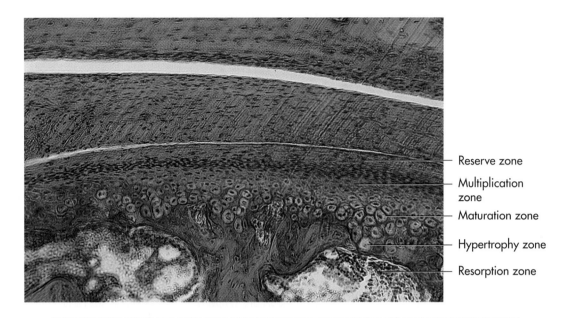

Reserve zone

Multiplication zone

Maturation zone

Hypertrophy zone

Resorption zone

FIG. 13-18   Histologic view of head of condyle and overlying articular disk. Head of condyle exhibits a perichondrium and zones of cartilage formation and resorption. Reserve cartilage cell zone overlies multiplication zone, zone of cartilage cell hypertrophy, and zones of cartilage resorption and bone replacement.

(Courtesy Dr S Bernick. From Avery JK: *Oral development and histology*, New York, 1994, Thieme Medical.)

REMODELING OF TEMPOROMANDIBULAR JOINT ARTICULATION

Articular remodeling is the morphologic adaption of the joint in response to environmental stress. The articular surfaces of the TMJ have been shown to adapt to minimize the effects of the stressful mandibular function. Presence of cartilage on the condyle and the fossa allows the TMJ to withstand stress better than other fibrous joints. Progressive remodeling occurs with proliferation of the articular cartilage and production of intercellular matrix followed by its mineralization. The cartilage is then resorbed as it is replaced by bone (Fig. 13-18). This may happen in one or both of the condylar heads and articular eminences and may relate to any changes in structure of the articular surfaces. In some cases, remodeling may begin in the proliferative zone, causing an increase of cartilage on the surface, which may then become mineralized and be replaced by bone at the zone of resorption. Functional adaption is the response of chondrogenesis and osteogenesis to withstand the effects of mastication resulting from compression. In aging, with decreased proliferation, these changes may be degenerative.

CLINICAL COMMENT

Myofacial pain dysfunction (MPD) continues to be an area of concern because of varying opinions about treatment. Because much remains to be learned about both the normal and abnormal functions of the TMJ, more progress in the treatment of MPD is expected.

CONSIDER THE PATIENT . . .

Discussion: Several approaches exist, but occlusal adjustment is usually the treatment of choice because of the prevalence of malocclusion. The administration of a mandibular anesthetic could help alleviate the pain. During this injection the needle pathway is through the mucosa and the buccinator muscle and lateral to the medial pterygoid muscle and the anesthetic is deposited near the mandibular foramen.

SELF-EVALUATION QUESTIONS

1. Name the three supporting ligaments of the TMJ.
2. What is the role of the TMJ capsule?
3. Describe the two different functions of the upper and lower compartments of the TMJ.
4. How do the heads of the condyles change as a person grows and matures?
5. What are the functions of the two heads of the lateral pterygoid muscle?
6. What is the significance of the sling muscles, and is this a function of the muscles' location and innervation?
7. What are the location and function of the temporalis muscle?
8. What is the significance of the TMJ's and the masticatory muscles' having the same innervation?
9. What are the major blood vessels supplying the TMJ?
10. What is the function of the synovial cells?

SUGGESTED READING

Baume LJ: Cephalo-facial growth patterns and the functional adaption of the temporomandibular joint structures, *Europ Orthodont Soc Trans* 45 Cong '69, 1970.

Blackwood HJ: Adaptive changes in the mandibular joints with function, *Dent Clin North Am*, vol 10, Nov 1966.

Boyer CC, Williams W, Stephens F: Blood supply of the temporomandibular joint, *J Dent Res* 43:2, 1963.

Dixon AD: Structural and functional significance of the inter-articular disk of the human temporomandibular joint, *Oral Surg Oral Med Oral Pathol* 15:1, 48-61, 1962.

Griffin CJ, Hawthorne R, Harris R: Anatomy and histology of the human temporomandibular joint, *Monograph Oral Sci* 4:1, 1975.

McNamara JA Jr: Functional adaptions of the temporomandibular joint, symposium on an alterable centric relation in dentistry, *Dent Clin North Am* 18:3, 1975.

Meikie C: The role of the condyle in the postnatal growth of the mandible, *Am J Orthod* 64:50, 1973.

Sarnat BG, Laskin DM: *Temporomandibular joint: biological basis for clinical practice,* Springfield, Ill, 1979, Charles C Thomas.

Thilander B: The structure of the collagen in the temporomandibular disc of man, *Acta Odontol Scand* 22:1, 135-149, 1964.

Wright DM, Moffett B Jr: The postnatal development of the human temporomandibular joint, *Am J Anat* 141:235-250, 1974.

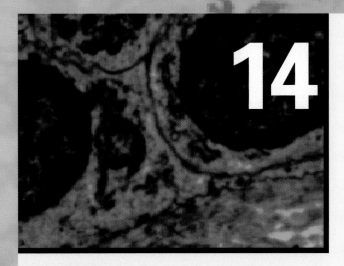

14 Oral Mucosa

OVERVIEW

The structure of stratified squamous epithelium of the oral mucosa includes both the nonkeratinized lining mucosa of the cheeks, lips, soft palate, and floor of the mouth and the keratinized epithelium covering the palate and alveolar ridges. Masticatory mucosa consists of multiple layers of epithelial cells associated with the lamina dura layer, which contains blood vessels, nerve endings, and serous, mucous, or mixed glands. A third type of mucosa found on the surface of the tongue is specialized mucosa, consisting of four types of papillae, which are filiform, fungiform, foliate, and circumvallate.

Taste is associated with the latter three types of papillae, which are located on the tongue, soft palate, and pharynx. Four types of taste are regionally associated with the tongue. At the tip, sweet and salty tastes are perceived; sour taste is associated with the sides of the tongue; and bitter taste is at the back of the tongue.

Masticatory mucosa includes the gingiva, which is composed of the tissue surrounding the necks of the teeth. The gingiva consists of three areas, which are free, attached, and interdental. The free gingiva is characterized by the gingival sulcus. The attached gingiva has junctional epithelium, which binds the gingiva to the necks of the teeth. The interdental area is that tissue between the teeth below their contact point. The hard palate is covered by masticatory mucosa, which is firmly attached to the underlying bone.

Cells of the oral mucosa are termed keratinocytes and can be distinguished from the nonkeratinocytes, which are Langerhans' cells, Merkel's cells, and melanocytes. In case of inflammation, lymphocytes and leukocytes may appear in the mucosa. They are commonly found in gingival epithelium.

Four types of nerve receptors—heat, cold, pain, and touch—are located in the lips and oral cavity. They are most numerous in the lips and in the tip of the tongue. With age, the oral mucosa becomes thinner and may be lower on the necks of the teeth. Also, it can become less moist because of the decrease in activity of the salivary glands.

STRUCTURE OF ORAL MUCOSA

The oral cavity is lined with stratified squamous epithelium, which is divided into three types of tissue. **Lining mucosa** covers the floor of the mouth and the cheeks, lips, and soft palate. It does not function in mastication and therefore has little attrition. **Masticatory mucosa** covers the hard palate and alveolar ridges and is so named because it comes in primary contact with food during mastication. **Specialized mucosa,** which covers the surface of the tongue, is quite different in structure and appearance from the two previous tissues.

Each type of tissue has structural differences: the lining mucosa is soft, pliable, and nonkeratinized; the masticatory mucosa is keratinized, indicative of the attrition that takes place during mastication. Specialized mucosa on the tongue surface is composed largely of cornified epithelial papillae, which function in mastication. The mucosa of the oral cavity has several features common to epithelium elsewhere in the body. One of these features is the lamina propria, the connective tissue layer immediately below the epithelium. It is composed of the papillary layer and deeper reticular layer (Fig. 14-1). In the papillary layer the connective tissue extends into pockets in the epithelium. This increases the surface of the epithelium for contact with vascular supply and nerves. The reticular layer contains the deeper plexi of vessels and nerves supported by the connective tissue. These two layers, papillary and reticular, contribute the lamina propria or dermis. Beneath this zone is the submucosa or subcutaneous tissue.

CONSIDER THE PATIENT . . .

A patient mentions that she heard the oral cavity is a logical location to place medication because the medication can be resorbed and taken into the bloodstream. She asks if this is true for all medications.

Lining Mucosa

Lining mucosa is composed of a thin layer of epithelium and an underlying lamina propria. The epithelium is composed of a basal layer of cuboidal cells, termed the **stratum basale.** The next cell layer is called the **stratum intermedium** or **stratum spinosum.** The cells in this layer appear oval and somewhat flattened. The third or superficial layer is termed the **stratum superficiale,** and its cells are flattened, with many containing small oval nuclei (Fig. 14-1). These three cell layers of the epidermis form the nonkeratinized epithelium of the oral mucosa and appear similar to the lining of the pharynx. Another component of the mucosa is the dermis or lamina propria, composed of the papillary and reticular connective tissue layers.

Lips

The inner oral surface of the lips is lined with moist-surface, stratified squamous cells, nonkeratinized

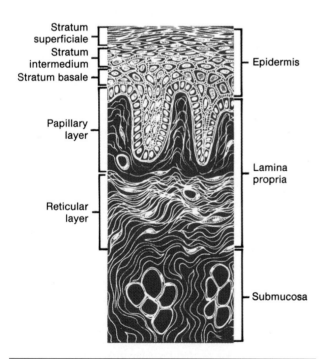

FIG. 14-1   Relationships among oral epidermis, dermis (lamina propria), and submucosal tissue. Names of layers of epidermis and dermis are noted on left.

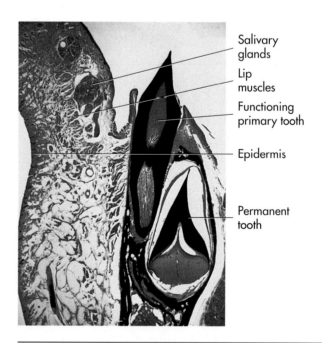

FIG. 14-2   Histology of lip and alveolar bone, which contains functioning primary and developing permanent teeth.

epithelium and is associated with small, round seromucous glands of the lamina propria. These glands are part of the minor salivary glands found throughout the oral cavity. Beneath the lamina propria is the submucosa, in which fibers of the orbicularis oris muscle are located (Fig. 14-2). Nonkeratinized mucosa of the lips is distinguished by a red border known as the **vermilion border.** This area is at the junction between the oral mucosa and the skin of the lips, becoming modified into keratinized epithelium, which is different from skin or mucosa. There are three reasons that the vermilion border is red, which are the following: the epithelium is thin; this epithelium contains **eleidin,** which is transparent; and the blood vessels are near the surface of the papillary layer, revealing the red blood cells' color (Fig. 14-3). Also observable in the skin of the lips are hair follicles and their associated sebaceous glands, erector pili muscles, and sweat glands. Sebaceous glands can be seen at the angles of the mouth. They are not associated with hair follicles. These glands are known as **Fordyce's spots** (Fig. 14-4).

Soft Palate

Lining mucosa of the highly vascularized soft palate is more pink than the mucosa of the keratinized epithelium of the hard palate (Fig. 14-5). This tissue is pink because the lamina propria contains many small blood vessels. Beneath the connective tissue of the lamina propria is the submucosa, which contains muscles of the soft palate and mucous glands.

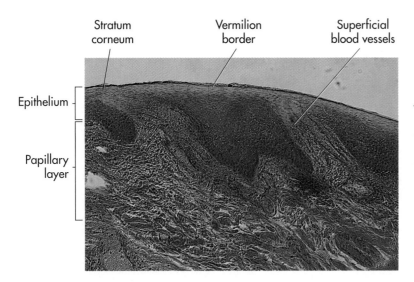

FIG. 14-3 Vermilion border of lip illustrating thin and lucent stratum corneum and presence of capillaries in papillary layer. Observe close relationship of blood supply to surface of vermilion border epithelium.

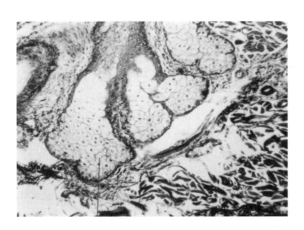

FIG. 14-4 Fordyce's spots, sebaceous glands not related to hair follicles, are found at angles of mouth.

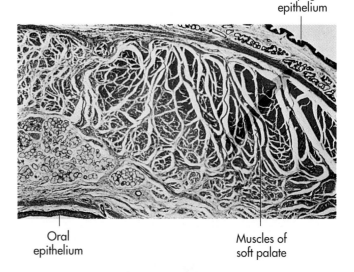

FIG. 14-5 Sagittal plane of soft palate *(anterior on left)*. Nasal cavity is above, and respiratory epithelium covers superior part of soft palate. Oral cavity is below this tissue and is covered with squamous epithelium. Observe glands underlying oral mucosa and muscle throughout submucosa.

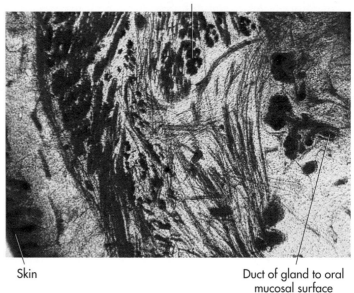

Seromucous glands between
muscle fibers

FIG. 14-6 Histology of cheek tissues. Skin is on far left, and oral mucosa on far right. Observe glands intermingling with muscle fibers in subcutaneous zone of cheek.

Skin

Duct of gland to oral
mucosal surface

Cheeks

The mucosa of the cheeks is like that of the lips or soft palate because each has stratified squamous epithelium that is nonkeratinized, lamina propria, and underlying submucosa. In the cheeks, however, the submucosa contains fat cells and mixed glands (seromucous) located within and between the muscle fibers. The presence of these glands and fat cells is a unique feature of the cheeks (Fig. 14-6).

Ventral Surface of the Tongue

Lining mucosa also contains a lamina propria and submucosa. In the submucosa, muscle fibers are located under the surface of the tongue. The entire area exhibits dense, interlaced muscle and connective tissue fibers. Limits of the submucosa are not distinct because the submucosa continues with the deep muscles of the tongue along with connective tissue fibers (Fig. 14-7).

Floor of the Mouth

Nonkeratinized mucous membrane covers the floor of the mouth and appears loosely attached to the lamina

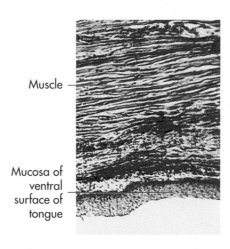

Muscle

Mucosa of
ventral
surface of
tongue

FIG. 14-7 Histology of ventral surface of tongue showing density of muscle fibers intermingling in lamina propria.

propria. In contrast, the adjacent undersurface of the tongue mucosa is firmly attached (Figs. 14-7 and 14-8). In the floor of the mouth are minor salivary glands (Fig. 14-8) and the right and left major mucous glands, the sublingual glands.

Masticatory Mucosa

Masticatory mucosa is the epithelium covering the gingiva and hard palate. This mucosa is thicker than the nonkeratinized mucosa with the addition of a keratinized surface of flat, hornified cells offering resistance to attrition. The basal and intermediate stratum (**stratum spinosum**) layers are the same as those of nonkeratinized epithelium. The granular layer (**stratum granulosum**) and the surface layer (**stratum corneum**) are the

 CLINICAL COMMENT

Recognition of change in a patient's mucosa is based in part on knowledge of the individual's normal characteristics and on evaluation of the patient's history. Among the basic conditions of the mucosa to be considered are variations in tissue color, dryness, smoothness, or firmness and whether the gingiva bleeds easily.

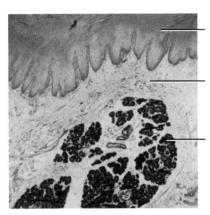

Epithelium of floor of mouth

Connective tissue fibers

Salivary gland (minor)

FIG. 14-8 Histology of mucosa lining floor of mouth. Observe lack of muscle fibers and delicate appearance of connective tissue fibers. Scattered glands of minor serous and mucous salivary glands are near tip of tongue.

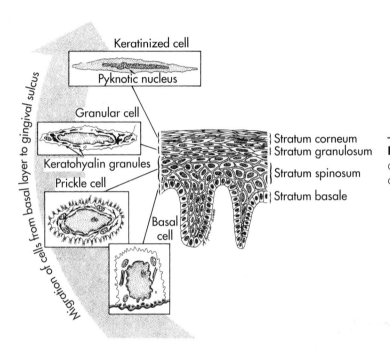

Keratinized cell

Pyknotic nucleus

Granular cell

Keratohyalin granules

Prickle cell

Basal cell

Stratum corneum
Stratum granulosum

Stratum spinosum

Stratum basale

Migration of cells from basal layer to gingival sulcus

FIG. 14-9 Keratinized stratified squamous epithelium of oral cavity. Observe characteristics of four cell types of this epithelium, from basal to surface layers.

two other layers (Fig. 14-9). The cells of the basal layer are cuboidal or columnar. Their nuclei are irregularly oval and exhibit numerous mitotic figures as they undergo constant cell division. These basal cells gradually migrate to the surface of the mucosa. Fig. 14-9 shows the differences in each cell layer. The second layer, stratum spinosum, is several cells thick. These cells are oval to polygonal, and mitotic figures can be seen in this layer.

Basal cells interface with a membrane separating the epithelium and connective tissue. This membrane is called the **basal lamina** (Fig. 14-10). The basal cells are attached to the basal lamina by minute disks termed **hemidesmosomes** (Fig. 14-10). These thickenings of the cell membrane are supported by filaments from within the cells, anchoring fibrils that attach the basal lamina and the epithelial cells to the collagen fibers of the lamina propria. Fig. 14-11 shows these structures.

The next layer of cells superficially is the stratum granulosum, so named because the cells contain many kera-

tohyalin granules (Fig. 14-12). The surface layer of cells, the stratum corneum, is characterized by thin, flattened, nonnucleated cells. These cells are filled with a soft keratin that replaces the cell cytoplasm. This soft keratin may be compared to hard keratin of the nails and hair. Keratin is tough, nonliving material that is resistant to friction and impervious to bacterial invasion.

To permit cell movement and loss of individual cells along the surface, the superficial layers have surface interdigitations rather than desmosomes. These cells are continually becoming lost and replaced by cells of the underlying layers.

As each cell moves to the surface of the epithelium, it does so by means of cell attachments to neighboring cells that hold until the cell has reached a specific stage of development. When that stage occurs, the cell attachment releases, which allows that cell to move to a higher level where it reattaches. All epithelial cells function with **desmosomes.** In the oral mucosa, desmosomes are discoid and are called **macula adherens** (Fig. 14-13). The

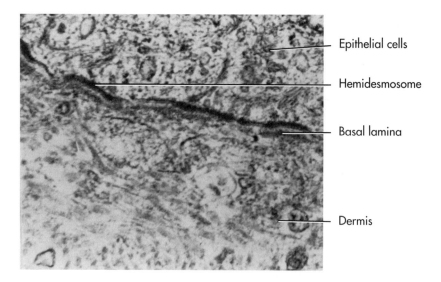

FIG. 14-10 Ultrastructure of junction of epithelium and lamina propria as seen in electron micrograph. Extending across field from left to right is basal lamina, to which epithelial cells are attached by hemidesmosomes.

(Courtesy Dr D Turner, University of Michigan, School of Dentistry.)

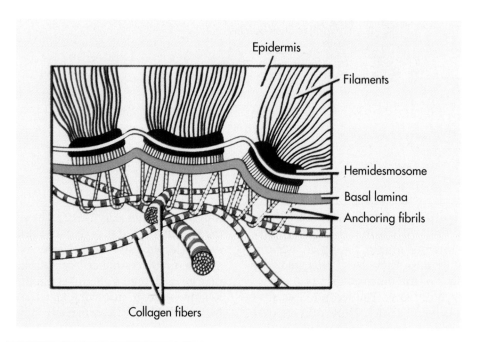

FIG. 14-11 Diagram of hemidesmosomes of oral mucosa showing how hemidesmosomes of epithelial cells attach to basal lamina membrane. Anchoring collagen fibers of connective tissue attach to basal lamina and fibers of hemidesmosome.

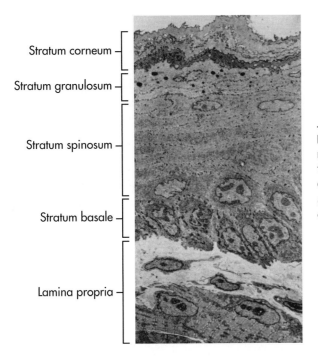

Stratum corneum

Stratum granulosum

Stratum spinosum

Stratum basale

Lamina propria

FIG. 14-12   Histology of oral epithelium. This is an electron micrograph of keratinized oral epithelium that shows relative thickness of each cell layer from stratum basale to stratum corneum and lamina propria beneath epithelium.

(Courtesy Dr D MacCullum, University of Michigan, School of Medicine.)

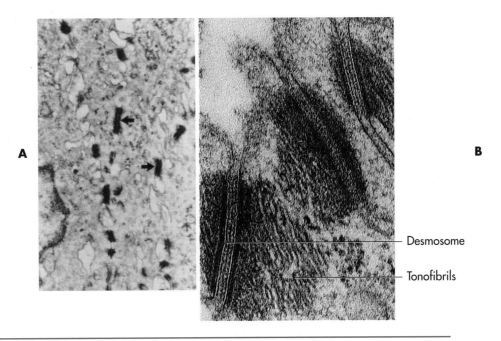

A

B

Desmosome

Tonofibrils

FIG. 14-13   Electron micrographs of cell junctions of oral epithelial cells. These are termed desmosomes or macula adherens. **A,** At low magnification, arrows indicate buttonlike attachments between each cell. **B,** At higher magnification, multilayer arrangement of desmosomes can be seen. Tonofibrils of cell attach to these platelike junctions.

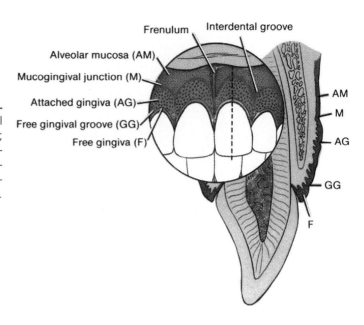

FIG. 14-14 Gingiva shown in both facial and longitudinal views. Shown are free gingiva *(F)* along the crest of gingiva; free gingival groove *(GG)* at junction between free and attached gingiva; stippled attached gingiva *(AG)*; mucogingival junction *(M)*, which separates gingiva from alveolar mucosa; and alveolar mucosa *(AM)* above attached gingiva. Frenulum and interdental zones (grooves) are also shown.

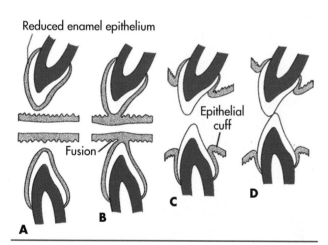

FIG. 14-15 Gingiva develops from reduced enamel epithelium of tooth combined with oral epithelium. The two meet, fuse, and rupture to allow tooth to erupt.

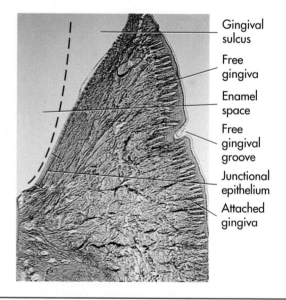

FIG. 14-16 Histology of gingiva illustrating gingival sulcus, junctional epithelium, and free gingiva. Enamel space is created by loss (decalcification) of enamel.

junctions are composed of thin protein adhesion disks located between the cells. These disks are anchored by means of intracellular filaments, termed **tonofibrils**, which arise in the cell and project to the surface, where they attach to the cell junction. The disks temporarily hold the cells in contact but later release them, allowing the cells to move superficially and reattach to a cell in another location (Figs. 14-12 and 14-13).

Gingiva and Epithelial Attachment

In the oral mucosa the gingiva surrounds the necks of the teeth and extends apically to the mucogingival junc-

tion (Fig. 14-14). The gingiva develops as a coalescence of the oral and reduced enamel organ epithelium when the tooth first emerges into the oral cavity (Fig. 14-15, *A* to *C*). The reduced enamel organ epithelium makes contact with the undersurface of the oral epithelium, and the two fuse. Then the tooth penetrates this combined layer to enter the mouth and produces the gingiva as the epithelium continues to separate from the enamel surface (Fig. 14-15, *C*) until occlusion of the teeth is reached (Fig. 14-15, *D*). At this point the gingiva covers only the cervical area of the enamel where it is attached (Fig. 14-15, *D*).

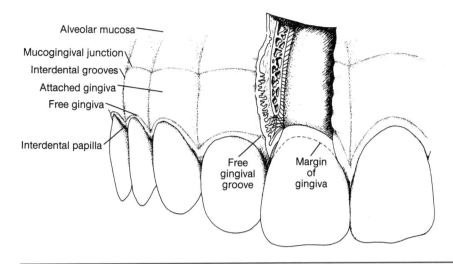

FIG. 14-17   Location of free and attached gingivae and location of mucogingival junction, which separates keratinized gingiva from nonkeratinized alveolar mucosa.

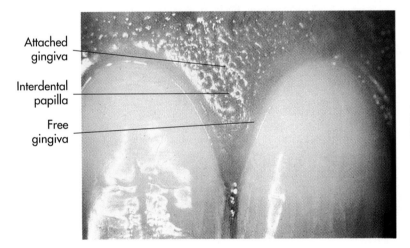

FIG. 14-18   View of normal gingiva illustrating free and attached (stippled) gingivae.

The gingiva is divided into three zones. They are (1) the **free** or **marginal zone,** which encloses the tooth and defines the gingival sulcus; (2) the **attached gingiva,** that portion of the epithelium attached to the neck of the tooth by means of junctional epithelium; and (3) the **interdental zone** (groove), the area between the two adjacent teeth beneath their contact point (Fig. 14-14). The free and attached gingivae have an indistinct groove on the surface of the epithelium separating them. This groove is termed the **free gingival groove** (Figs. 14-14 and 14-16).

Free and Attached Gingiva

The free or marginal gingiva is bound on its inner margin by the gingival sulcus, which separates it from the tooth; on its outer margin by the oral cavity; and apically at its free surface by the **free gingival groove** (Fig. 14-17). This groove separates the free and attached gin-

givae. Therefore the attached gingiva lies adjacent to the free gingiva and is separated from the alveolar mucosa by the **mucogingival junction** (Fig. 14-17). The free and attached gingivae are keratinized, but the alveolar mucosa is not. The attached gingiva is stippled, but the free gingiva has a smooth surface (Fig. 14-18). In some instances the free gingiva may be covered with parakeratinized mucosa, which contains keratinized cells modified by the presence of nuclei in the cells of the surface layer. The unique feature of attached gingiva is the junctional epithelium.

Junctional Epithelium

Junctional epithelium provides attachment for the gingiva to the tooth in the cervical area and forms the epithelium-lined floor of the gingival sulcus (Fig. 14-19). Cells of the attached epithelium are cytologically different from other cells of the gingival epithelium.

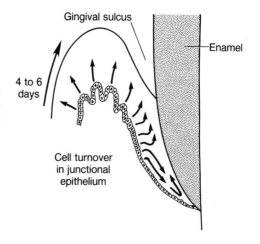

FIG. 14-19 Epithelial cell turnover in gingiva. Note the direction of epithelial cell maturation from basal cell to surface in attachment zone and in the margin of gingiva.

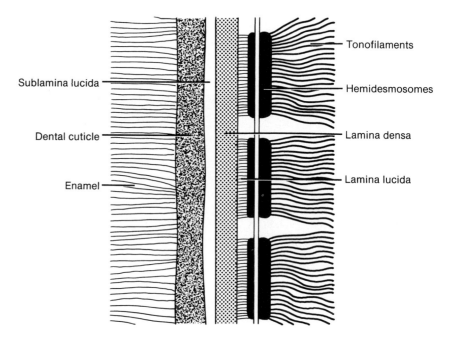

FIG. 14-20 The means of gingival attachment with tooth's surface. Hemidesmosome is a specialized attachment plaque that attaches to protein (cuticle or pellicle) on tooth's surface. Protein of enamel surface is composed of dense and lucent layers. If hemidesmosome is disturbed, reattachment can take place.

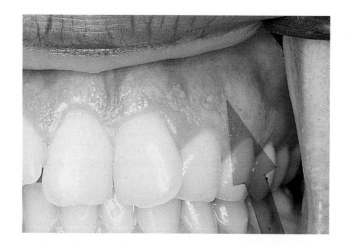

FIG. 14-21 Clinical view of gingiva showing free and attached gingiva and interdental groove *(arrow)*. The col is found in this area.

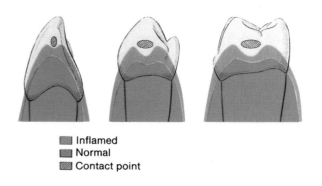

FIG. 14-22 Positional relationship of col in health and disease. Col is accentuated in inflammation and swelling of gingiva. Col is pointed anteriorly and flat or concave posteriorly. Contact point on each tooth is represented by oval above col.

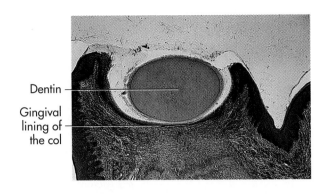

FIG. 14-23 Histology of col, a concave nonkeratinized epithelial lining of gingival col between teeth. Contact point is represented by dentin shown above col.

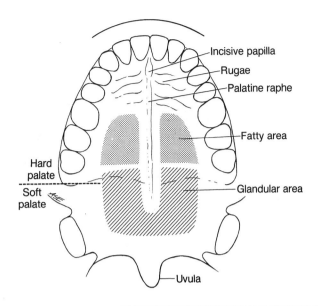

FIG. 14-24 Palate. After noting landmarks, observe location of glandular zone anteriorly and fatty zone posteriorly. These tissues are found in subcutaneous tissue underlying lamina propria. Midline of palate has no subcutaneous zone; only lamina propria exists in midline and gingiva of lateral palate.

They have fewer desmosomes (cell attachment buttons). This indicates a higher rate of turnover than occurs in the other gingival epithelial cells (Fig. 14-19). These cells have been reported to turn over in approximately 6 days, from the time of their appearance in the stratum basale to the time when they are sloughed in the free surface. The cells have many organelles, such as rough surface endoplasmic reticulum, Golgi's apparatus, and mitochondria, indicating high metabolic activity.

Stratum basale cells also contain **hemidesmosomes**, the mechanism for the attachment of cells to the salivary protein layer, which covers the cervical area of the enamel (Fig. 14-20). The half a desmosome in these junctional epithelial cells is like the hemidesmosome of the basal cells of the squamous epithelium, which attaches to the basal lamina and lamina propria of the gingiva (Fig. 14-12). Disturbance of this attachment to the tooth by infection, food impaction, calculus, or other irritants results in a deepening of the gingival sulcus.

Interdental Papilla and Col

Gingiva located between the teeth and extending high on the interproximal area of the crowns on the labial and lingual surfaces is known as the **interdental papilla** (Fig. 14-18). This tissue fills the space created by the constricted cervical areas of the adjacent crowns. In the interproximal area, between the lingual and vestibular papilla, is a concave zone of the gingiva that follows the contour of each crown (Fig. 14-21). The junctional epithelium of this zone is known as the **col**. The col is char-

acterized as a thin, nonkeratinized epithelium. These basal epithelial cells invade the connective tissue where inflammatory cells of the lamina propria may appear (Figs. 14-22 and 14-23). The col is more inclined in a peak between anterior teeth and more flattened or concave between posterior teeth. When the interproximal gingiva becomes inflamed or hyperemic, the col is exaggerated and is positioned higher on the neck of the tooth (Fig. 14-22).

Hard Palate

The roof of the mouth, or hard palate, is covered with keratinized stratified squamous epithelium. This epithelium is similar to that of the gingiva in the middling area, where there is no submucosa. The midline is known as the **median raphe,** which may only be barely discernible, except anteriorly, where an incisive papilla can be seen. On each side of the median raphe are ridges of tissue called **rugae** (Fig. 14-24). These folds of epithelium are supported by dense lamina propria (Fig. 14-25). In the anterior lateral palate a zone of fatty tissue is located in the submucosa. However, in the posterior lateral hard palate is mucous glandular tissue (Fig. 14-24). Both the hard and soft palates have mucous glands. **Traction bands** (Fig. 14-26) exist in the lamina propria of the rugae. These bands also exist between the lobules of fatty tissue and glands of the anterior and posterior hard palate. Traction bands are bundles of collagen fibers that insert into the papillary fibers of the lamina propria and extend into the bony palate. These

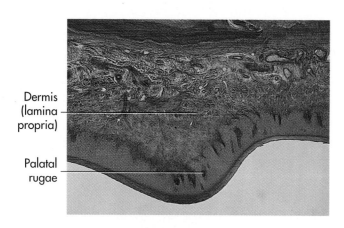

FIG. 14-25   Histologic section of anterior palate showing rugae. Rugae are epithelium-covered ridges in lamina propria of anterior palate.

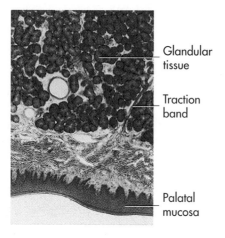

FIG. 14-26   Histologic section of palate in glandular zone. Traction bands of collagen fibers bind palatal epithelium to underlying bone.

collagen fibers anchor the palatal mucosa to the underlying bone, and the hard palate assists in mastication.

Specialized Mucosa

Types of Papilla

The dorsum or superior surface of the tongue (anterior two thirds) is covered with a specialized mucosa. This mucosa consists of four types of epithelial structures called **papillae** (Fig. 14-27). The majority of these papillae are **filiform papillae,** which are slender, threadlike keratinized extensions of the surface epithelial cells. The entire roughened surface of the tongue is covered with this papillae (Figs. 14-27 through 14-29). They project

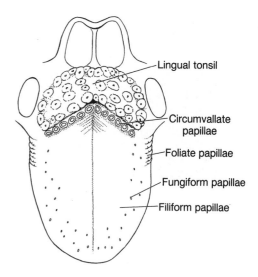

FIG. 14-27   Dorsal surface of tongue showing papillae. Filiform papillae are scattered over surface of tongue body. Fungiform papillae are few in number, round, and pink, but larger than filiform papillae. Foliate papillae are 4 to 11 in number along posterior sides of tongue. Circumvallate papillae are 8 to 10 in number along junction of body and base of tonsillar area of tongue.

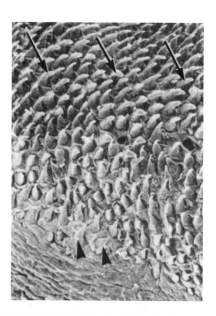

FIG. 14-28   A scanning electron micrograph of tongue's surface showing filiform papillae *(arrows).* These pointed papillae are directed toward the throat and assist in moving food in that direction as the tongue moves.

(Courtesy Dr M Pirbazane.)

about 2 to 3 mm high from the surface of the tongue. These papillae facilitate mastication and movement of the food on the surface of the tongue.

Interspersed between the filiform papillae are the **fungiform papillae,** which are few in number but more

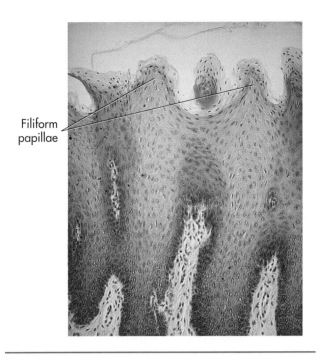

FIG. 14-29   Histologic picture of filiform papillae of tongue's dorsal surface. Pointed keratinized projections are shown.

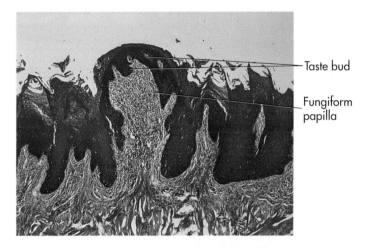

FIG. 14-30   Histologic section of fungiform papilla, with connective tissue core and epithelial covering. Two taste buds are located on papilla surface.

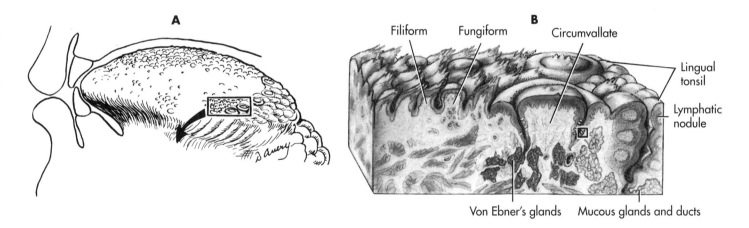

FIG. 14-31   **A,** Circumvallate papillae. Note large (2-mm) papillae with trench around each and underlying serous (von Ebner's) glands, which wash out taste from area of taste buds. **B,** Rectangle in **A** is enlarged. Dorsal appearance of tongue with filiform, fungiform, and circumvallate papillae. A taste bud is shown within small, rectangular area.

numerous near the tip of the tongue. The fungiform papillae are mushroom shaped with the cap usually larger than the stalk (Fig. 14-30). The covering epithelium of the fungiform papillae is thin and nonkeratinized, so the papillae appear pink or reddish because blood vessels are near the surface. Taste buds are occasionally found on the superior surface of the fungiform papillae (Figs. 14-30 and 14-31, *B*). A third type of papilla is the **circumvallate papilla.** Only 10 to 14 in

number, the circumvallate papillae are located along the V-shaped sulcus between the body and base of the tongue (Fig. 14-31). These papillae are level with the surface of the tongue, and each has a surrounding groove. They are large, 3 mm in diameter.

Ducts of the underlying serous glands (von Ebner's glands) are seen opening into the grooves surrounding these papillae. Taste buds line the walls of the papillae (Fig. 14-31, *B*). The watery secretion of these glands washes out substances so that new tastes can be perceived. On the lateral posterior sides of the tongue are 4 to 11 vertical grooves or furrows containing taste buds (Fig. 14-31, *A*). These furrows are termed **foliate papillae.** Like circumvallate papilla, they contain serous glands underlying the taste buds, which cleanse the trenches of the foliate papillae (Fig. 14-31, *B*).

Table 14-1	
Taste Buds in the Human Adult	
Location	Number
Tongue	10,000
Soft palate	2,500
Epiglottis	900
Larynx and pharynx	600
Oropharynx	250

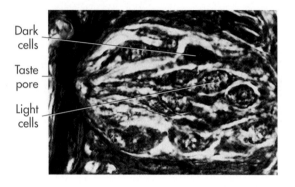

FIG. 14-32 Light microscope picture of a taste bud with its dark and light cells. Taste pore for reception of substances opens in wall of trench.

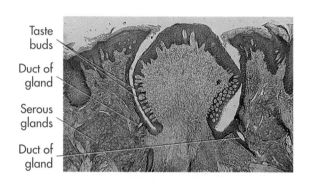

FIG. 14-33 Histology of circumvallate papilla with taste buds located on its walls in trench. Serous gland and its ducts are emptying into trench from lower left and right.

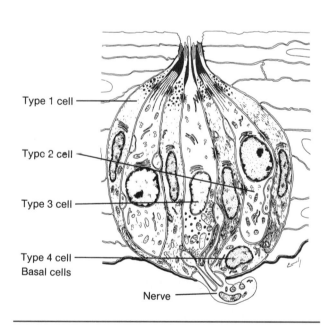

FIG. 14-34 Typical taste bud. Four types of cells can be noted. Type 1, dark cells, represents 60% of the cells. Type 2, light cells, represents 30%. Type 3 represents 7%. Type 4, basal cells, represents 3%.

(Courtesy Dr R Murray, University of Indiana, School of Medicine.)

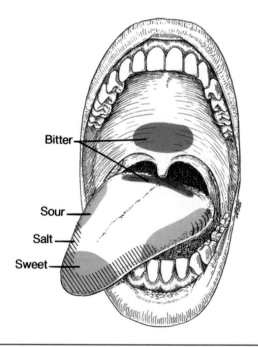

FIG. 14-35 Location of taste perception on tongue and soft palate. Tip of tongue has sweet receptors; along front sides are salty receptors; on posterior sides are sour receptors; and on posterior center and soft palate are bitter receptors.

Taste Buds

Taste buds are microscopically visible barrel-shaped bodies found in the oral epithelium. These discrete sense organs contain the chemical sense of taste. They are generally associated with the papillae of the tongue, the circumvallate, foliate, and fungiform, although some are distributed in the soft palate, epiglottis, larynx, and pharynx (Figs. 14-32 to 14-34 and Table 14-1).

Taste buds are easily recognized under the microscope as barrel-shaped structures; their epithelial cells appear ovoid (Fig. 14-32). Although they have been referred to as neuroepithelial structures, they are more correctly referred to as epithelial cells closely associated with club-shaped sensory nerve endings. These nerves arise from the chorda tympani and come to lie among the taste cells.

Several types of taste cells are found among the 10 to 14 cells in a taste bud. Each taste bud contains a few **supporting** or sustentacular cells (several types) that lie in the periphery of the taste bud. The majority of **taste cells** bear either elongated microvilli that project into the taste pore or ones with shortened villi that open into the base of the pore. Each cell is associated with nerves that penetrate the taste bud. Another type of cell found in the taste bud is the **basal cell.** These basal cells are in close contact with the basal lamina (Fig. 14-34). There is a rapid turnover of these cells, approximately 10 days. They are believed to arise from the surrounding epithelial cells.

Four types of taste sensation can be detected, and evidence of regional sensitivity for these tastes is on the tongue and palate. The four taste sensations are **sweet,** **salty, sour,** and **bitter.** Sensations of sweet and salty are perceived at the tongue's tip, sour on the sides, and bitter in the region of the circumvallate papillae (Fig. 14-35). These areas overlap, and evidence indicates that all papillae respond to all four types of taste sensations. However, the levels of sensitivity differ. For example, with higher concentrations of a bitter taste, the sensation is perceived most notably on the posterior segment of the tongue. This indicates a regional selectivity of taste in the mouth, which may be caused in part by the origin of the nerve supply.

Nerves for taste buds of the anterior two thirds of the tongue pass to the chorda tympani branch of the facial nerve; those of the posterior one third pass to the glossopharyngeal nerve; and those from the epiglottis and larynx pass to the vagus nerve.

Mixing the four basic modalities of taste cannot explain all of the flavors that humans are capable of experiencing. Factors such as odors and temperature also contribute to flavors. In addition, taste buds can discriminate between subtleties in flavor, such as the difference between citric or acetic acid. This enables taste buds to identify specific substances even when they are mixed.

CLINICAL COMMENT

The distribution of nerve endings in the oral cavity is greatest in the lips and anterior oral mucosa and least in the more posterior regions of the oral cavity. Therefore the mouth tastes food and beverages before they are taken farther into the alimentary canal. The one exception to this anterior sensitivity is that of cold and pain nerve endings, which are numerous in the posterior palate.

NERVES AND BLOOD VESSELS

The nerves and blood vessels appear in the lamina propria. Terminal endings of nerves and loops of blood vessels appear in the dermal papillae. There blood vessels consist of a deep plexus of larger vessels in the submucosa underlying the lamina propria, and capillary loops extend into a secondary plexus in the dermal papillae. The overlying epithelium is avascular, and its metabolic needs come from the vessels of the lamina propria. Nutrition passes from these vessels through the connective tissue and basal lamina and then enters the epithelium. Throughout the gingiva, nerves and nerve endings are prevalent. The encapsulated touch and temperature endings are located in the papillary tissue of the lamina propria and axons associated with Merkel's cells (Fig. 14-36). Free endings associated with pain can be seen entering the epithelium between the cells (Fig. 14-36). Table 14-2 shows the areas and levels of sensitivity.

Table 14-2			
Levels of Sensitivity of the Oral Region			
	Sensation	Greatest Sensitivity	Moderate Sensitivity
	Pain	Lips, pharynx, base of tongue	Anterior tongue
	Heat	Lips	Tip of tongue
	Cold	Lips, posterior palate	Base of tongue, ventral tongue
	Touch	Lips, tip of tongue	Gingiva

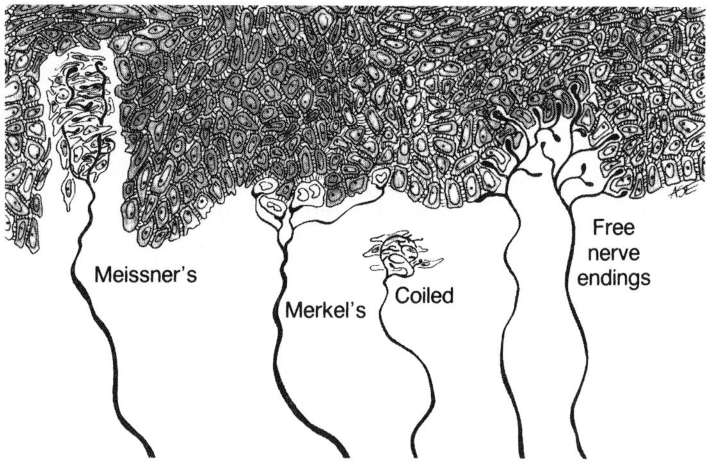

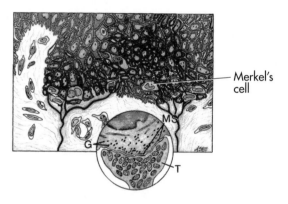

FIG. 14-36 Nerve endings in oral mucosa showing location of various types in epithelium or lamina propria.

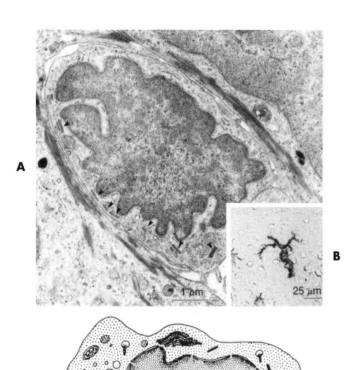

FIG. 14-38 Merkel's cells are located in basal cell layer and their relationship to a nerve ending (MS). Inset shows nerve terminals (T) and secretory granules in Merkel's cell (G).

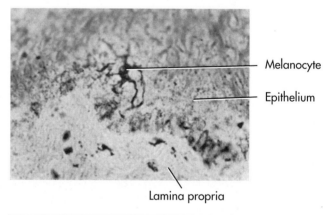

FIG. 14-37 Three histologic views of a nonkeratinocyte. **A,** In electron micrograph of Langerhans' cell, the rodlike granules are indicated by arrows. **B,** Appearance of cell under light microscopy. **C,** Diagram of Langerhans' cell.

(Courtesy Dr I Mackenzie, University of Iowa.)

FIG. 14-39 Histology of another type of nonkeratinocyte. Dendritic melanocyte is in the stratum basale of oral epithelium.

EPITHELIAL NONKERATINOCYTES

In contrast to the epithelial cells or keratinocytes, the nonkeratinocytes constitute about 10% of the mucosal cell population. These cells have a clear halo around their nuclei and have been called "clear cells." The three types of these cells are **Langerhans' cells, Merkel's cells,** and **melanocytes.** Two other nonkeratinocytes, lymphocytes and polymorphonuclear leukocytes, appear in the epithelium in cases of inflammation.

Langerhans' Cells

Langerhans' cells are found in the stratum spinosum and are believed to function in the processing of antigenic

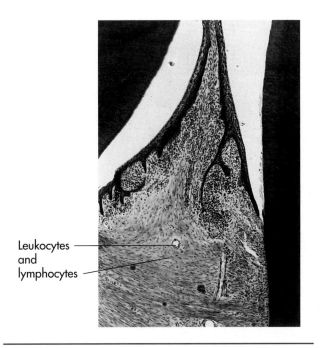

Leukocytes
and
lymphocytes

FIG. 14-40 Inflamed gingiva with many leukocytes and lymphocytes in connective tissue of gingiva.

 CLINICAL COMMENT

Halitosis can be caused by multiple factors. If the ingestion of offensive foods is ruled out as a cause, possible food impaction, plaque, or the need for an oral prophylaxis should be considered. Disease of tooth origin or the periodontium is another factor. Diseased tonsils or sinuses and systemic factors, such as lung problems, are also possible causes.

material. They are therefore in an ideal location to make contact with invading bacteria and establish response mechanisms to protect the body. The cells appear to have processes but do not have desmosomes or tonofilaments. This type of cell has unique racket-shaped organelles (Fig. 14-37).

Merkel's Cells

Merkel's cells are located in the basal layer of the gingival epithelium. Unlike keratinocytes, these cells are associated with the terminal axon. However, they may contain round electron-dense granules in their cytoplasms adjacent to their axons. These cells and their axons are believed to function as touch receptors (Fig. 14-38).

Melanocytes

Melanocytes are melanin-producing cells in the basal layer of the gingival epithelium. Melanocytes lack desmosomes and tonofilaments and are dendritic. A characteristic feature of the melanocyte is the melanin granules (melanosomes) in the cytoplasm. Such cells may inject melanosomes into nearby keratinocytes (Fig. 14-39).

Lymphocytes and Leukocytes

Lymphocytes, leukocytes, and mast cells, which are associated with gingival inflammation, may be found in the gingival epithelium and connective tissue. They may be found in the gingival epithelium and underlying connective tissue. They may be located anywhere in the gingiva but most often underlie the junctional epithelium. Their appearance is different from keratinocytes because they have no desmosomes, tonofilaments, or organelles. These lymphocytes appear typical, with a large oval nucleus occupying most of the cytoplasmic space (Fig. 14-40). Granule-bearing mast cells may also be seen in the gingival mucosa during inflammation.

CHANGES WITH AGING

Recognition of changes in the oral mucosa associated with aging is important. With age the oral epithelium becomes thinner and more fragile. A flattening of the surface ridges and surface cells causes the oral mucosa to appear smoother. Because of gradual atrophy of the minor salivary glands and less activity of the major glands, the oral mucosa appears less moist. In aging, cellular activity decreases and fibrosis increases. Also, calcifications appear in the lamina propria of the gingiva and the periodontal ligament. The ability to repair is reduced, and the length of healing time is increased. Apical migration of the gingiva usually is associated with periodontal disease but appears routinely in the aging oral mucosa. Some patients may be taking blood thinners or other medications that will affect gingival bleeding. Compare Figs. 14-41 and 14-42.

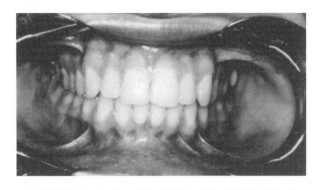

FIG. 14-41 Healthy gingiva in 25-year-old shows normal color, form, and density.

(Courtesy Dr R Courtney, University of Michigan, School of Dentistry.)

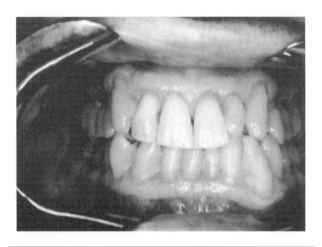

FIG. 14-42 Healthy gingiva of 80-year-old differs from that of 25-year-old shown in Fig. 14-41. Normal form and contours are altered in older person.

(Courtesy Dr R Courtney, University of Michigan, School of Dentistry.)

SELF-EVALUATION QUESTIONS

1. Describe the three areas of the gingiva and the characteristics of each.
2. Name the areas covered with lining mucosa and masticatory mucosa.

3. Where are taste buds most numerous in the oral cavity, and in what other areas are they located?
4. What are the locations and functions of traction bands?
5. Describe junctional epithelium and state its turnover time.
6. What are the location and function of Langerhans' cells?
7. Name four types of nerve sensation found in the oral cavity and where they are located.
8. What taste sensations are located on the tip, anterior sides, posterior sides, and posterior center of the tongue?
9. What is the name and type of gland found at the corners of the mouth?
10. Describe the structure and function of a hemidesmosome.

 CONSIDER THE PATIENT . . .

Discussion: The floor of the mouth is an appropriate area for absorption of some medications, such as for the relief of angina, because it is a rapid route. The epithelium is thin and nonkeratinized, with capillaries present in the dermis, which are near the surface of the mucosa.

SUGGESTED READING

Bhaskar SN, editor: *Orban's oral histology and embryology,* ed 11, St Louis, 1991, Mosby.

Kobayashi K, Rose GG, Mahan CL: Ultrastructure of the dentoepithelial junction, *J Periodont Res* 11:313-330, 1976.

Listgarten, MA: Electron microscopic study of the gingivodental junction in man, *Am J Anat* 119:147-177, 1966.

Schroeder HE, Listgarten MA: *Fine structure of the developing epithelial attachment of human teeth,* vol 2, ed 2, New York, 1977, S Karger, 1977.

Waterhouse JP, Squier CA: The Langerhans' cell in human gingival epithelium, *Arch Oral Biol* 12:341-348, 1967.

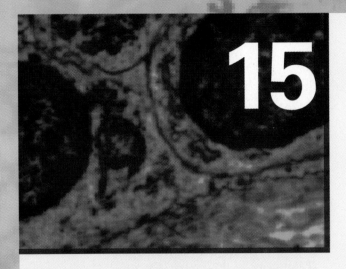

15 Salivary Glands and Tonsils

OVERVIEW

This chapter discusses the structure and function of the salivary glands, saliva, and tonsils. Despite different structures and functions, these soft tissues all contribute significantly to oral health. Saliva is a balanced secretion resulting from both (1) the composition of the secretion and (2) the location of the salivary gland secretions into the oral cavity. The two cell types are serous, which is high protein and low carbohydrate, and mucous, which is low protein and high carbohydrate. Glands of the lips, cheeks, and anterior floor of the mouth produce a watery mixture of a serous and mucous secretion, whereas other glands of the posterior palate, pharynx, and tongue contribute a viscous mucous solution that protects the membranes in those regions. The major salivary glands contribute 85% to 90% of the saliva into the more anterior area of the mouth. In addition to protein and carbohydrate, the parotid, which is the largest gland, secretes the enzyme amylase, which aids in digestion of carbohydrates. Therefore the buffering ability of saliva is due to ionic secretions by the salivary glands. These secretions are collected and modified through an elaborate secretory duct system.

Tonsils, like the salivary glands, have locations that maximally affect and protect the oral environment. These lymph node–like organs are positioned in the oropharynx at the entrance to the alimentary canal. They produce lymphocytes and, with the assistance of macrophages, protect against microbes, foreign cells, and cancer cells. Lymphocytes can recognize foreign cells and respond to them either by becoming T cells, which destroy the foreign cells directly, or by forming B cells, which transform into plasma cells that secrete antibodies to eliminate the foreign cells.

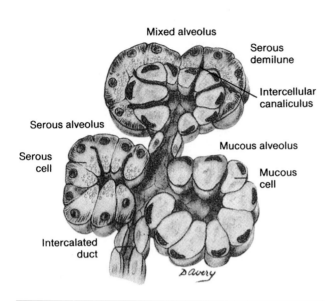

FIG. 15-1   Salivary acinar cells. The serous, mixed, and mucous alveoli are displayed. Observe cell size, shape, and position relative to collecting tubules (intercalated duct).

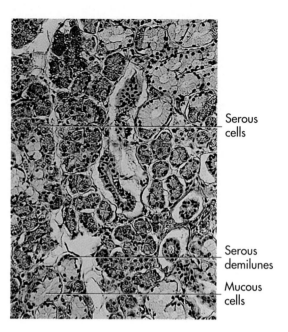

FIG. 15-3   Histologic features of submandibular gland. Serous cells are at upper left and mucous cells at lower left. A few mucous cells are capped with serous cells (serous demilunes).

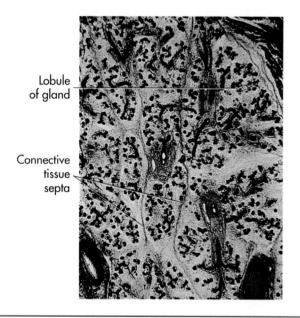

FIG. 15-2   Histology of developing salivary gland at a stage in which lobules can be seen outlined by connective tissue fibers (septa).

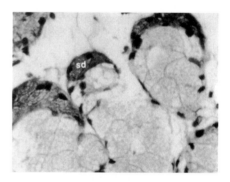

FIG. 15-4   Histology of serous demilune *(sd)* cap on mucous cells in mixed acinus of submandibular gland.

CLASSIFICATION OF SALIVARY GLANDS

Salivary glands are classified as either major or minor depending on their size and the amount of their secretion. The **major glands** carry their secretion some distance to the oral cavity by means of a main duct. The smaller **minor glands** empty their products directly into the mouth

by means of short ducts. Both are composed, however, of the same type of cells, either **serous** or **mucous** or a combination of the two called **serous demilunes** (Fig. 15-1).

The functional unit of the salivary gland is the **alveolus** or **acinus**. An acinus is a cluster of pyramidal cells, either mucous or serous or a combination of the two, that secretes into a terminal collecting duct (Fig. 15-1). The collecting duct is termed the **secretory end piece** or **intercalated duct**. Both the large and small glands are composed of many acini, although the larger glands contain more acini or units arranged in lobules and lobes (Fig. 15-2). Each cell type provides a different type of secretion. Serous cells secrete mostly proteins and small amounts of carbohydrates. Their secretion also contains **zymogen granules**, precursors of the enzyme **amylase**, which functions in the breakdown of carbohydrates. Serous cell secretion has a watery consistency. Mucous

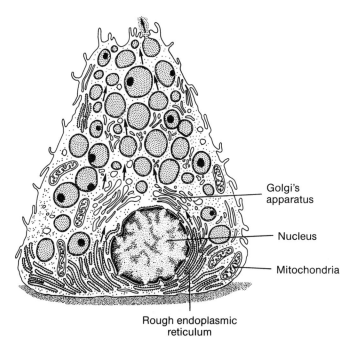

FIG. 15-5   Ultrastructure diagram of serous cell with vesicles developing and migrating to cell apex above. Note the round nucleus, Golgi's apparatus, and rough endoplasmic reticulum that are characteristic of a protein-secreting cell. Arrows point to vesicles arising from Golgi's zone and migrating to cell surface.

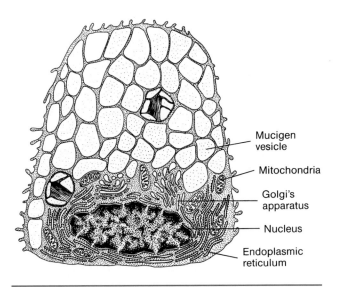

FIG. 15-6   Ultrastructure design of mucous cell. Compare shape of this cell and its nucleus to serous cell. Shown are Golgi's apparatus, rough surface endoplasmic reticulum, and mucous accumulation (mucigen vesicles) in cell.

cells are high in carbohydrates and low in proteins and discharge a viscous product called **mucin** (Fig. 15-3). When mucin mixes with watery oral fluids, it becomes mucous, causing the saliva to be thick and viscous.

Both types of acinar cells are pyramidal. The nucleus of the serous cell is oval to round, and that of the mucous cell is oval to spindle shaped (Fig. 15-1). In each of these cell types, the nuclei appear in the basal part of the cell. The cytoplasm of the serous cell stains deeply because it is filled with albumin, whereas the mucous cell

appears light and foamy because of the presence of carbohydrates in mucin (Figs. 15-3 and 15-4).

Ultrastructurally, the serous cell is filled with secretory granules in the apical region, rough surface endoplasmic reticulum, Golgi's apparatus, mitochondria, and an oval nucleus (Fig. 15-5). The mucous cells contain larger droplets of mucin apically and a prominent Golgi's apparatus and rough endoplasmic reticulum around the flattened nucleus (Fig. 15-6). A third cell-type arrangement is a terminal alveolus of mucous cells with a cap of serous cells (Fig. 15-4). This configuration is termed a **serous demilune,** with the secretion of the serous cells' passing down a duct between the terminal mucous cells to the lumen of the alveolus (Fig. 15-1).

Salivary glands are termed **merocrine glands** because the basic mode of product excretion is through membrane vesicles passing to the cell's apex. These vesicles fuse with the cell plasma membrane and are then exteriorized (Fig. 15-6).

    CLINICAL COMMENT

The serous and mucous cells of the major glands secrete 85% to 90% of saliva. Their combined secretions produce the viscosity as well as the important buffering actions of saliva. These properties are due in part to the actions of protein, carbohydrate, carbonate, and phosphate that are contributed by the secretory ducts of the glands.

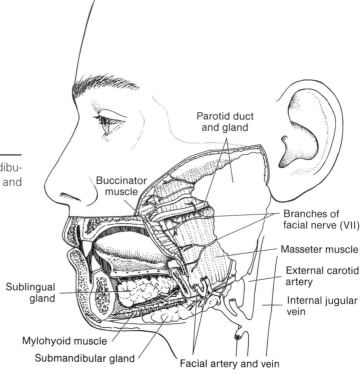

FIG. 15-7 Location of major glands—parotid, submandibular, and sublingual—and relationship of facial nerves and blood vessels to parotid gland.

Table 15-1

Major Salivary Glands and Contribution to Saliva

Gland	Size	Location	Type Cells	Amount Secretion (%)	Duct Type Striated/ Intercalated
Parotid	Largest	Anterior ear	Serous	25	Long/long
Submandibular	Intermediate	Angle of mandible	Mixed serous demilune	60	Long/short
Sublingual	Smallest	Anterior floor of mouth	Mucous	5	Short/none

MAJOR SALIVARY GLANDS

The major salivary glands are present as three bilateral pairs. The **parotid glands** are located on the sides of the face in front of the ears; the second pair, the **submandibular,** are inside the angle of the mandible; and the third pair, the **sublingual,** are on either side of the midline beneath the mucosa of the anterior floor of the mouth (Fig. 15-7).

Each major gland secretes a different product. The parotids produce a nearly pure serous secretion, the submandibular a mixed serous and mucous secretion, and the sublingual nearly pure mucous.

The parotids are the largest glands, although they contribute only 25% of the total saliva. The submandibular glands are intermediate in size, but they produce 60% of the saliva. The sublingual glands are the smallest, contributing only about 5% of the saliva. The **minor salivary glands** located throughout the oral cavity contribute about the same amount as the sublingual.

These salivary glands are organized like grapes on a vine. The acini are the grapes, and they are arranged in groups or **lobules** invested in connective tissue. These groups of lobules form larger **lobes.** In turn the lobes are surrounded by connective tissue containing the ducts that drain the glands and the blood vessels that supply the glands (Fig. 15-8).

The parotid ducts extend anteriorly across the masseter muscles and then bend toward the mouth, opening adjacent to the crowns of the maxillary molar teeth (Fig. 15-7). The ducts of the submandibular and sublingual glands have a common opening in the anterior floor of the mouth, located at the sublingual papillae on either side of the frenulum and at the tongue's tip (Fig. 15-7).

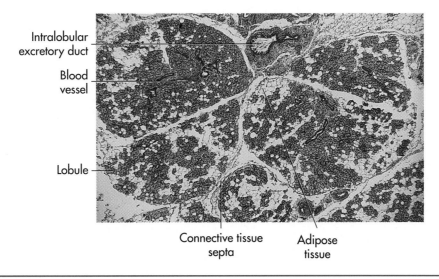

FIG. 15-8 Photomicrograph of lobular nature of parotid gland. Blood vessels can be seen within lobule. Light lines that surround each lobule are connective tissue fibers that support lobules. Parotid gland contains many adipose cells *(light-stained cells)*.

Table 15-2

Minor Salivary Glands' Contribution to Saliva		
Name	**Location**	**Type Secretion**
Labial	Lips	Mixed
Buccal	Cheeks	Mixed
Palatine	Hard and soft	Pure mucous
Lingual	Anterior	Mixed
	Middle	Serous
	Posterior	Pure mucous

MINOR SALIVARY GLANDS

The minor salivary glands are classified as serous, mucous, and mixed types, the same as the major glands. These glands are located throughout the oral cavity and are named for their location. The glands of the cheeks and lips are termed the **buccal** and **labial glands.** They contain a combination of serous and mucous secretions and are thus known as **mixed glands.** The glands of both the posterior hard palate and soft palate are called **palatine glands,** and those of the tonsillar folds are the **glossopalatine glands.** These glands are referred to as **pure mucous glands.** The tongue contains **lingual glands,** which are mixed glands at the tongue's tip. **Serous glands** are located at the junction of the tongue's body and base, where the watery secretion washes out the taste buds of the circumvallate papillae. The tongue also has mucous glands in the posterior region under the lingual tonsillar tissue. Fig. 15-9 shows all these minor glands. Each minor gland is small, consisting of a cluster of acini, and each is drained by a short duct.

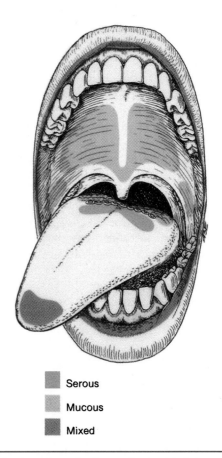

■ Serous

■ Mucous

■ Mixed

FIG. 15-9 Location of minor salivary glands in oral cavity. Serous glands are located in midtongue, mucous glands in the palate, and mixed glands in lips, cheeks, and tongue tip.

CLINICAL COMMENT

The locations of various minor glands in the oral cavity are important to oral functions. In the palate, where keratinized epithelium is present, mucous glands provide adequate lubrication to the epithelium. The lips and cheeks have similar mixed glands that assist in mastication, swallowing, and speech. These minor glands assist in swallowing and speech. Contributions of the three bilateral major glands provide the other 90% of oral fluids.

SALIVA

Composition

All of the major and minor salivary glands contribute to the composition of saliva. This composition varies according to the rate of secretion, which is low during sleep and high (1 ml per minute ±) during stimulation. Secretion is controlled by the salivary center in the brain, and flow is generated by taste (gustatory). Masticatory function is controlled through receptors in the periodontium and muscles of mastication. Oral and pharyngeal pain and irritation can also induce secretion.

Saliva has fewer proteins and ions than blood. Saliva contains potassium, sodium chloride, calcium, magnesium, phosphorus, carbonate, urea, and traces of ammonia, uric acid, glucose, and lipids. The major salivary protein is amylase, which is present in the parotid gland and to a lesser extent (20%) in the submandibular gland. The sublingual or minor glands do not have any amylase. Saliva also contains the proteins lysozyme and albumin. The viscous nature of saliva is due to the presence of salivary mucin, which is a mixture of glycoproteins. Saliva contains epithelial cells shed by the oral epithelium as well as leukocytes from the gingival crevices and lymphocytes from the tonsils. The latter two are known as **salivary corpuscles.**

CLINICAL COMMENT

Saliva is important in mastication, swallowing, and speech. In addition, saliva contains amylase, an important enzyme that functions in the breakdown of carbohydrates and initiates digestive action in the oral cavity.

Functions

The three pints of saliva secreted each day serve several important functions, some of which are the following:
1. To wash the surfaces of the teeth and reduce the possibility of acid etching's leading to dental caries
2. To keep the oral tissues moist and protect against irritants and desiccation
3. To aid in mastication and swallowing of food
4. To provide antibacterial action
5. To assist in the formation of the pellicle, which is a protective membrane on the tooth's surface
6. To provide protection in acid-neutralizing and acid-buffering actions, which prevent dissolution of enamel

The presence of calcium and phosphate ions in saliva increases enamel surface hardness of newly erupted teeth and may assist in enamel remineralization. Through the action of amylase, starches are broken down to more easily digestible carbohydrates. Saliva also enhances taste by breaking down food molecules into a solution that is then brought into contact with the taste buds.

Saliva has numerous proteins—such as lysozymes, lactoperoxidase, and lactoferrin—that have antimicrobial properties. Additionally, saliva has antibodies or immunoglobulin, such as IgA. Saliva also contains an **epidermal growth factor,** which may assist in the healing of injured oral mucosa.

During most of the day and night, salivary flow is minimal. Secretion depends on gustatory and masticatory stimulation. Both taste and smell perform a major role in determining salivary flow as do the nerve endings in the periodontal ligament and the muscles of mastication.

Duct Systems

Ducts of the smallest diameter are in direct contact with salivary acini. They become much larger as other acini empty into a collecting duct, which continues increasing in size until it enters the oral cavity. The ducts of the major glands are long, and various types of ducts are within the glands. Many of these ducts are so small that it is difficult to visualize them microscopically.

The duct system consists of a **secretory portion,** which lies among the acinar cells, and an **excretory portion,** which lies in the connective tissue septa between the lobules and lobes of the glands. These ducts continue beyond the glands, emptying into the oral cavity (Fig. 15-10). The difference between the secretory and excretory ducts is that substances enter and leave the cells of the secretory duct by ion exchange with the adjacent blood vessels, whereas the excretory duct is simply a saliva-collecting tube. Acinar cells drain directly into **intercalated ducts,** which are low cuboidal cells (Fig. 15-10). These secretory cells have metabolic function and contain mitochondria, rough endoplasmic reticulum, and secretory granules.

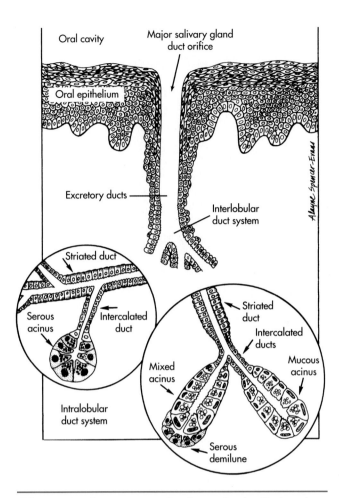

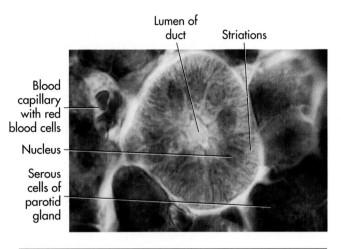

FIG. 15-11 Histology of a striated duct in center of field surrounded by parotid acinar cells. In duct cell is the centrally located nucleus with basal striations on the periphery of each cell. These striations are due to enfolding of outer cell membrane, which provides a larger area for exchange of nutrients with adjacent vascular supply. Blood capillary is on left.

FIG. 15-10 Duct system of salivary glands. Circles show the duct system of intralobular ducts, that is, intercalated and striated secretory ducts located within the lobule. Above are interlobular and multicelled excretory ducts located outside lobules and lobes.

 CLINICAL COMMENT

The action of saliva provides an important protective function on the tooth's surface and the oral epithelium, where acids contribute to changing conditions. Saliva also contains calcium and phosphate, which may aid in the demineralization of the enamel surface and reverse the action of dental caries.

The intercalated duct opens directly into a larger duct called the **striated duct**. The cells of the striated duct are slightly taller and more columnar than the intercalated (Fig. 15-10). These cells have striations caused by enfolding of the basal membrane, which increases the sur-face area of the cell and allows increased exchange of ions with the nearby blood vessels (Fig. 15-11). Sodium resorption and potassium secretion occur in these cells, causing changes in the saliva composition.

Both intercalated and striated ducts are part of the **intralobular duct system**, located inside the lobules. In contrast, the remaining **interlobular excretory ducts** are located in the connective tissue septa between the lobules and lobes of the gland (Fig. 15-10). As the ducts enlarge, their walls contain larger and more numerous cells, such as stratified columnar cells. Near its orifice the duct becomes lined with stratified squamous epithelium, which is continuous with the oral epithelium. **Stensen's duct** drains the parotid gland, and **Wharton's duct** drains the submandibular gland.

 CONSIDER THE PATIENT . . .

A patient complains of pain and tenderness on the right side of the floor of the mouth. What is the best approach in determining the cause?

MYOEPITHELIAL CELLS

Myoepithelial cells originate from the oral epithelium at the time that the oral epithelial cells of the salivary gland

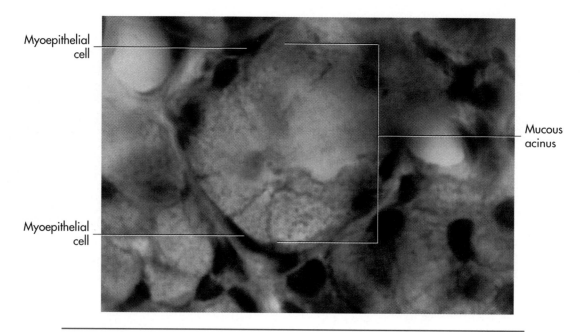

Myoepithelial cell

Myoepithelial cell

Mucous acinus

FIG. 15-12   Histology of light-stained mucous acinus that contains mucous cells surrounded by myoepithelial cell.

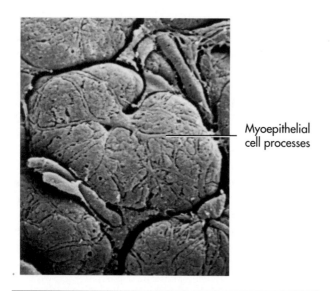

Myoepithelial cell processes

FIG. 15-13   Scanning electron micrograph of myoepithelial cell illustrating cell and its cytoplasmic processes wrapping around acinus of submandibular gland.

(Courtesy Dr TM Nagato.)

grow into the mesenchyme. The cells remain on the outside of the secretory end pieces and function as muscle cells to contract and squeeze the acinus, facilitating secretion. Therefore the term *myoepithelial cells* is used because these cells have an epithelial origin and a muscle function. These cells have long processes that wrap around the acinar and intercalated duct cells (Figs. 15-12 and 15-13). Their large nuclei and cytoplasms, containing microfilaments, enable them to act as muscle cells.

 CLINICAL COMMENT

Drugs such as tranquilizers, barbiturates, and antihistamines decrease salivary flow. In some older patients, who may already have deficient salivary flow, this could be a cause of dry mouth (xerostomia).

CLASSIFICATION OF TONSILLAR TISSUE

Tonsillar tissue surrounds the oropharynx in a ring called **Waldeyer's ring**. In the oropharyngeal midline is the single **pharyngeal tonsil** or **adenoid**; adjacent to the posterior molars are the bilateral **palatine tonsils**; and in the floor of the mouth are the bilateral **lingual tonsils** (Fig. 15-14). Tonsils are part of the lymphatic system, which also includes lymph nodes, thymus, spleen, and diffuse lymphatic tissue. Each tonsil is composed of lymphatic tissue or nodules. The lymphatic nodules in turn may have **germinal centers**, which are active sites of lymphocyte formation. These centers are common in the lingual and palatine tonsils. The tonsils are covered with epithelium. In the pharyngeal tonsil the epithelium is respiratory because the tonsil is in the nasopharynx. In the orally located palatine and lingual tonsils it is stratified squamous epithelium. This epithelial covering lines the grooves or clefts of each gland. Tonsils, unlike lymph nodes, have no afferent lymphatic vessels that lead to them. However, both tonsils and lymph nodes do have efferent lymphatic vessels draining them. Each tonsil is

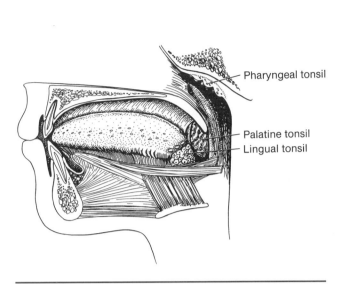

FIG. 15-14   Location of three tonsillar groups. Palatine tonsil is in lateral wall of oropharynx, lingual in midline of floor of mouth, and pharyngeal in midline posterior pharyngeal wall.

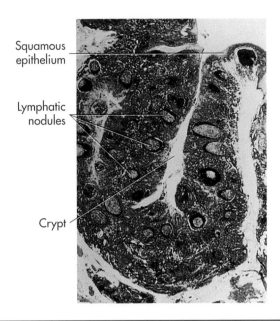

FIG. 15-16   Histology of palatine tonsil showing the investing squamous epithelium, deep branching crypts, and organized lymphatic nodules.

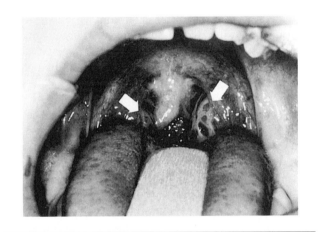

FIG. 15-15   Oral view of palatine tonsils *(arrows)*. These inflamed, swollen tonsils project into oropharyngeal cavity.

supported by connective tissue and has associated glands underlying it.

Palatine Tonsils

The palatine tonsils are large in children and best recognized when they become infected and bulge into the throat, causing difficulty in swallowing. When the tonsils are infected and swollen, they appear red with streaks of white, purulent material on their surfaces (Fig. 15-15). They become infected largely as a result of their structure. Because palatine tonsils have deep, branching crypts in which oral bacteria may become lodged, these crypts may become plugged with lymphocyte discharge and desqua-

mated epithelial cells. Beneath the palatine tonsils are seromucous glands, which assist in flushing out these crypts. Their ducts, however, do not open into the tonsillar crypts but onto the surface of the glands. This lack of flushing action in the crypts may account for the accumulation of foreign debris and bacteria that causes tissue inflammation. Structurally these are the largest tonsils of the three types and are divided into lobules by the crypts. Each lobule contains numerous lymphatic nodules, which contain **germinal centers** (Fig. 15-16). Septa of connective tissue support the nodules of lymphatic tissue and invest the gland in a capsule.

Lingual Tonsils

Lingual tonsils are located on the surface of the posterior third of the tongue (Fig. 15-14). The tonsillar mass is bilateral as it is divided in the midline, reflecting the bilateral origin of the tongue. The lingual tonsils are composed of wide-mouthed crypts and are nonbranching. They form rows of lymphatic nodules supported by connective tissue septa that are present in each lobule of the gland (Fig. 15-17). These tonsils also have a connective tissue capsule investing them. The capsule is covered with nonkeratinized stratified squamous epithelium. Underlying these tonsils, between the mucous glands, are skeletal muscles and adipose tissue of the tongue. These mucous glands, with their ducts opening into the crypt, function in a cleansing action. Also, because these tonsils are located in the posterior floor of the mouth, the washing action of saliva provides effective cleansing. Therefore this tonsillar mass is rarely inflamed.

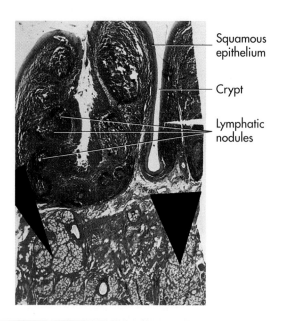

FIG. 15-17 Histology of posterior tongue tonsil (lingual tonsil) showing the investing squamous epithelium, short crypts, and lymphatic nodules. Arrows denote underlying mucous glands.

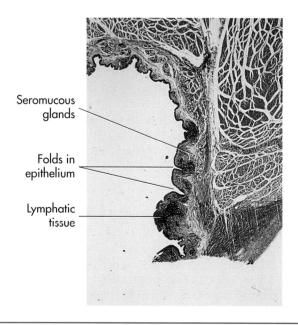

FIG. 15-18 Histologic appearance of pharyngeal tonsil with folds in epithelium rather than crypts in tissue, diffuse lymphatic tissue rather than nodules, and seromucous glands underlying the tonsillar tissue.

Pharyngeal Tonsil

The pharyngeal tonsil, or **adenoid,** is located in the posterior wall of the superior portion of the nasopharynx. It is subject to infection in childhood. The pharyngeal tonsil may grow laterally from the midline location to surround the opening of the eustachian tubes. Tonsillar tissue at this location is called the tubal tonsil and can be the source of infection to the eustachian tubes. The pharyngeal tonsil is unlike the other tonsils in that it is an aggregation of lymphocytes that does not have crypts but has occasional folds that appear as clefts in the mucosa (Fig. 15-18). This tonsil is variable in structure because only occasionally are there lymphoid nodules, which are usually only on a surface accumulation of diffuse lymphoid tissue. The covering epithelium is transformed either into respiratory or into stratified squamous epithelium. Underlying the tonsil are mixed glands that drain the surface of the epithelium overlying the gland tissue. This tonsil overlies the muscles of the pharynx.

FUNCTION OF TONSILS

The most notable function of tonsils is the production of lymphocytes that protect the body from foreign microorganisms inhaled or swallowed. Allergens may be sensed by these cells, which start the complex process of coding for antibody production. Because of their ability to retain this information, the lymphocytes have been called **memory cells.** Some lymphocytes transform into **T cells** and engulf bacteria or discharge substances to destroy them. Other lymphocytes become **B cells,** which differentiate into plasma cells. Plasma cells secrete antibodies that destroy antigens. Plasma cells and lymphocytes are found in chronic infections, such as periodontal disease. Plasma cells found in the area of the salivary glands produce IgA, which joins in the end piece of the intercellular area to form secretory IgA. Some foreign substances are absorbed from the crypts of the glands into the gland proper and then destroyed.

 CLINICAL COMMENT

Tonsils are ideally positioned around the entrance to the alimentary canal to aid in protecting the body from invasion of microorganisms. They are important in the antibacterial action of the B and T lymphocytes and in the action of the plasma cells in the formation of secretory IgA, which neutralizes viruses and can be an antibody to food antigens.

SELF-EVALUATION QUESTIONS

1. Discuss the location and function of the myoepithelial cells.
2. Describe the types of secretory duct cells and their functions.
3. What are the contributions of the major and minor salivary glands to the total volume of saliva?
4. Compare the appearance and function of serous and mucous cells.
5. Where are most serous demilune cells found?
6. What is the origin of secretory IgA?
7. Name and describe the various types of minor salivary glands.
8. Describe the gland type underlying each tonsil.
9. How does gland structure relate to the causes of tonsillitis?
10. What is the function of B and T cells in the tonsils?

 CONSIDER THE PATIENT . . .

Discussion: The dentist must examine the mouth carefully, and radiographs should be taken. Radiographs may reveal a stone in the submandibular duct, which is the most common site for a stone. Such a stone will interfere with salivary gland function and should be removed. Palpation by the dentist could assist the stone in passing through the duct.

SUGGESTED READING

Bradley RM: Salivary secretion. In Getchell TV et al, editors: *Smell and taste in health and disease*, New York, 1991, Raven Press, pp 127-144.

Castle D: Cell biology of salivary protein. In Dobrosielski-Vergona K, editor: *Biology of the salivary glands*, Boca Raton, Fla, 1993, CRC Press, pp 81-104.

Drummond JR, Chrisholm DM: A quantitative and qualitative study of the aging human salivary glands, *Arch Oral Biol* 29:151, 1984.

Field A, Scot J: Changes in the structure of salivary glands with age. In Dobrosielski-Vergona K, editor: *Biology of the salivary glands*, Boca Raton, Fla, 1993, CRC Press, pp 397-439.

Quissell DO: Stimulus exocytosis coupling mechanism in salivary gland cells. In Dobrosielski-Vergona K, editor: *Biology of the salivary glands*, Boca Raton, Fla, 1993, CRC Press, pp 105-127.

Rice DH, Becker TS: *The salivary glands*, New York, 1994, Thieme Medical.

Turner RJ: Mechanisms and secretion by salivary glands, *Ann NY Acad Sci* 694:24-35, 1993.

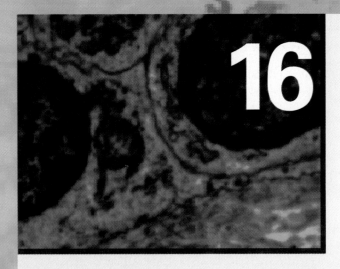

16 Pellicle, Plaque, and Calculus

OVERVIEW

This chapter describes substances that form on the surface of the teeth and explains how they develop. The primary cuticle is of cellular origin and is formed before tooth eruption. All other products originate from saliva. The primary cuticle forms the zone of junctional epithelium; the remaining epithelium is lost soon after the teeth erupt into incisal or occlusal contact. Saliva contains salivary proteins and glycoproteins that attach to enamel or exposed cementum or dentin. Saliva then deposits a thin protein coat or membrane, called a pellicle, on the surface of the tooth. The pellicle, although protective to the tooth, allows plaque to form on the surface of the tooth. This plaque is composed of bacteria and salivary proteins that will become a dense layer that gradually accumulates on the tooth's surface if not removed. The bacteria in plaque may produce acid that can cause etching and disintegration of the tooth's surface. This leads to the initiation of dental caries. Dental caries therefore develops in areas where brushing or washing of the tooth's surface does not occur. In other instances, plaque may not produce acid but may become mineralized into calculus. Calculus forms by mineralization of the remaining plaque bacteria into a hydroxyapatite deposit on the enamel and exposed cementum surfaces. Continuous acquisition of calculus forms a thick deposit that should be removed because the potential for inflammation or infection of gingival tissue could lead to destructive periodontal disease.

CUTICLE

The **primary** or **developmental cuticle** is deposited on the enamel's surface by the ameloblasts as their last function, shortly before the tooth crown erupts into the oral cavity. At this time, the formed enamel has reached a thickness of 2 to 2.5 mm over the cusps and is fully mineralized. In their final action the ameloblasts secrete a thin, structureless protein membrane on the tooth's surface. On the outer surface of this cuticle is the remainder of the enamel organ cells, termed the **reduced enamel epithelium.** This cellular membrane on the tooth's surface includes the ameloblasts and other remnants of the enamel organ. Ameloblasts form the primary cuticle. The reduced enamel epithelium is lost during eruption of the teeth in the oral cavity (Fig. 16-1). Only the developmental cuticle remains on the surface of the tooth as it erupts into occlusal function. However, this cuticle is not present long on the enamel because abrasion from contact of the opposing teeth causes it to wear away. Only that part covering the enamel in the gingival crevice remains (Fig. 16-2). This membrane serves as an attachment of the gingival junctional epithelial cells to the tooth. The sulcular epithelium is continually forming protein, which renews the gingival attachment throughout its life. Cuticular protein, which initiates attachment of the junctional epithelium to enamel, is the most important function of the primary cuticle.

ACQUIRED PELLICLE

When the tooth's surface is cleansed, salivary proteins and glycoproteins are quickly deposited with their strong attraction for the enamel surface. The resulting layer forms a thin, structureless membrane about 0.5 to 1.0 μm thick, which is in contrast to the previously formed cuticular layer. This membrane is termed the **pel-**

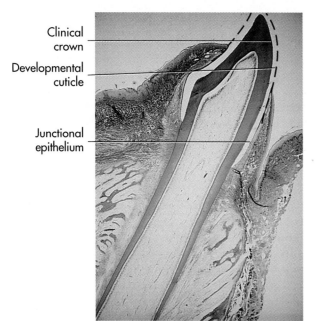

Clinical crown

Developmental cuticle

Junctional epithelium

FIG. 16-1 Crown's clinical appearance at time enamel is covered with developmental cuticle.

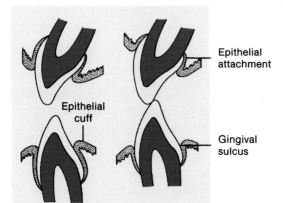

Epithelial attachment

Epithelial cuff

Gingival sulcus

FIG. 16-2 Diagram of erupting tooth showing ultimate position of gingiva and epithelial attachment on cervical enamel.

(Courtesy Dr RM Frank, Professor and Dean, and Dr A Brendel, Professor, Faculty de Chirurgie Dentaire, Strasbourg, France. From Avery JK, editor: *Oral development and histology,* New York, 1994, Thieme Medical.)

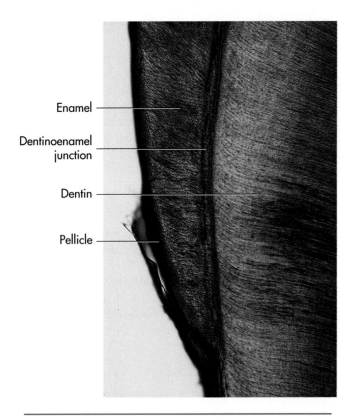

FIG. 16-3 Histology of enamel surface and structureless organic pellicle, which covers enamel rods, in this case at the cervical area.

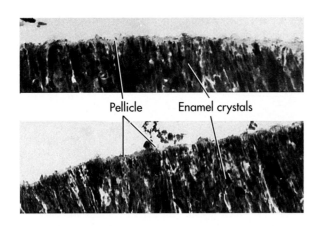

FIG. 16-4 Electron micrograph showing two areas of newly formed bacteria-free acquired pellicle on enamel's surface (prismless zone).

licle or **acquired pellicle** (Fig. 16-3). Although the pellicle is bacteria free when formed, bacteria rapidly attach to its surface. The pellicle covers the entire free surface of the enamel and may penetrate any convenient defect in the tooth's surface, such as a crack, a pit, or an overhanging restoration (Fig. 16-4).

Normally, surface layers of enamel rods are straight and at right angles to the tooth surface. The zone is about 30 μm thick, with the long axis of the apa-

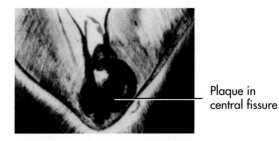

FIG. 16-5 Incipient carious lesion in central fissure of enamel in human molar. Plaque has accumulated in this area.

(Courtesy Dr Knut S Selvig, Professor and Head, Department of Dental Research, School of Dentistry, University of Bergen, Bergen, Norway. From Avery JK, editor: *Oral development and histology*, New York, 1994, Thieme Medical.)

CLINICAL COMMENT

The bathing of the tooth's surface with saliva causes formation of a thin organic membrane, the pellicle, which in part protects the tooth's surface from the action of oral bacteria. Oral bacteria lodge anywhere there is a crevice or other defect and can attach and penetrate the pellicle, causing enamel dissolution by acid production.

tite crystals oriented nearly perpendicular to the enamel surface (Fig. 16-4). This area is termed the **prismless zone** of enamel. The acquired pellicle overlying this zone has a fine, granular appearance and is approximately 500 Å thick when viewed in ultrastructure (Fig. 16-4).

If the pellicle is lost as a result of an oral prophylaxis, it forms again in a few minutes. Although the acquired pellicle is considered protective to the enamel surface, it does provide an attachment site for bacteria, which form plaque.

PLAQUE

The central fissure of a molar, premolar, or cervical margin of any tooth is the site for accumulation and colonization of oral organisms (Fig. 16-5). In addition to bacteria that attach to the pellicle, lymphocytes, leukocytes, desquamated epithelial cells, and clumps of mucin may lodge in any of these sites (Figs. 16-6 and 16-7). Organisms attach to the pellicle and utilize the presence of debris in acid formation.

In gingival or tonsillar inflammation, the number of lymphocytes and leukocytes increases (Fig. 16-8). If a

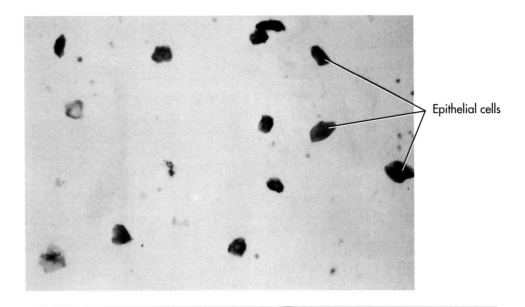

FIG. 16-6 A salivary smear viewed microscopically showing presence of desquamated epithelial cells.

Epithelial cells

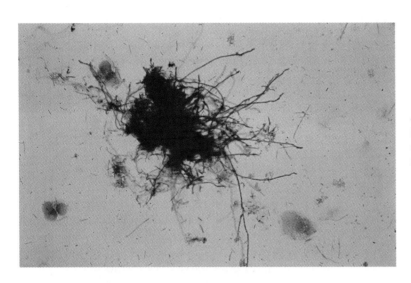

FIG. 16-7 Clumps of mucin from saliva that may adhere to crevices or imperfections in enamel's surface.

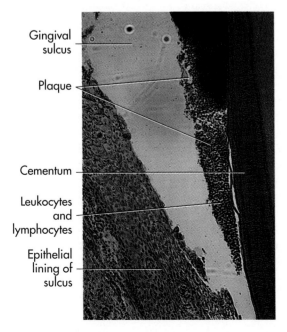

Gingival sulcus

Plaque

Cementum

Leukocytes and lymphocytes

Epithelial lining of sulcus

FIG. 16-8 The gingival sulcus viewed microscopically. Leukocytes and lymphocytes appear along surface of sulcus and tooth.

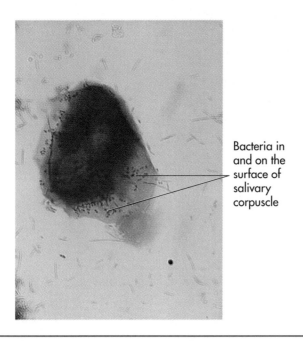

FIG. 16-9 Salivary corpuscle: lymphocyte with bacteria on its surface as present in saliva.

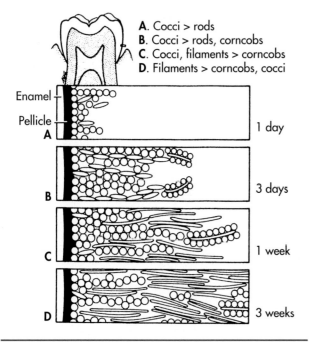

FIG. 16-10 Changes in plaque composition over a 3-week period. **A,** At 1 day. **B,** At 3 days, the cocci and a few filaments characterize the plaque. **C,** After 1 week, the filamentous organisms increase in number. **D,** By 3 weeks, the filamentous organisms predominate in the plaque.

(Courtesy Dr Walter Loesche, Professor of Biologic and Material Science, University of Michigan School of Dentistry, Ann Arbor. From Avery JK, editor: *Oral development and histology,* New York, 1994, Thieme Medical.)

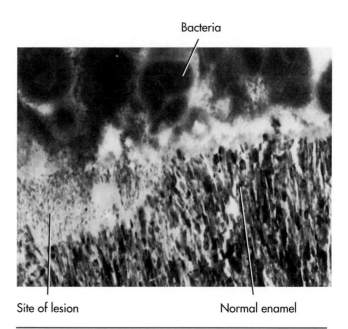

FIG. 16-11 Electron micrograph of bacterial effects on enamel surface. Initial lesion is shown in enamel surface (at left). Notice loss of enamel crystals.

(Courtesy Dr RM Frank, Professor and Dean, and Dr A Brendel, Professor, Faculty de Chirurgie Dentaire, Strasbourg, France. From Avery JK, editor: *Oral development and histology,* New York, 1994, Thieme Medical.)

microscopic analysis of a saliva sample reveals many lymphocytes, tonsillitis is indicated. However, an increase in leukocytes in saliva is indicative of gingival inflammation. These cells are called **salivary corpuscles** (Fig. 16-9). At first only a few bacteria are on the pellicle, but they rapidly grow into a thick **plaque** that contains a variety of microorganisms. The initial plaque quickly changes in composition to include rods and filamentous organisms. These appear after a few days, as shown in Fig. 16-10.

The composition of plaque depends also on the extent of gingival disease and whether the location of the plaque is supragingival or subgingival. The initial carious lesions affect the prismless zone of enamel because plaque bacteria cause dissolution of these surface crystals. A breakdown of enamel crystals is seen clinically as a brown spot on the tooth's surface. Fig. 16-11 shows a microscopic view of the loss of enamel rod structure. The enamel pellicle may overlie the area of an early lesion on the tooth's surface and be covered by plaque bacteria. Such a lesion may become filled with organic debris and bacteria (Fig. 16-12). Crystals appear to dissolve in one area and be intact in an adjacent area of enamel. Plaque can best be seen when a **disclosing solution** (0.2% basic fuchsin or erythrosin red #3 dye) is used to

Bacteria   Pellicle   Enamel dissolution   Normal enamel

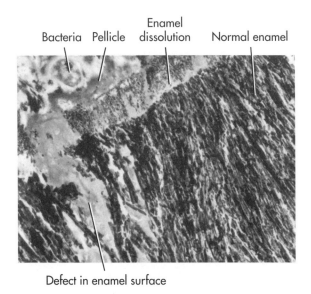

Defect in enamel surface

FIG. 16-12 Electron micrograph of a penetrating carious lesion appearing in the enamel *(left)*. Initial enamel dissolution and normal enamel under the pellicle and plaque are shown *(upper right)*.

(Courtesy Dr RM Frank, Professor and Dean, and Dr A Brendel, Professor, Faculty de Chirurgie Dentaire, Strasbourg, France. From Avery JK, editor: *Oral development and histology,* New York, 1994, Thieme Medical.)

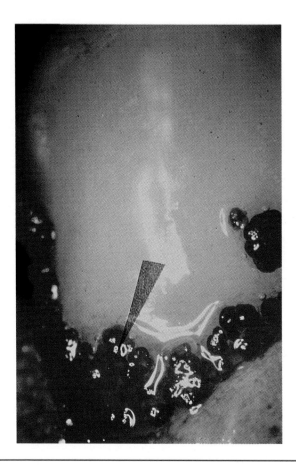

FIG. 16-13 View of gingival crevice area and tooth surface after use of disclosing solution with areas of stained plaque indicated by arrow.

determine if all the plaque has been removed. The advantage of using #3 dye is that it does not permanently discolor composite restorations or clothing. The stain left after a quick rinsing reveals any remaining plaque deposits, as observed in Fig. 16-13. These visible deposits can be removed by further polishing.

 CONSIDER THE PATIENT . . .

A patient appears who is suffering from tonsillitis. The dentist also finds a high level of lymphocytes in the saliva. Why is saliva important in determining oral health?

CALCULUS

Calculus is a stonelike concretion that forms on teeth or dental prostheses. It is primarily composed of calcium phosphate in the form of **hydroxyapatite,** which develops on the organic cell walls of bacterial plaque. Calculus formation is the reverse of enamel surface demineralization.

 CLINICAL COMMENT

Deposition of calculus can occur when the bacteria become calcified, forming a stonelike deposit. A disclosing agent can expose plaque bacteria to facilitate its removal, but plaque will reappear unless appropriate oral hygiene prevention is practiced. The removal of plaque is therefore important in the prevention of gingival and periodontal disease.

Calculus appears most often near the opening of the parotid excretory duct on the buccal surfaces of maxillary molars and on the lingual surfaces of the lingual incisors near the openings of the submandibular and lingual ducts. After plaque accumulates, mineralization begins in the inner layer of the pellicle and then spreads into the overlying plaque. Plaque continues to thicken

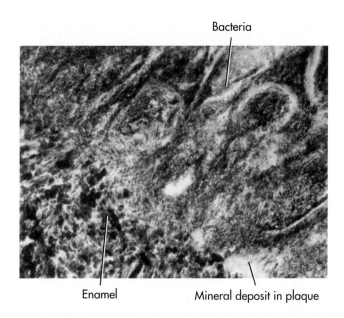

FIG. 16-14 Calculus formation viewed by electron microscopy. Minute mineral crystals fill circular bacterial ghosts on enamel surface.

(Courtesy Dr RM Frank, Professor and Dean, and Dr A Brendel, Professor, Faculty de Chirurgie Dentaire, Strasbourg, France. From Avery JK, editor: *Oral development and histology,* New York, 1994, Thieme Medical.)

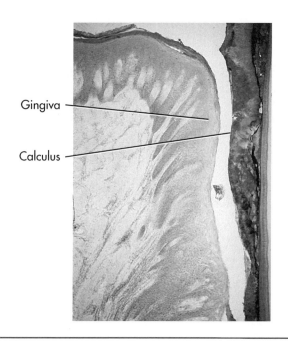

FIG. 16-16 Calculus appearing in this gingival crevice will relate to pocket formation.

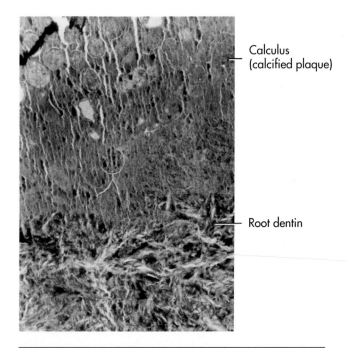

FIG. 16-15 Calculus on irregular surface of dentin. Minute mineral crystals are in calculus *(above)* with larger crystals in dentin *(below)*.

with further deposition of plaque protein. The calcified bacteria appear as circular profiles (Fig. 16-14) and are known as bacterial ghosts.

Calculus deposition follows any surface irregularity of the tooth, such as enamel or cementum (Fig. 16-15). Therefore calculus forms in a calcospherite manner as the calcium salts derived from saliva organize in the organic skeletons of plaque bacteria. As the plaque calcifies, it loses its ability to produce an acid environment.

Calculus varies in both composition and hardness. Harder calculus contains more mineral matter. Calculus may develop above the gingival margin or within the gingival crevice. Subgingival calculus is much harder and forms more slowly than supragingival calculus. Subgingival calculus is referred to as **serumal calculus** and is usually darker because it contains serum and blood pigments.

Typical bacteria and calculus appear in the gingival crevice (Fig. 16-16). Gram-positive organisms appear in the supragingival area, and gram-negative organisms are in the subgingival area (Fig. 16-17). This is because gram-positive organisms are aerobic or live in air, whereas gram-negative organisms are anaerobic or function best without air. Bacterial action and the deposits result in gingival inflammation, affecting the location of the gingival attachment to the cementum rather than the cervical enamel.

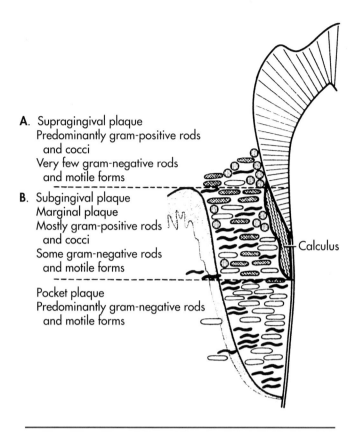

A. Supragingival plaque
   Predominantly gram-positive rods
   and cocci
   Very few gram-negative rods
   and motile forms

B. Subgingival plaque
   Marginal plaque
   Mostly gram-positive rods
   and cocci
   Some gram-negative rods
   and motile forms

   Pocket plaque
   Predominantly gram-negative rods
   and motile forms

Calculus

FIG. 16-17 Diagram comparing composition of supragingival plaque organisms with subgingival organisms. Deep in the pocket are gram-negative rods and motile spirochetes. Gram-positive rods are in the area of the supragingival and gingival margin.

(Courtesy Dr Walter Loesche, Professor of Biologic and Material Science, University of Michigan School of Dentistry, Ann Arbor. From Avery JK, editor: *Oral development and histology,* New York, 1994, Thieme Medical.)

CLINICAL COMMENT

Salivary calculus is damaging to the gingival tissues and should be removed by scaling. This scaling is frequently accompanied by bleeding of the gingival tissues. The gingiva heals rapidly, however, and the bleeding soon abates.

SELF-EVALUATION QUESTIONS

1. Describe the changes that occur in plaque from 1 day to 3 weeks.
2. Define salivary corpuscles.
3. On what matrix does calculus form?
4. Name and characterize the outermost layer of enamel.
5. What types of bacteria are seen supragingivally and subgingivally?
6. Where does plaque usually form?
7. What are the components of a pellicle?
8. How long does it take an acquired pellicle to form?
9. Discuss the purpose of using a disclosing solution.
10. What is the difference between serumal and salivary calculus?

CONSIDER THE PATIENT . . .

Discussion: Saliva may reveal other information, such as the presence of bacterial flora, lymphocytes, and leukocytes. Microscopic examination of saliva will disclose the health of the oral tissues. This condition can be indicative of infection in the gingival crevice, especially if bacterial plaque is present.

SUGGESTED READING

Frank RM, Brendel A: Ultrastructure of the approximal dental plaque and underlying normal and carious enamel, *Arch Oral Biol* 11:783-812, 1966.

Listgarten MA: Structure of the microbial flora associated with periodontal health and disease in man, *J Periodontol* 47:1, 1976.

McHugh WD, editor: *Dental plaque,* Edinburgh, 1970, E&S Livingstone.

Newman HN: Update on plaque and periodontal disease, *J Clin Periodontol* 7:251, 1980.

Selvig KA: Attachment of plaque and calculus to tooth surfaces, *J Periodont Res* 5:8-18, 1970.

Glossary

Accessory root canal   Secondary canal extending from the pulp to the surface of the root, usually found near apices of the root.

Acellular cementum   That part of the cementum covering one third to one half of the root of a tooth adjacent to the cementoenamel junction. It consists of collagenous fibers and ground substance.

Acinus (alveolus)   A small, terminal, saclike dilation particular to glands such as the salivary glands.

Acquired pellicle   An acellular, organic, thin skin or film deposited on the surface of teeth from salivary proteins (saliva) that bathe the surface of the teeth after eruption.

Alveolar bone   Ridge of bone; refers to tooth-bearing part of the mandible and maxilla because it contains the tooth sockets.

Alveolar bone proper   A thin lamina of bone that lines the tooth sockets, supports the roots of the teeth, and gives attachment to principal fibers of the periodontal ligament.

Alveolar crest fibers   Principal fibers of the periodontal ligament extending between the crest of the alveolar bone and the neck of the tooth.

Alveoli   See *Dental alveoli.*

Ameloblast   One of the differentiated cells of the inner layer of the enamel organ. From the cells there comes the enamel of the teeth.

Amelogenesis   The process of production and development of enamel.

Amelogenin   Protein found in newly deposited enamel matrix. Amelogenins are lost during maturation of enamel.

Amylase   Enzyme that catalyzes the hydrolysis of starch into smaller water-soluble carbohydrates.

Anatomic crown   That portion of the tooth covered by enamel.

Angioblasts   Cells that give rise to blood cells and blood vessels.

Angstrom   Unit of wavelength equivalent to 0.1 millimicron (10^{-7} mm). Abbreviated Å.

Antibody   A protein that is produced in the body in response to invasion by a foreign agent or antigen and that has a specific reaction.

Aortic arches   A series of arterial channels encircling the embryonic pharynx within the mesenchyme of the branchial arches.

Apical foramen   Opening at the apex of the tooth's root giving passage to the nerves and blood vessels.

Appositional growth (exogenous)   Deposition of successive cell products laid down upon those already present.

Articular disk (of the temporomandibular joint)   The fibrous disk that separates the upper and lower joint cavities.

Attached gingiva   The part of the oral mucosa that is firmly bound at the neck of the tooth and the alveolar process.

Attached pulpal stones or denticles   Mineralized tissues that are partly fused with the dentin of the coronal pulp or root canal.

B cells   Lymphocytes that have differentiated into plasma cells. Plasma cells secrete antibodies that destroy antigens.

Basal lamina   Membrane separating the epidermis and dermis that is a product of both.

Bell stage   Developmental stage of the tooth characterized by the differentiation of inner enamel epithelial cells into ameloblasts and the formation of the outline of the future crown by these cells.

Blastocyst   The postmorula stage of development; a blastula with a fluid-filled cavity.

Bone   Mineralized animal tissue consisting of an organic matrix, cells, and fibers of collagen impregnated with mineral matter, chiefly calcium phosphate and calcium carbonate. See also *Bundle bone, Cancellous bone, Compact bone, Haversian bone.*

Branchial   Barlike, resembling the gills of a fish.

Branchial arch   One of a series of mesodermal bars located between the branchial clefts. During embryonic stages, the arches contribute to the formation of the face, jaws, and neck. They appear in higher forms only vestigially.

Branchial arch cartilages   The cartilages found in the branchial arches of the embryo.

Bud stage   Initial stage of tooth development; the enamel organ develops from this structure. The dental papilla lies adjacent to the epithelial bud, and the dental sac encloses both.

Bundle bone   Specialized bone lining the tooth socket into which the fibers of the periodontal ligament penetrate. The radiographic term *lamina dura* is synonymous with bundle bone.

Calcification   See *Diffuse calcification.*

Calcospherite   One of the small globular bodies formed during the process of calcification by chemical union between the calcium particles and the albuminous organic matter of the intercellular substance.

Calculus   An abnormal concretion within the body, usually formed of mineral salts and often deposited around a minute fragment of inorganic material, the nucleus. See also *Dental calculus, Serumal calculus.*

Canals   See *Haversian canals.*

Cancellous bone   Spongy or latticelike structure composed mainly of bone tissue.

Cap stage   Part of tooth development, an early stage in enamel organ formation. It follows the bud stage.

Cartilage   Fibrous connective tissue characterized by nonvascularity and a firm consistency. Forms most of the temporary skeleton of the embryo. See also *Hyaline cartilage.*

Cell   Smallest unit of living structure capable of independent existence.

Cell-free zone   Relatively cell-free layer of the dental pulp adjacent to odontoblasts and overlying the cell-rich zone. Composed of delicate fibrils in ground substance.

Cell-rich zone   Layer of the dental pulp situated between the pulp core and the cell-free zone, which is richly supplied with cellular elements, blood vessels, and nerves.

Cellular cementum   That part of the cementum covering the apical one half to two thirds of the root of a tooth. This cementum is most abundant on the root tip.

Cementicles   Calcified spherical bodies composed of cementum lying free within the periodontal ligament, attached to the cementum, or embedded within it.

Cementoblast   A large cuboidal cell lying on the surface of the bone that is active in cementum formation.

Cementocyte   A cell found in the lacuna of cellular cementum. Numerous cytoplasmic processes extend from its free surface.

Cementoid layer   See *Intermediate cementum*.

Cementum   Bonelike connective tissue that covers the tooth from the cementoenamel junction to and surrounding the apical foramen. See also *Acellular cementum, Cellular cementum*.

Central nervous system (CNS)   Composed of the brain and spinal cord.

Centriole   Either of two short cylinders appearing near the nucleus that migrate to opposite poles of the cell during cell division.

Cervical loop   Growing free border of the enamel organ. Here the outer and inner enamel epithelial cell layers are continuous with each other.

Chromosome   A structure in the nucleus containing a thread of DNA during cell division and providing genetic information.

Circumpulpal dentin   Inner portion of the dentin located near the pulp organ of the tooth.

Clinical crown   That portion of the crown exposed and visible in the oral cavity.

CNS   See *Central nervous system (CNS)*.

Col   Valleylike depression in the facial lingual plane of the interdental gingiva. It conforms to the shape of the interproximal contact area.

Collagen   White fibers of the corium of the skin, tendon, and other connective tissue. The fiber is composed of fibrils bound with interfibrillar cement.

Collagen fiber   High-molecular-weight protein composed of several structural types that vary in diameter and usually are arranged in bundles.

Compact bone   Dense bone more highly calcified than cancellous (spongy) bone.

Condyle   See *Mandibular condyle*.

Coronal pulp   Pulp present in the crown of a tooth.

Cranial   Pertaining to the cranium, specifically those bones covering the brain.

Cranial base   Lower portion of the skull constituting the floor of the cranial cavity.

Crypts   Pitlike depressions or tubular recesses on a free surface.

Cuticle   See *Primary cuticle*.

Cytoplasm   Protoplasm of a cell located in the area surrounding the nucleus.

Cytosol   Semifluid part of cytoplasm in which organelles are suspended and solutes dissolved.

Dead tracts   Empty tubules resulting from loss of the odontoblastic processes.

Deciduous dentition   Primary teeth that function during the first 8 years of life and then exfoliate, providing space for the permanent teeth.

Dehiscence   Alveolar bone loss in the coronal root.

Demilune   A crescent-shaped structure or cell. See also *Serous demilune*.

Dendrite   Component of the neuron that receives impulses and conducts them to the cell body.

Dental alveoli   The alveoli or sockets in which the roots of teeth are embedded.

Dental calculus   Stonelike concretion formed on the teeth, on a prosthesis, or in salivary ducts. It varies in color from creamy yellow to black and is composed mostly of calcium phosphate.

Dental lamina   Horseshoe-shaped epithelial bands that traverse the upper and lower jaws and give rise to the ectodermal portions of the teeth.

Dental papilla   Part of the formative organ of the teeth that forms the dentin and the pulp.

Dental plaque   Organic deposit on the surface of teeth. Site of bacterial growth and formation of dental calculus.

Dental pulp   The soft tissue contained within the pulp chamber. Consists of connective tissue, blood vessels, nerves, and lymphatics.

Dental sac (follicle)   Area of mesenchymal cells and fibers that surround the dental papilla and the enamel organ of the developing teeth. It produces the periodontal ligament, alveolar bone, and cementum.

Dentin   Yellowish body of the tooth. It surrounds the pulp and underlies the enamel on the crown and the cementum on the roots of the teeth. Composed of 20% organic matrix, which is mostly collagen, and 10% water. The inorganic fraction (70%) is hydroxyapatite, with some carbonate, magnesium, and fluoride. See also *Intratubular or peritubular dentin* and *Mantle dentin*.

Dentinoenamel junction   Interface of the enamel and dentin of the crown of a tooth.

Dentinogenesis   The process of dentin formation in the development of teeth.

Dermatomes   Dorsal lateral portion of the somite of the embryo. These cells form the dermis, subcutaneous tissue, and supporting tissue of the gastrointestinal tract.

Dermis   Arises from the mesoderm underlying the epidermis. The dermis and the epidermis together form the skin.

Desmosome   Cell junction. It consists of a dense plate near the cell surface that relates to a similar structure on an adjacent cell, between which are thin layers of extracellular material.

Diaphysis   The shaft of the long bone.

Differentiation   Process by which cells acquire individual cellular characteristics from an undifferentiated state, that is, specialization.

Diffuse calcification   Irregular calcified deposits along collagen fiber bundles or blood vessels in the pulp or elsewhere. It is considered a pathologic condition.

Diphyodont   Species that develops two separate dentitions during a lifetime.

Direct innervation   Theory based on the belief that nerves may extend to the dentinoenamel junction from the pulp.

DNA (deoxyribonucleic acid)   Contains the genetic information in the cell.

Drift   Movement of a tooth to a position of greater stability.

Duct   Tube with well-defined walls for passage of excretions or secretions.

Dystrophy   A disorder arising from defective or faulty nutrition.

Ectomesenchyme   Neural crest cells, mesoderm. Forms spinal ganglia.

Edentulous jaw   Alveolar bone without teeth.

Eleidin   A protein allied to keratin and protoplasm but more transparent than protein keratin.

Embryonic period   The second to eighth weeks of prenatal life.

Enamel   See *Gnarled enamel.*

Enamel crystals   Hydroxyapatite crystals found in enamel rods. They are formed during tooth mineralization.

Enamel lamellae   Thin, leaflike spaces that extend from the enamel surface toward the dentinoenamel junction. They represent defects or organically filled spaces in the enamel.

Enamel organ   Originates from the dental lamina and consists of four distinct layers.

Enamel pearls   Enameloma, a developmental anomaly in which a small nodule of enamel is formed near the cementoenamel junction, usually at the bifurcation zone of molar teeth.

Enamel rod   One of the structural units of enamel, extending from the dentinoenamel junction to the surface of the tooth and normally having a translucent crystalline appearance.

Enamel spindles   Tubular spaces in enamel found at the dentinoenamel junction in which a terminal extension of the odontoblastic processes can be found.

Enamel tuft   Narrow, ribbonlike structures whose constricted inner end arises at or near right angles to the dentinoenamel junction and extends a third of the way into the thickness of the enamel. Tufts consist of hypocalcified spaces that may be filled with organic substance.

Enamelin   The organic protein component of enamel.

Enameloid   A thin, structureless layer of substance that may be a form of enamel that is deposited by the root sheath.

Endochondral   Relating to the type of bone formation that occurs within cartilage and replaces it.

Endocrine   Refers to glands of internal secretion that release their secretory product(s) hormones directly into the bloodstream rather than through a duct system.

Endometrium   The mucous membrane lining the uterus.

Endoplasmic reticulum (ER)   An ultrastructural organelle consisting of membrane-bound cavities in the cytoplasm of the cell.

Epidermis   The surface nonvascular cell layer of the skin that develops from the surface ectodermal cells. It consists of five layers; from the inner to the outer layer, they are (1) basal, (2) spinous, (3) granular, (4) clear (lucidum), and (5) horny (corneum).

Epiphysis   The extremity of a long bone as opposed to the shaft (diaphysis).

Epithelial attachment   Attachment of the gingival epithelium to the tooth's surface at the dentogingival junction.

Epithelial cell rests   Origin from the epithelial root sheath that covers the roots during root development. As the sheath develops further, it breaks up into epithelial cell rests, which migrate into the periodontal ligament. Occasionally they may develop into dental cysts. The cell groups are of these types: (1) resting, (2) proliferating, and (3) degenerating.

Epithelial diaphragm   Formed by the root sheath at the beginning of root development, important during root formation. It narrows the width of the cervical opening of the root.

Epithelial pearls   Discrete rounded or ovoid groups of epithelial cells, frequently keratinized, found in the lamina propria.

Epithelial root sheath   Cervical loop enamel organ cells that proliferate, forming a double layer of cells (Hertwig's) that function in root formation.

Epithelium   Cellular avascular layer covering all the free surfaces of the body, internal and external, and the lining of vessels. Consists of cells and small amounts of intercellular substance. See also *Inner enamel epithelium.*

ER   See *Endoplasmic reticulum.*

Exfoliate   To shed or eliminate something from the surface of the body, as in the loss of teeth from the jaws.

Exocrine   Denotes glands that release their secretory product(s) into a duct system.

Exocytosis   Discharge of secretory product(s) from the cell, preserving the cell membrane through fusion of the secretory vesicles with the cell membrane.

Fenestration   The area of alveolar bone loss where an apical root penetrates the bone.

Fetal period   The embryo from the eighth prenatal week to birth.

Fibroblastoclasts   Those fibroblasts that can both form and destroy collagen fibers.

Fibroblasts   Elongated, ovoid, spindle-shaped, or flattened cells found in connective tissue.

Filiform papillae   The most numerous papillae appearing on the dorsum of the tongue. These threadlike elevations point dorsally and toward the throat.

Fontanelle   One of several membrane-covered spaces found in the incompletely ossified skull of the fetus or newborn.

Fordyce's spots   A condition characterized by minute yellowish white papules (sebaceous glands) on the oral mucosa.

Free gingiva   The portion of the gingiva that surrounds the tooth and is not directly attached to the tooth surface; the outer wall of the gingival sulcus.

Fundic bone   Bone enclosing the apex of the tooth root.

Fungiform papillae   Minute elevations on the dorsum, tip, and sides of the tongue. The papillae are mushroom shaped with the top being broader than the base.

Ganglion   A group of nerve cell bodies located outside the central nervous system.

Gap junctions   Specialized communicating junction between cells with pores permeable to ions and small molecules.

Gingiva   Soft tissue surrounding the necks of erupted teeth that cover the alveolar process. The gingiva consists of fibrous connective tissue enveloped by mucous membrane. See also *Attached gingiva, Free gingiva, Interdental gingiva.*

Gingival sulcus   The shallow V-shaped trench around each tooth, bound by the tooth on one surface and the epithelium-lined free margin on the other.

Ginglymoarthrodial A type of synovial joint that allows opening and closing, symmetrical protrusion and retrusion, and asymmetrical lateral movement of the mandible.

Gland See *Merocrine gland.*

Globular dentin Areas of defective growth with interglobular spaces that underlie the enamel and surface of the root.

Gnarled enamel The enamel located at the tips of the cusps, in which the rods or groups of rods are twisted, bent, and intertwined. It is seen ultrastructurally.

Golgi's apparatus or complex A continuation of the endoplasmic reticulum. A cuplike structure within cells made up of saccules where carbohydrate side chains of glycoproteins form.

Granular layer of Tomes A thin, granular-appearing layer of defective dentin located along the root surface adjacent to the cementum.

Gubernacular cord A fibrous tissue band connecting the tooth sac with the alveolar mucosa. This cord may function in tooth eruption.

Hard palate Anterior part of the palate consisting of the bony palate bound above by the nasal cavity and below by the mouth. It is covered by keratinized stratified squamous epithelium. In addition, the hard palate contains palatine vessels and nerves, adipose tissue, and mucous glands.

Haversian bone Compact bone containing tubular channels with blood vessels, nerves, and bone cells surrounded by concentrically located lacunae. These structures are termed the haversian system.

Haversian canals These nutrient canals are located in cortical bone and extend in the direction of the tooth's long axis.

Hemidesmosome Half of a desmosome that forms a site of attachment between epithelial cells and the basal lamina or between epithelial cells (junctional cells) and the tooth's surface.

Hormone Chemical substance formed in one organ or part of the body and carried by the bloodstream to another part where it stimulates or depresses activity.

Howship's lacunae Absorption lacunae. Tiny cup-shaped depressions on the resorbing front of any hard tissue, the result of resorptive activity by osteoclasts.

Hunter-Schreger bands Alternating dark and light bands in enamel that result from absorption and reflection of light caused by differences in orientation of adjacent groups of enamel rods originating at the dentinoenamel junction and extending toward the outer enamel surface.

Hyaline cartilage A flexible, semitransparent, elastic substance composed of a collagen fibrillar matrix and chondrocytes in lacunae.

Hydrodynamics Science of factors determining the flow of liquids. In dentistry, it refers to a theory that pain conduction through dentin results from odontoblastic movement making contact with nerve endings.

Hydroxyapatite An inorganic compound that constitutes bone and teeth.

IgA A distinct class of immunoglobulins. A protein of animal origin with known antibody activity, synthesized by lymphocytes and plasma cells; found in serum, other body fluids, and tissues.

Imbrication lines Also known as von Ebner's lines, incremental lines in dentin that run at right angles to the tubules. These lines, which represent the daily growth pattern, indicate layers of dentin that are less calcified and appear darker than adjacent dentin.

Impaction Position of a tooth in the alveolus that makes it incapable of eruption into the oral cavity.

Incisor liability The succession of larger permanent incisors replacing primary ones. The size ratio of the two incisors of the two dentitions.

Increment The amount by which a given quantity is increased. A measurable amount.

Incremental deposition Deposition of material in discrete amounts rather than constant deposition. Rhythmic recurrent deposition of enamel, bone, dentin, or cementum.

Incremental line An evident line produced through a rhythmic, recurrent deposition of successive layers upon present layers.

Inner enamel epithelium Cells that line the concavity of the enamel organ in the cap and early bell stages of tooth development and differentiate into ameloblasts.

Innervation Presence and distribution of nerves within a part or the supply of nerves stimulating a part.

Intercellular tissue Tissue located between or among cells of any structure.

Interdental gingiva The soft tissue between adjacent contacting teeth in the same arch.

Interdental septa Bony partitions that project into the alveoli between the teeth, interalveolar.

Intermediate cementum A deposition by the epithelial root sheath cells on the root surface formed during root formation. May be termed *enameloid.*

Interstitial growth (endogenous) Growth by expansion of the matrix by cell deposits within the matrix.

Interstitial spaces Spaces between groups or bundles of periodontal fibers.

Intramembranous Within a membrane. Bone formation occurring within or among connective tissue fibers. It does not replace cartilage, as does endochondral bone.

Intratubular or peritubular dentin The dentinal matrix that immediately surrounds the dentinal tubule.

Junctional epithelium Epithelial attachment. That epithelium adhering to the tooth surface at the bottom of the gingival crevice and consisting of one or more layers of nonkeratinizing cells.

Keratinized Having developed a horny layer of flattened epithelial cells containing keratin.

Keratinized mucosa Stratified surface of cornified epithelial cells that lack a nucleus and whose cytoplasm is replaced by large amounts of keratohyalin protein.

Keratinocytes Cells of the oral mucosa. These epidermal cells synthesize keratin.

Lacunae The very small cavities in bone that are filled with bone cells. See *Howship's lacunae.*

Lamella Thin leaf or plate, as of bone. See also *Enamel lamellae.*

Lamina dura A thin layer of hard compact bone lining the tooth sockets. Used in radiography to designate a thin radiopaque line.

Lamina propria Layer of connective tissue underlying the epithelium of skin or a mucous membrane.

Langerhans' cells   Clear or dendritic cells found in both superficial and deep layers of the epidermis and oral epithelium.

Leeway space   The difference in the space in the arch required for the two primary molars and the successional permanent premolars replacing them. The leeway space in the maxilla is 1.3 mm and in the mandible is 3.1 mm.

Lingula   The sharp medial boundary of the mandibular foramen, to which is attached the sphenomandibular ligament.

Lining mucosa   Nonkeratinized oral mucosa that covers the surface of the cheeks, lips, soft palate, floor of the mouth, and ventral surface of the tongue.

Lysosome   Small membrane-bound body that contains a variety of acid hydrolases, which function in breaking down substances both inside and outside the cell. It is visible through electron microscopy.

Macroglossia   Enlargement of the tongue that can be caused by muscular hypertrophy.

Macrognathia   Excessive size of the jaw.

Macrophages   Any of the large mononuclear phagocytic cells found in various tissues and organs of the body. These cells are a normal constituent of the pulp and function in tissue maintenance.

Malassez's rests   Epithelial cell remnants of Hertwig's sheath in the periodontal ligament. These cell groups appear near the surface of the cementum; they may develop into dental cysts.

Mandible   Horseshoe-shaped bone forming the lower jaw and articulating the condyles with the temporal bone on either side. The mandible is composed of the horizontal body and inclined ramus. The body includes the alveolar process, which contains the teeth.

Mandibular condyle   The rounded bony projections of the mandible that articulates with the temporal fossa of the temporal bone in the temporomandibular fossa.

Mantle dentin   The initially deposited portions of the dentin formed immediately adjacent to the enamel.

Masticatory mucosa   The mucosa that functions in mastication. It tends to be bound to bone and is therefore immovable. This mucosa covers the hard palate and the gingiva.

Maturation zone   Zone of cartilage characterized by chondrocyte enlargement.

Maxilla   Upper jaw bone, an irregularly shaped bone articulating with the nasal, lacrimal, zygomatic, palatine, ethmoid, sphenoid, and frontal bones of the face and containing teeth.

Maxillary sinus   Paired sinus cavities occupying the space beneath the floor of the orbit and above the roots of the posterior maxillary molars.

Meckel's cartilage   The initial skeletal component of the first branchial arch. It is the supporting cartilage of the mandibular arch in the embryo.

Medial nasal process   The area of the nose in the embryo. The tissue medial to the naris.

Median raphe   The line denoting union of the palatine bones in the midline of the palate. No submucosa is under the palatal mucosa in this area.

Meiosis   Process of reduction division of chromosomes in the daughter cell with half as many as in the parent cell.

Melanocytes   Cells responsible for synthesis of melanin that provide pigmentation to the skin.

Merkel's cells   Cells located in the basal layer of the gingival epithelium and thought to be epithelial in origin. They function as touch receptors.

Merocrine gland   The secreting cells that remain intact during the formation and release of the secretory product.

Mesenchyme   Loose, undifferentiated embryonic connective tissue that is a mixture of mesodermal and neural crest cells. The connective tissues of the body form from this tissue.

Mesial drift   General movement of a tooth or teeth anteriorly toward the midline of the jaw.

Mesoderm   The third primary germ layer of the embryo to differentiate. It is positioned between the ectoderm and the endoderm. From mesoderm are derived connective tissues, bone, cartilage, muscle, blood and blood vessels, lymphatics, notochord, pleura, and peritoneum.

Microglossia   Smallness of the tongue.

Micrognathia   Smallness of the jaw, especially the mandible.

Microtubules   Small tubular structures found in the cytoplasm and composed of the protein tubulin. They are cylindrical and hollow.

Mitochondrion   Small spherical organelle that is a membrane-bound structure lying free in the cytoplasm and present in all cells. This structure is the principal site of energy generation in the cell.

Mixed dentition   Simultaneous possession of both primary and permanent teeth.

Morula   Mass of blastomeres resulting from the early cleavage divisions of the zygote.

MPD   Myofacial pain dysfunction.

Mucin   A glycoprotein that is the primary constituent of mucus.

Mucoceles   Retention cysts of the minor salivary gland ducts, which contain mucous secretion. They usually result from rupture of the excretory duct of a minor salivary gland, causing pooling of saliva in the tissues. The resulting vesicular elevation is a mucocele.

Mucous acinus   Minute saclike secretory portion of a mucous gland. This is the functional unit of the gland.

Mucous glands   Glands that produce viscous proteinaceous secretions, such as the sublingual gland and glands of the hard palate.

Myoblast   An embryonic cell that becomes a cell of muscle fiber.

Myoepithelial cells   Spindle-shaped, contractile epithelial cells with stellate bodies and processes found in salivary and sweat glands. They are located in the terminal portion of the salivary gland acini and are believed to have contractile ability that facilitates movement of the glandular secretion into the ducts.

Myofibrils   Fine longitudinal fibrils (parallel to the long axis) found in a muscle fiber. They are composed of numerous myofilaments.

Nasal fin   A zone of epithelial contact of the medial nasal and maxillary processes during development.

Neonatal line   Accentuated incremental or hesitation line seen in bone, dentin, and enamel, probably caused by changes occurring at or near birth.

Nerves   Whitish cords composed of fibers arranged in bundles (fascicles) and held together by a connective tissue sheath, the perineurium. The fascicles are surrounded by epineurium. Nerves transmit stimuli from the central nervous system to the periphery by the efferent motor system or from the periphery to the central nervous system by the afferent sensory system.

Neural crest   Ganglionic crest, a band of ectodermal cells that appear along either side of the embryonic neural tube at the time of closure.

Neuroblasts   Primitive nerve cells that develop into adult nerve cells, the neurons. They are the functional cells of the brain, spinal cord, and peripheral nerves.

Neurocranium   That part of the skull enclosing the brain, as distinguished from the bones of the face.

Neuroglia   The supporting structure of the brain and spinal cord, which is composed of specialized cells and their processes.

Neuron   A nerve cell, which is any of the conducting cells of the nervous system, consisting of a cell body and containing the nucleus and its surrounding cytoplasm; the dendrite, which carries impulses to the cell body; and the axon that conducts impulses away from the cell body to the area of synapse.

Nonkeratinized mucosa   Lining mucosa, in which the stratified squamous epithelial cells retain their nuclei and cytoplasm. Lining mucosa is found on the inner lips, cheeks, soft palate, vestibular fornix, alveolar mucosa, floor of the mouth, and undersurface of the tongue.

Nonkeratinocytes   Cells not producing keratin. Clear or dendritic cells found in oral epithelium, such as pigment cells (melanocytes), Langerhans' cells, Merkel's cells, and inflammatory cells such as lymphocytes.

Nucleolus   A round vacuole-like achromatic body rich in RNA found within the nucleus of a cell.

Nucleus   A spheroid body within a cell, containing the genetic matter DNA, organelles, nucleoli, chromatin, linin, and nucleoplasm. It has a thin nuclear membrane vital to protein synthesis.

Occlusion   Relation of the functional contact of the maxillary and mandibular teeth during activity of the mandible.

Odontoblast   One of a layer of columnar cells with long processes extending into the dentinal tubules and lining the peripheral pulp of a tooth. These cells function in dentin formation and vitalize this tissue.

Odontoblastic process   A cytoplasmic extension of the cell body of the odontoblasts, some of which extend from the cell as far as the dentinoenamel junction or the cementoenamel junction.

Odontogenic zone   This area is peripherally adjacent to the dentin in both the coronal and radicular pulp. It contains the formative cells of dentin known as odontoblasts.

Olfactory mucosa   Site of most receptors for the sense of smell. It occupies the superior aspect of the nasal cavity between the superior nasal conchae, roof of the nose, and upper part of the nasal septum.

Organelles   Living particles located in the cytoplasm of cells. They include mitochondria, Golgi's complex, centrosomes, lysosomes, ribosomes, centrioles, endoplasmic reticulum, microtubules, and microfilaments.

Organic matrix   Formative portion of a tooth or bone as opposed to mineralized hydroxyapatite.

Osteoblasts   Bone-forming cells derived from mesenchyme. They form the osseous matrix, in which they may become enclosed to become osteocytes.

Osteoclasts   Multinucleated cells larger than osteoblasts and derived from monocytes from the bloodstream. Osteoclasts contain abundant acidophilic cytoplasm formed in bone marrow and function in the absorption and removal of osseous tissue.

Osteocytes   Cells of the bone located within lacunae, functioning in maintenance and vitality of bone.

Osteodentin   Dentin that appears more like bone than dentin because it contains cells.

Oxytalan fibers   Type of connective tissue fibers chemically different from collagen fibers and found in the periodontal ligament and gingiva. They appear similar to immature elastic fibers. These fibers are believed to support blood vessels and the principal fibers of the ligament.

Paciniform (Pacinian) corpuscle   Laminated nerve ending that functions in the perception of pressure.

Palatal rugae   Transverse ridges located in the mucous membrane of the anterior part of the hard palate. They extend laterally from the incisive papillae and have a core of dense connective tissue.

Palate   See *Primary palate, Secondary palate.*

Palatine tonsils   Two large oval masses of lymphoid tissue embedded in the lateral wall of the oropharynx and bilaterally located between the pillars of the fauces.

Papillae   Small protuberances on the tongue that are sensitive eminences, possessing a tactile function.

Parasympathetic nervous system   The craniosacral portion of the autonomic nervous system, its preganglionic fibers traveling with cranial nerves II, VII, IX, X, and XI and with the second to fourth sacral ventral roots. It innervates the heart, smooth muscle and glands of the head and neck, and thoracic, abdominal, and pelvic viscera.

Parenchyma   The functional elements of an organ rather than the supporting framework (stroma) of the organ.

Parotid   Serous-secreting salivary gland anterior to the ear. It is encapsulated and produces 26% of the secretions of the major salivary glands.

Pellicle   See *Acquired pellicle.*

Perforating fibers (Sharpey's fibers)   Penetrating connective tissue fibers by which the tooth is attached to the adjacent alveolar bone. These bundles of collagen fibers penetrate both the cementum and the alveolar bone.

Perikymata   Wavelike transverse grooves and ridges believed to be manifestations of the striae of Retzius on the surface of the enamel. They appear transverse to the long axis of the crown.

Perimysium   Connective tissue demarcating a fascicle of skeletal muscle fibers.

Periodontal ligament   Connective tissue ligament that is a mode of attachment of the tooth to the alveolus and that consists of collagenous fiber bundles. Between the bundles are loose connective tissue, blood vessels, and nerves.

Periodontium   Tissue surrounding and supporting the teeth. The tissue has two distinct components: the gingival unit, composed of the free and attached gingivae and the alveolar mucosa, and the component known as the attachment apparatus of the teeth, which includes the cementum, periodontal ligament, and alveolar bone.

Peritubular dentin The zone of dentin forming the wall of the dentinal tubules. This dentin has a 9% higher mineral content than does the remainder of the intertubular dentin.

Phagocytose To engulf and destroy bacteria and other foreign substances, denoting the action of the phagocytic cells.

Pharyngeal tonsils A collection of more or less closely aggregated lymphoid cells located superficially in the posterior wall of the nasopharynx, the hypertrophy of which results in the condition called adenoids.

Plaque See *Dental plaque.*

Plasma cells Cells derived from B lymphocytes, which actively synthesize and secrete immunoglobulins from an extensive rough endoplasmic reticulum. Under appropriate conditions, antigen stimulation induces proliferation and morphologic alteration in B lymphocytes to form plasma cells.

Plasma membrane or plasmalemma (cell membrane). Envelops the entire cell and provides a selective barrier that regulates transport of substances into and out of the cell.

Predentin Band of newly formed, and as yet unmineralized, matrix of dentin located at the pulpal border of the dentin.

Preeruptive phase Developmental stage preparatory to eruption of teeth and characterized by movements of the growing teeth within the alveolar process.

Primary cuticle A thin film on the enamel surface of an unerupted tooth. It is the product of the degenerating ameloblasts.

Primary palate That part of the palate formed from the median nasal process. The first palate to form is anterior to the secondary palate.

Prismless enamel Enamel formed without any rods or prism pattern.

Proliferative period Time during which cells grow and increase in number by cell division.

Ptyalin Synonymous term for salivary amylase, the enzyme in saliva that catalyzes the hydrolysis of starch into water-soluble carbohydrates.

Pulp bifurcation Zone of branching of the pulp organ, as found in multirooted teeth.

Pulp organ Soft tissue within the tooth, consisting of connective tissue, blood vessels, nerves, and lymphatics.

Pulpal blood vessels Characteristic thin-walled blood vessels of the dental pulp.

Pulpal stones or denticles Calcified masses of dentinlike substance located within the pulp or embedded in or attached to the dentinal wall. These stones may appear as a result of aging or trauma. They may be free, embedded, or attached to the dentin.

Quiescent stage A period of inactivity.

Radiation Transmission of rays, such as light rays, short radiowaves, ultraviolet rays, or x-rays.

Radicular pulp The pulp occupying the root canals that extend from the cervical coronal region to the apex of the root.

Ramus General term to designate a smaller structure given off by a larger one or one into which a larger structure divides.

Ramus of mandible Quadrilateral process projecting posteriorly and superiorly from the body of the mandible.

Raphe See *Median raphe.*

Red blood cell (corpuscle, erythrocyte) A nonnucleated biconcave hemoglobin that bears cells and is responsible for transport of oxygen to tissues via the circulatory system.

Reduced enamel epithelium The layers of the epithelial enamel organ compacted and remaining on the surface of enamel after enamel formation is complete.

Remodeling Alteration of the structure by reconstruction. The continuous process of turnover of bone carried out by osteoblasts and osteoclasts.

Reparative dentin (tertiary dentin) Deposited after trauma to the tooth by the original odontoblasts. A defensive reaction whereby hard tissue formation walls off the pulp from the site of injury.

RER See *Rough endoplasmic reticulum (RER).*

Response dentin Deposited after trauma to the tooth by newly recruited odontoblasts.

Reticulum A system of membrane-bound cavities in the cytoplasm of a cell. It occurs in two types, granular and agranular surface.

Retzius' striae Lines reflecting successive incremental deposition of mineralized enamel.

Reversal lines Lines separating layers of bone or cementum deposited in a resorption site distinguishing it from the scalloped outline of Howship's lacunae.

Ribosomes Particles that translate genetic codes for proteins and activate mechanisms for their production.

RNA (ribonucleic acid) Carries information to sites of actual protein synthesis located in the cell cytoplasm.

Root canal Extension of the pulp from the coronal zone to the root apex. See also *Accessory root canal.*

Root resorption Dissolution of the root of a tooth by action of osteoclasts. This may occur anywhere along the surface of the tooth root in response to caries or trauma or during the loss of a primary tooth.

Root sheath cells (Hertwig's sheath) Merged outer and inner epithelial layers of the enamel organ, extending beyond the region of the crown to invest the developing root.

Root trunk The part of the tooth immediately below the crown neck before division into the roots, covered by cementum and fixed in the alveolus.

Rough endoplasmic reticulum (RER) (granular) The ribosomes attached to the endoplasmic reticulum that function in synthesis of secretory protein.

Ruffled border An area enfolding the plasma membrane of the osteoclast that borders the resorptive zone.

Saliva Clear, slightly alkaline, somewhat viscid mixture of secretions of the salivary glands and gingival fluid exudate. It moistens the mucous membranes and food, facilitating speech and mastication. Consists of water and 0.58% solids.

Salivary calculi Calcium phosphate concentrations (salivary stones or sialolithiasis) found within a salivary gland or duct, most commonly in the main excretory duct of the submandibular gland (Wharton's duct).

Salivary corpuscle One of the leukocytes or lymphocytes found in saliva.

Salivary glands   Exocrine glands whose secretions flow into the oral cavity.

Schwann's cell   Cell forming the myelin sheath of nerves and seen in association with all nerves of the pulp.

Sclerotic (transparent) dentin   Dentin in which the tubules are occluded with mineral. Occurs mostly in elderly people, especially in the roots of the teeth.

Sclerotomes   Part of the somite consisting of mesenchymal tissue that develops into vertebrae and ribs.

Secondary dentin   Circumpulpal deposition of dentin formed after tooth eruption.

Secondary palate   The palate proper formed by fusion of the lateral palatine processes of the maxilla.

Serous   Relating to, containing, or producing a serum substance with a watery consistency.

Serous demilunes   Half-moon or crescent-shaped serous cells associated with the terminal external surface or mucous alveoli.

Serous glands of tongue (von Ebner's)   Serous glands opening into the bottom of the trough surrounding the circumvallate papillae and functioning in a cleansing action.

Serumal calculus   Subgingival calculus so termed because it results in part from exudation of serum.

Sharpey's fibers   See *Perforating fibers (Sharpey's fibers)*.

Sialography   Diagnostic x-ray technology used to visualize salivary gland ducts by injection of a radiopaque substance into the main excretory duct.

Smear layer   The fine particles of cut dentinal debris in dentinal tubules that are produced by cavity preparation.

Smooth muscle cells   Cells whose contractility is under control of the autonomic nervous system.

Soft palate   Posterior muscular portion of the palate, forming an incomplete septum between the nasopharynx and the oral cavity.

Somites   Paired blocklike masses of mesoderm arranged segmentally along the neural tube in the embryo and forming the dermis, vertebral column, and musculature.

Specialized mucosa   Mucosa found on the dorsum of the tongue. It consists of four types of papillae, which are filiform, fungiform, circumvallate, and foliate.

Spindles   The termination of dentinal tubules in inner enamel.

Squamous.   Relating to the flat squama, as of the temporal bone.

Squamous epithelium   Composed of a single layer of flat scalelike cells, as in the lining of the pulmonary alveoli, or stratified, as in oral epithelium.

Stellate reticulum   A network of star-shaped cells in the center of the enamel organ between the outer and inner enamel epithelia.

Stensen's duct   The epithelium-lined duct that drains the parotid gland.

Stomodeum   The embryo's future oral cavity, an invagination lined by surface ectoderm.

Stratified epithelium   A type of epithelium composed of a series of layers. The cells of each may vary in size and shape, as seen in skin and some mucous membranes.

Stratum intermedium   Epithelial cell layer of the enamel organ that lies external and adjacent to the inner enamel epithelium and is attached to it by desmosomes. Stratum intermedium also refers to the intermediate layer of nonkeratinizing epithelia.

Striae of Retzius   See *Retzius' striae*.

Striated duct   An intralobular gland duct that secretes saliva and is involved in ionic transport. The duct is located between the intercalated and interlobular ducts and is named for the basal striations produced by the enfolding of the basal membrane within the cells.

Stroma   Supporting framework of a gland, such as the capsule and trabeculae, rather than the functional parenchyma.

Sublingual   Refers to the area beneath the anterior lower jaw.

Sublingual gland   The smallest of the three pairs of major salivary glands. A pure mucous gland located in the anterior floor of the mouth.

Submandibular   Refers to the area beneath the angle of the mandible.

Submandibular gland   One of the three paired major salivary glands. The submandibular glands contribute 65% of saliva. These bilateral glands are a mixed seromucous type.

Submucosa   Layer of tissue that lies beneath the lamina propria underlying the mucous membrane of the lip, cheek, palate, and floor of the mouth.

Successional lamina   That portion of the dental lamina lingual to the developing deciduous teeth, which gives rise to the enamel organs of permanent teeth.

Supporting bone   Bone tissue functionally related to supporting the roots of the teeth. It surrounds, protects, and supports the tooth roots through the alveolar bone proper.

Sympathetic nervous system   The thoracolumbar part of the autonomic nervous system. Preganglionic fibers arise from cell bodies in the thoracic and first three lumbar segments of the spinal cord. Postganglionic fibers are distributed to the heart, smooth muscle, and glands of the entire body.

Synapse   The region of the junction between two nerve cells where an impulse passes between the axon of one cell and the dendrite of another cell.

Synchondrosis   A type of cartilaginous joint that usually is temporary.

Syndesmosis   A type of fibrous joint in which opposing surfaces are united in fibrous connective tissue, as in the union between most facial bones.

Synovial membranes   Membranes that line joint cavities and secrete a small amount of transparent alkaline fluid (synovial fluid) in the articular spaces. Synovial fluid acts as a lubricant and nutrient for the avascular tissue cover, that is, the condyle and articular tubercle for the temporomandibular joint.

T cells   Cells, produced by the thymus, that destroy invading microbes and are therefore important to the body's immune system.

Taste bud   Receptor of taste on the tongue and in the oropharynx. One of several goblet-shaped cells oriented at right angles to the surface by the epithelium. The taste buds consist of supporting and gustatory cells.

Temporomandibular joint (TMJ)   Joint formed between the condyle of the mandible and the mandibular fossa (concavity of the temporal bone).

Temporomandibular ligaments   Four ligaments that include the sphenomandibular on the medial surface, the stylomandibular on the posterior surface, the temporomandibular on the lateral surface, and the capsular surrounding the joint.

Teratogen Agent or factor that produces physical defects in the developing embryo.

Terminal bar apparatus Localized condensations of cytoplasmic substance associated with the cell membrane of the apical area of the functional ameloblast.

Tertiary dentin See *Reparative dentin.*

TMJ See *Temporomandibular joint.*

Tomes' granular layer This layer of dentin is found only in the tooth root. It is adjacent to the peripheral zone of hyalinized root dentin as a thin, hypomineralized layer.

Tomes' process Specialized apical zone of the ameloblasts. Tomes' process is conical and interdigitates with the forming enamel rods.

Tonofibrils Systems of fibrils found in the cytoplasm of epithelial cells, which function with the desmosomal plaque to hold adjacent cells together.

Tooth crypt Space filled by the dental follicle and developing tooth within the alveolar process.

Tooth eruption Process by which teeth emerge into the oral cavity, a stage coordinated with root growth and maturation of tissues surrounding the tooth.

Traction bands of the palate Bundles of collagen fibers that firmly attach the oral mucosa to the underlying bone of the hard palate.

Transduction theory Proposal that odontoblasts are sensory receptors for pain stimuli that are transmitted through the dentin.

Transparent dentin See *Sclerotic (transparent) dentin.*

Tuft See *Enamel tuft.*

Vasculature Refers to the blood vessels and circulating blood system.

Vermilion border The exposed red portion of the lips. This color is due to a thin epithelium with the presence of eleidin in the cells and the superficial position of blood vessels.

Vestibular lamina Lip furrow band located labial and buccal to the dental lamina that forms the oral vestibule between the alveolar portions of the jaws, the lips, and the cheeks.

Viscerocranial Refers to those parts of the facial cranial skeleton originating from the branchial arch.

Volkmann's canals "Perforating canals" that enter the bone at right or oblique angles and establish a continuous system that contains the nerves and blood vessels of the bone.

Vomer Flat, unpaired bone located in the midline of the face, shaped like a trapezoid, and forming the inferior and posterior portions of the nasal septum. It articulates with the sphenoid, ethmoid, two maxillary, and two palatine bones.

Von Ebner's lines See *Imbrication lines.*

Waldeyer's ring A ring of tonsillary tissue surrounding the oropharynx. It is composed of palatine tonsils located laterally, the lingual in the floor of the mouth, and the pharyngeal in the posterior area of the pharynx.

Weil's basal layer See *Cell-free zone.*

Wharton's duct The duct that drains the submandibular gland.

Zygoma The process of the temporal bone that connects with the zygomatic bone.

Zygote The fertilized cell produced by the union of two gametes.

Zymogen An inactive precursor that is activated to an enzyme. Granules in serous cells of enzyme-secreting glands, such as the salivary glands and the pancreas.

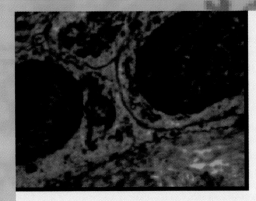

Index